HEALTH
AGAINST
WEALTH

HEALTH
AGAINST
WEALTH

HMOs and the Breakdown
of Medical Trust

GEORGE ANDERS

HOUGHTON MIFFLIN COMPANY
Boston   New York   1996

For information about permission to reproduce selections
from this book, write Permissions, Houghton Mifflin Company,
215 Park Avenue South, New York, NY 10003

For information about this and other Houghton Mifflin
trade and reference books and multimedia products, visit
The Bookstore at Houghton Mifflin on the World Wide Web
at http://www.hmco.com/trade/.

Library of Congress Cataloging-in-Publication Data
Anders, George, date.
    Health against wealth: HMOs and the breakdown of
medical trust / George Anders.
        p.   cm.
    Includes bibliographical references and index.
ISBN 0-395-82283-1
    1. Health maintenance organization — United States.   I. Title.
RA413.5.U5A55   1996
362.1'0425 — dc20   96-24869   CIP

Printed in the United States of America

QUM 10 9 8 7 6 5 4 3 2 1

FOR MY PARENTS,

AND FOR BETSY

Preface

Every November my wife and I participate in a small American ritual: we sit down at the kitchen table, surround ourselves with insurance-company brochures, and choose a health plan. In the first few years of our marriage, we made our decision quickly, almost frivolously. We were in our early 30s and healthy; our medical needs were minimal. We dabbled in HMOs, PPOs, MedSpend plans, and fee-for-service coverage, picking plans mostly on the basis of what piqued my curiosity as a staff writer at the *Wall Street Journal*. I even was without insurance for nine months in 1989–90, because we were tardy in filling out the forms. At that stage in life, health insurance didn't seem to matter much.

The past two years have been very different. Some of the people closest to us have confronted a difficult childbirth, an unexpected bout with cancer, a losing battle with diabetes. We have seen first-hand what happens when the medical/insurance system fails; we also have seen the life-saving power of the right doctor at the right time. As a result, our most recent kitchen-table sessions have been a lot longer. We have explored a series of "What if . . . ?" questions we had never asked before. "What if we become parents? What if our child has special needs? What if we have an emergency at night? What if we need to see a top specialist?"

Millions of other Americans find themselves in the same situation. New health plans offering some form of "managed care" beckon to workers and retirees alike. These plans are frequently known as health maintenance organizations (HMOs) or preferred provider organizations (PPOs). Not only are such plans cheaper than traditional insurance, they offer reduced paperwork and assurances that they can guard members against overtreatment. The advantages sound irresistible. But the choice isn't that simple. Managed-care plans save money by limiting patients' choices and by installing overseers who restrain what doctors can do. These restrictions can lead to painful breakdowns in medical care just when patients need help the most.

This book is meant for anyone who has tried to make sensible choices in the fast-changing world of medical insurance. There are no automatic answers that will be best for everyone. Within our own household, in fact, we are split: I'm willing to gamble that I can make managed care work; my wife is not, especially as she anticipates motherhood. But for everyone considering these choices, it helps tremendously to know how the game is played and where the greatest dangers lie. The middle chapters of the book talk about what managed care does well — and what it does badly — in treating major diseases. The final chapter offers some remedies to make the system work in patients' interests.

This book also is meant for people who make their living in health care: doctors, nurses, hospital administrators, and employees in allied fields. For most of the years after World War II, health care was a booming industry with almost unlimited resources for the effort to fight disease. Now the cost-minded dictates of managed care have drastically transformed the health-care market, and many providers find the new rules alarming and bewildering. The early chapters of this book explain why this transformation occurred; Chapters 12 and 13 spell out the factors that will determine what forces prevail in the continuing struggle over the future of American medicine.

Finally, this book is written for people with the power to change how we pay for medical care: legislators, regulators, investigative reporters, and ordinary citizens. When I started writing about health care for the *Wall Street Journal* in 1993, America was consumed by the idea that a single, sweeping national health plan could correct all the flaws in our medical system. That idea never was realized; the Clinton health plan and its offshoots collapsed in the summer of 1994. But as I worked on this book, the health-care debate moved to the states. By one estimate some 400 bills pertaining to managed care were introduced in state legislatures in early 1996. Some of those bills may be flawed, but many of them point the way toward a better health-care system, one that is both cost-effective and compassionate.

Each chapter of this book is meant to contribute to the discussion about creating such a system.

People in the HMO industry may view this book as a tough critique of their work. My mission was never to be hostile but always to be forthright. Over the next five years managed care undeniably will become the dominant form of American health insurance, if it isn't already. For all the theoretical appeal of managed care, however, there are too many instances in which lofty principles have been compromised or ignored on the way to the exam room or the patient's bedside. To avoid more such mistakes, we must identify the worst problem areas and start focusing on them. The cautionary examples in this book are meant as a first step.

Hundreds of people interrupted their lives to talk candidly with me about what managed care has meant to them. The bravest of all were the patients and their families, particularly Lamona Adams, Edmund Popiden, Stephen Bosworth, and Terry Lusignan. Doctors across the United States added their insights, hopes, and frustrations. Among HMO executives, Hyman Kahn, Joe Gerstein, Bill Popik, and Malik Hasan were thoughtful advocates for managed care, even in the face of difficult questions. Some HMO officials chose not to comment; their silence should not be interpreted as having any negative implications.

At the *Journal,* managing editor Paul Steiger encouraged me several years ago to learn about the intersecting worlds of medicine and money — and then cleared the way for me to write this book. Ron Winslow, Mike Waldholz, and Jerry Bishop taught me a lot about the subtleties of medical reporting. Colleagues, including Laura Johannes, Laurie McGinley, Hilary Stout, Elyse Tanouye, and Rhonda Rundle, freely shared ideas and sources. Neil Ulman, Dennis Kneale, Dan Hertzberg, Barney Calame, and Alan Murray also helped make this book happen.

Many outside readers and advisers helped me with quick feedback and wise advice. Edward and Joan Anders, Jack Corcoran, Ira Wilson, M.D., and Deborah Shlian, M.D., reviewed innumerable drafts of chapters. Each of them nudged me to explain things better while sharpening my thinking about what managed care does well and poorly. Tina Erickson opened doors in rural Tennessee. Nina Youngstrom, Adam Lilienfeld, and Mary Agnes Carey performed crucial research. Tom Petzinger, Arnie Milstein, M.D., Chuck Stevens, Jerome Kassirer, M.D., David Golub, Martin Kessler, Jeff Taylor, David Hilzenrath, David Schiman, and Nanci Schiman all provided helpful ideas.

At Houghton Mifflin, Steve Fraser proved once again to be a terrific editor. Lenora Todaro, Peg Anderson, and Glenn Kaye guided a bulky manuscript with skill and good cheer. My agent, Kim Witherspoon, and her colleague, Maria Massie, handled every negotiation well and honorably.

Once again my wife, Elizabeth Corcoran, was a special partner in completing the book. She was the first reader of every draft. She also was a selfless colleague, interrupting her own work at the *Washington Post* to help research a chapter in Tennessee, just when my deadline crunch seemed most overwhelming. Her support was a wonderful blessing.

Contents

HEALTH
AGAINST
WEALTH

1

A Baby's Struggle

THIS WASN'T THE WAY Lamona Adams wanted to spend the night. Resting her infant son on her shoulder, she paced to the edge of her garage and peered into the darkness, looking for the first sign of the headlights of her husband's car. It was 4:35 A.M. on a chilly March morning. All the other houses on Fireleaf Way were dark and still. Families in Fairburn, Georgia, were enjoying a few more hours of sleep before Saturday began. In a few hours the streets and lawns would be filled with the typical sights of an American suburb on a weekend: children bicycling, Rollerblading, or playing catch; parents going shopping or driving into Atlanta.

But Lamona Adams was already wide awake and very worried about her six-month-old son. What had started the day before as a moderate fever was steadily worsening. She had skipped work on Friday and taken the boy to the doctor, who recommended giving him Tylenol every four hours. That had helped for a while. By nighttime the Tylenol wasn't subduing his fever anymore. At 3:30 A.M., Lamona had awakened to find her son, James III, feeling unusually hot, panting and moaning. His temperature: 104 degrees Fahrenheit.

Alarmed, Lamona called her health plan's after-hours hotline at 3:50, asking what to do next. That was standard procedure for her; like millions of other Americans, she belonged to a "managed-care" plan, which required members to have most medical treatment approved in advance and to use only the most cost-effective doctors and hospitals if they wanted their bills covered. Only if a grave emergency arose were those restrictions waived.

It took a few minutes for Lamona's health plan, Kaiser Permanente, to log in the baby's symptoms and relay information from an operator to a nurse, from the nurse to a doctor, and then back to the nurse again. But by 4:05, word had come back: take the baby to the emergency room of Scottish Rite Children's Medical Center.

"That's the only hospital I can send you to," the hotline nurse added.

"How do we get there?" Lamona asked. She and her husband had moved to Georgia just a few months earlier and were still learning their way around.

"I don't know," the nurse replied. "I'm not good with directions." Rather than guess, the nurse passed along the hospital's phone number and suggested that Lamona call for directions herself.

For the next 20 minutes, Lamona hurried to get ready. She phoned her husband, James Jr., who was working as a night security guard, and implored him to come home at once. She called Scottish Rite and got directions. She told her sister, who was staying with her, to remove the baby from the cool bath that had been started moments earlier. The two women dried the infant and got him dressed. Around 4:25, Lamona slipped her baby into his shoes, grabbed his blanket, and scrambled downstairs to the garage. A few minutes later, she saw the first flicker of her husband's headlights. As her husband arrived, Lamona jumped into the back seat of their Plymouth Acclaim, holding the baby.

Her husband asked for directions, and she gave them. They had to drive three miles to reach Interstate 85 just south of Atlanta, then travel north on I-85 for more than 30 miles — past downtown Atlanta and on to the northern outskirts of the city. After that a junction, west six more miles on I-285, and about another mile on local streets.

"That's way up north!" James said. "I know," Lamona replied. "But that's the hospital that they told us to go to." With the streets deserted, James picked out a favorite shortcut that got them onto I-85 a little faster than usual. A former army sergeant who had served in Saudi Arabia as part of Operation Desert Storm, he was accustomed to making cool decisions in a crisis. As James started the long northward journey on I-85, Lamona urged him to drive faster. The speedometer nudged up to 75 m.p.h., then 80. James might have driven even faster, but it started to rain. What began as a drizzle quickly turned into a hard, torrential downpour. The small Plymouth slid across lanes, barely under control, then hydroplaned briefly on one of the curves.

Afraid that he might crash the car, James had no choice but to slow down.

About 20 miles into their drive, the Adamses passed the skyscrapers of downtown Atlanta. A few miles off the highway was the Egleston Children's Division of Emory University Hospital, a renowned pediatric center that could handle almost any crisis. Nearby were two more of Atlanta's leading hospitals: Georgia Baptist and Grady Memorial. Without permission to use any of those institutions, the Adamses kept driving. They had 22 more miles to travel. In the back seat of the car, Lamona kept looking into her baby's eyes, trying to reassure herself about his illness while making the baby aware that his mother was very close. For the first two thirds of the drive, the boy blinked back at her. As the car continued north, his eyes fell shut.

"Budé!" his mother snapped, calling her child briskly by a favorite nickname. "Budé!" The boy's eyes opened again. Lamona leaned forward and told her husband, "James, hurry!" The father accelerated as much as he dared, and he began to grow nervous too. A few minutes later he realized he had shot past the junction for I-285, the road leading toward Scottish Rite.

"I don't care, just go, go, go!" Lamona replied. They spotted a large blue "H" road sign, directing them to a closer hospital. As they neared the exit, the boy's eyes closed again. A few moments later his heart stopped. At 5:29 A.M. the parents pulled into the parking lot of Kennestone Hospital at Windy Hill. Lamona bolted out of the car holding her son and ran into the emergency room, crying, "Help my baby! Help my baby!"

A nurse grabbed the infant and gave two breaths of mouth-to-mouth resuscitation. A pediatric "crash cart" was wheeled into the area, stocked with emergency equipment designed to save a baby's life. Nurses and doctors began a whirlwind of rescue measures — inserting breathing tubes into baby James, beginning cardiopulmonary resuscitation and administering two doses of epinephrine, a powerful hormone and heart stimulant. As they started to work on the inert baby, his head lifted, then thudded against the emergency-room cot.

When she heard that thud, Lamona Adams screamed. She fell to her knees and, by her own account, became hysterical. Hospital employees took her arms and escorted her to the hospital's nearby chapel. A nurse came in and tried to soothe her. A few moments later her husband arrived, with grim news. "It doesn't look good," he said. "They've got all these tubes in him." Unable to move, Lamona stood in the chapel, praying, again and again, "Don't take my baby, God."

After nearly 20 minutes of resuscitation efforts, Kennestone's nurses reported the first sign of a renewed pulse. By 6 A.M. the baby's heartbeat was steady enough that CPR could stop. But blood tests showed that he was still profoundly sick, with carbon dioxide levels far above normal. Even more ominously, the original cause of his fever remained undiagnosed. Doctors administered antibiotics in the hope that they would help; they learned a day later that his body was ravaged by a potentially fatal infection: meningococcemia.

At 7 A.M. Kennestone's doctors decided to transfer the Adams baby to Scottish Rite, the hospital he originally was headed for, which could do far more for gravely ill children. This time, at last, an ambulance carried the boy. At Scottish Rite swarms of specialists clustered at the boy's bedside around the clock for days. Neurologists, surgeons, infectious-disease experts, and others tried to assess the damage. It was clear that antibiotics were subduing his fever and that the hospital could keep the infant alive for at least a few days. But the doctors' early assessments were full of foreboding. Meningococcemia had already caused vast, perhaps devastating, damage to little James. He was immobile and unresponsive. The blood flow in his hands and feet had essentially ceased.

One of the doctors, James Jose, began talking with the parents about whether it might be appropriate to withdraw life support at some stage. The crucial question, he said, was how badly the boy's brain had been damaged. Could he still see? Would he ever be able to move? To speak? To read? Even if his brain had withstood the double trauma of meningococcemia and heart stoppage, further crises lay ahead. Little James's skin had begun to turn black at his extremities, as blood cells and tissue died. It was clear that if he did survive, his ruined hands and feet would have to be amputated.

"We all understand that a tragic outcome is definitely in the future," Dr. Jose wrote in the boy's medical chart on March 31, 1993. "The parents are quite brave, intelligent and articulate issues well. But the best, or most acceptable, course isn't yet clear." The parents decided to wait a week to see if the boy's condition would improve at all. If not, they said, they would agree to withhold life support, let the boy die quickly, and be buried intact, without any surgery.

April 6 was the Adamses' self-imposed deadline. Early that morning they got an excited phone call from Dr. Jose: "He's following the bear!" As part of a routine neurological test, Dr. Jose had passed the boy's teddy bear back and forth in front of his eyes. For the first time, James's eyes tracked the stuffed animal and seemed to recognize it. His vision and at least part of his higher mental capacities were saved.

For the Adamses and their doctors, the next step was clear. Within an hour the boy was wheeled into a pediatric surgery unit, where he would undergo amputations to ward off further gangrene. From this point onward doctors would do everything they could to help the boy — though he would have to live with the catastrophic loss of both his hands and both his feet. The baby's medical chart, written in aloof clinical language, tried to mask the horror of what needed to be done. "Under general anesthesia, the patient's extremities were prepped and draped in the usual fashion," wrote Steven Cohen, a pediatric plastic surgeon at Scottish Rite. "The procedure took place very rapidly, beginning first at the right leg . . ."

Two months later James III had recovered enough to be discharged from Scottish Rite. His physical wounds had healed with incredible speed, as is generally true for babies. Scar tissue had formed at his extremities, cushioning the previously exposed muscle and bone. As his bandages came off, he began to move about in his hospital crib, smiling at his parents when they came to visit. He was not quite nine months old — too young to realize how different he was from any other child his age. In a whispered moment, a Scottish Rite doctor confided to the parents that only a tiny child could be so determined to live.

Back in Fairburn, the Adamses put their family life back together as best they could. Lamona kept her civilian job with the army, if only to secure health insurance for her little boy. Her husband quit his job to spend more time at home with his son and to handle the boy's frequent appointments with doctors and therapists. In the parents' hours at home together, away from the stares of strangers who didn't understand what had happened to the boy, they built their own sanctuary. Lamona resumed breast-feeding her baby, while her husband sang lullabies to him. To their great delight, it became clear that their son's energy and intelligence had somehow survived the ordeal. On weekend evenings the whole family — James Jr., Lamona, James III, and his older sister, Alysia — stretched out in the parents' bedroom and watched HBO movies while nibbling on popcorn. At such times they were almost happy.

When the Adamses told people about the events leading up to their little boy's amputations, however, a sense of outrage began to build. The parents had tried to win timely medical care for a very sick child, to no avail. They had been told to drive 42 miles to a remote hospital — a fact that grated on the parents each time they brought their baby back to Scottish Rite for physical therapy or further surgery. Each day hundreds of parents brought sick children to Egleston, Georgia Baptist, and Grady hospitals in downtown Atlanta. James Jr. and Lamona Adams kept asking themselves: why didn't Kaiser allow us that chance?

At the urging of Lamona's mother, the couple hired a lawyer and sued Kaiser in mid-1993, alleging negligence. It took 18 months for the case to come to trial, but in January 1995, proceedings began. Each day grim-faced doctors and nurses stepped into the Fulton County state courthouse in downtown Atlanta, ready to testify in *James and Lamona Adams v. Kaiser Foundation Health Plan of Georgia Inc.* What had begun as one family's tragedy soon grew into an exhaustive analysis of why a major managed-care plan had handled the case the way it had. The inquiry was especially striking because Kaiser generally was regarded as an industry leader in caring about its members' well-being. But as details about Kaiser's methods emerged, the case suggested that the margins of safety in a giant health plan are sometimes much thinner than people realize.

In court and in pretrial depositions, expert witnesses filled out the missing elements of the Adamses' story. Doctors testified about what modern medicine could do to fight the baby's illness. Other experts pulled back the curtain to explain what transpired at Kaiser at crucial stages. With that extra information, jurors could decide the trial's central questions: were the Adamses simply victims of catastrophic bad luck, as Kaiser maintained? Or was the big health plan — with all its controls and guidelines — to blame in some way?

The very word *meningococcemia* is enough to scare a pediatrician. It is a rare but not unheard-of bacterial infection, striking about 800 infants a year. Its early symptoms don't stand out much from those of ordinary flu episodes: fever, lethargy, irritability, and sometimes vomiting. With stunning speed, however, meningococcemia can become devastating. Bacterial infection can rapidly attack the membranes enclosing the brain and spinal cord, known as the meninges. Meanwhile, tiny blood vessels in almost any part of the body far enough from the heart can clot, shutting down blood circulation. In a standard warning to doctors, the 1992 edition of the *Merck Manual of Diagnosis and Therapy* declared: "Since acute bacterial meningitis, especially meningococcal, can be lethal in hours, accurate diagnosis and treatment are urgent. . . . When bacterial meningitis is seriously suspected, administration of antibiotics should not await the results of diagnostic tests."

At crucial stages, Kaiser had a chance to pinpoint the problem or summon help in a hurry. Each time, the health plan didn't realize that a dread disease was stalking the little boy. And in the carefully controlled world of a big health plan such as Kaiser, it isn't always easy for such realizations to occur. The great strength of such a managed-care plan is the ability to deliver reliable, cost-effective treatment in the areas of medicine that can be standardized and dealt with routinely. The system's great vulnerability is the unexpected case.

Kaiser's first chance to help baby James Adams came the morning of Friday, March 26, nearly 24 hours before the eventual crisis. When Lamona Adams started breast-feeding her son that morning, she noticed he was feverish. She called her health plan at about 6:45 A.M., relayed the symptoms, and asked for advice, as well as for a same-day appointment with a doctor. A Kaiser employee suggested using over-the-counter Tylenol to lower the baby's fever and scheduled an 11:50 A.M. pediatric exam at one of Kaiser's clinics in nearby Southwood. By the time the baby arrived, his temperature had risen to 102 degrees, enough to worry his mother, though still well below the fevers that infants sometimes run.

When pediatrician Cindy Juster began the 10-minute exam, she did what Kaiser later described as appropriate care. She checked the boy's ears for possible infection. She listened to his chest with a stethoscope. She recommended sticking with Tylenol to fight the fever and administering saline solution to help clear up his nasal congestion. All were standard approaches to treating a bout of the flu, the most likely diagnosis based on the baby's symptoms. Dr. Juster didn't take a blood sample or prescribe antibiotics, Lamona Adams recalled in a legal deposition a year later. Instead the pediatrician provided a classic piece of Kaiser-style preventive care: she urged Lamona Adams not to let her husband smoke cigarettes inside the house, for the baby's sake.

The Adamses never alleged any negligence in Dr. Juster's exam. Medical experts in the court case noted that it was highly unlikely that any doctor would have ordered a blood culture based on the baby's symptoms at the time — or that such a test would have yielded positive results in time to make a difference. Even so, a former Kaiser pediatrician raised questions about the HMO's priorities. She testified that the health plan in 1992 briefed its doctors on the importance of cost containment. The basic message: "We can practice good medicine without spending as much money." Kaiser around that time also had speeded up its routine pediatric exams from the previous 15 minutes to 10 minutes apiece. That saved money, but it left less time to consider the range of things that might be going on.

Kaiser's next chance came at 3:50 A.M. the following morning, by which time the Adams baby was very sick. Like many managed-care plans, Kaiser had set up an after-hours nurse advice line that members were supposed to call if they had a medical problem. In the most extreme emergencies, members were allowed to go directly to a nearby hospital. But Lamona Adams couldn't tell for certain how severely ill her son was. Like many people in a managed-care plan, she felt that her first obligation was to call the hotline and get advice from the plan's own nurses.

Such 24-hour advice lines are saving money for health plans; they also are profoundly changing emergency medicine. Nurses who staff these lines are meant to spot true crises quickly and point those patients toward the emergency room or an ambulance, while weeding out false alarms and recommending lesser care. Overall, ER visits and ambulance calls can be cut in half, according to advice-line specialists. A well-run line actually can improve patient care, medical experts say — as long as three conditions are met. Nurses must be fully briefed on emergency medicine for all kinds of patients. Telephone exchanges with patients or parents must mimic the thinking of a good emergency-room doctor. That means asking first about any evidence of life-threatening symptoms, no matter how remote, and proceeding to simpler problems only after ruling out the possibility of something grave. Finally, nurses need to relay information about tough cases quickly and accurately to a backup physician. If those conditions aren't met, experts say, the risk of a medical disaster rises.

In the predawn hours of March 27, 1993, Esther Nesbitt was working the night shift at Kaiser's nurse hotline. She had been a nurse for 20 years, working in New York City emergency rooms early in her career. After coming to Georgia in 1984, she became a nursing-home inspector, then joined Kaiser. Her career experience in pediatric units amounted to "maybe a year, a year and a half," she later said in a court deposition.

On Nesbitt's desk was a *Manual of Pediatric Protocols,* including a three-page tip sheet entitled "Fever." The tip sheet was arranged much like a set of college notes, with a nine-line definition of fever at the top, an explanation of fever's causes, and only then a series of questions that parents should be asked. Down near the bottom of the first page, ninth in a list of 11 questions, was a question that many emergency-room doctors would pose right away: "Is [the] child having problems breathing?"

From her perch at Kaiser's offices, Nesbitt decided after a few minutes that little James Adams wasn't in respiratory distress. The telephone operator who took Lamona Adams's initial call had handed Nesbitt a summary sheet that read: "moaning, panting breathing, no vomiting." Medical experts called by the Adamses' attorney said they would regard such symptoms as clear signs of breathing problems. Nesbitt talked briefly with Lamona Adams on the phone about the baby's problems. Based on that conversation, Nesbitt later testified, "I had no indication from my assessment that the child was in any distress in order to necessitate 911 being called." From her appraisal of the case, Nesbitt prepared to point the Adamses toward Kaiser's usual hospital, without knowing how far away it was.

One last chance remained for Kaiser to treat the case as an all-out emergency. Under the health plan's own rules, hotline nurses were supposed to check with an on-call doctor on the handling of many cases. After speaking to Lamona Adams, Nesbitt phoned Carol Herrmann, a Kaiser pediatrician who was sleeping at home but was available for consultations. The doctor and the nurse differ greatly about what was said. Nesbitt said she passed along a full summary of the case, including the initial phone-log assessment of the baby's panting and moaning. But in separate testimony Dr. Herrmann offered a decidedly different version. In a legal deposition she said Nesbitt didn't tell her that the child was moaning and panting. The physician added, "Had I gotten that information, I would have asked for Ms. Adams' phone number so I could call her. . . . If there was actual moaning, I would say I would like that child seen within 15 to 20 minutes. . . . If a child is having agonal respirations there would be a good likelihood that death would be imminent." Based on the information given, however, Dr. Herrmann concurred with nurse Nesbitt's treatment plan.

There would be no ambulance called, no authorization for the family to seek the closest hospital. Kaiser had given its instructions. It was up to Lamona Adams to stand in her driveway, holding her baby in the dark, and wait for her husband to come home.

The decision to send the Adamses to Scottish Rite — 42 miles from their home — was no whim on the part of the night nurse. It was the way Kaiser wanted most pediatric hospitalizations handled. Like most managed-care plans, Kaiser regularly dealt with only a handful of the hospitals in its area. The plan's financial managers regarded that as good business; they could get discounts in return for promising to steer many patients to their chosen hospitals. Kaiser's doctors generally saw value in selective contracting, too. The health plan could pick out hospitals it regarded as modern, efficient, and of high quality, then direct almost all its patients to those centers. For both those reasons, Kaiser in 1990 signed a multiyear contract with Scottish Rite. The health plan agreed to send most of its pediatric cases to the hospital in Atlanta's northern suburbs in return for a 10 percent discount on the first $5 million of business each year. If Kaiser's patient volume exceeded that amount, the discount would increase to 15 percent. When the Scottish Rite contract was signed, it could have been clear this would inconvenience some of the health plan's members. But to judge from the decision taken, that was not seen as an overriding factor.

In the final stages of the trial, medical experts clashed about whether the Adamses' long drive — and baby James's heart stoppage — ultimately changed his fate. Doctors summoned by Kaiser said that the delays and the heart attack hadn't worsened the outcome. Meningococcemia was rampant throughout the baby's body, these doctors contended; he was doomed to have the amputations regardless of how quickly he was seen after Lamona Adams's call to the nurse hotline.

But Roger Barkin, chairman of the department of pediatrics at Rose Medical Center in Denver, argued otherwise. Called as an expert witness on behalf of the Adamses, Dr. Barkin testified that if an ambulance had carried little James Adams to the nearest emergency room before his heart stopped, nearly all of the subsequent catastrophe could have been avoided. Antibiotics would have been administered 60 to 70 minutes earlier, Dr. Barkin calculated. The heart attack wouldn't have occurred; circulation damage from the infection would have been much less. In such circumstances, Dr. Barkin suggested, the boy might have "had some loss of part of a toe or part of a finger," but not much more. The Adamses' lawyer, Thomas Malone, built that assessment into his closing arguments in the case. In Malone's view, "We went from a 10 percent chance of the child losing his limbs to a 90 percent chance."

On February 1, 1995, legal arguments were finished. *Adams v. Kaiser* went to the jury. Kaiser asked that the suit be dismissed; Malone pressed for millions of dollars in damages. One of his damage estimates, he told the jury, amounted to $100 an hour for the rest of little James Adams's expected life. "That may seem like a lot of money," he said. "But would any of you want to change places with this little boy, even for $100 an hour?"

After one and a half days of deliberations, the jury found Kaiser guilty of medical negligence and awarded the plaintiffs more money than they had dared expect. The boy was awarded $40 million; his parents, an additional $5.5 million. That amount later was shrunk significantly when Kaiser reached an out-of-court settlement in return for forgoing its right to appeal. Still, the case ended up with a multimillion-dollar penalty for Kaiser — and an indelible emotional impression for jurors. One moist-eyed juror walked over to Lamona Adams after the verdict was announced and softly said, "You take good care of that baby, now." Another juror, unable to find the right words, simply threw her arms around Lamona and gave her a hug.

Once the publicity died down, Lamona Adams faced the much harder job of helping her son grow up. Some days brought smiles to her face as she shared the normal parts of parenting: letting the boy watch *Barney* videos, arguing over bedtime, sharing his joy when he looked at a mantelpiece portrait and declared: "Grandma!" Other days were heartbreaking as she realized how much would be maddeningly hard or impossible for her son to do.

Therapists fitted James with prostheses that helped him walk around the house. But sports, hiking, and most strenuous outdoor activities would never be possible. Doctors said his mental functioning was average or above average. Yet James Adams III was a "catastrophically handicapped child," as his case manager, Kathy Willard, observed. Extensive training with artificial hands lay ahead if he was to have any hope of doing what other children master without thinking: picking up a pencil, getting dressed, or playing with friends. More distant goals, such as living outside his parents' home or finding work, seemed even more daunting.

Within Kaiser the Adams tragedy caused considerable soul-searching. In a policy switch, the health plan told its hotline nurses in Georgia to ask repeat callers at the end of a conversation, "Is there anything that makes you think you should go to an emergency room right away?" Scottish Rite Medical Center added a new sentence to the start of its automated telephone greeting: "If this is a life-threatening medical emergency, please hang up and call 911." Carol Herrmann, the pediatrician who was phoned the night that Lamona Adams sought advice from the hotline, quit Kaiser and went to work for a different pediatric practice. She gave her home number to parents and told them to call her directly — at any hour of the night — if they were seriously worried about a sick child.

Kaiser administrators continued to deny that there were any fundamental flaws in their approach to medicine. "We feel this was not a managed-care systems issue," Kaiser spokesman Dan Danzig said a year after the Adams verdict. "Maybe it was an emergency access thing." In Georgia, Kaiser administrators weren't even prepared to concede that much. "The care that we gave this young patient was appropriate," the health plan declared in a one-page statement in January 1996. "While we recognize the jury's understandable sympathy for the child and his family, the judgment was not supported by medical evidence."

For Lamona Adams, however, Kaiser's way of doing things didn't allow for an adequate margin of safety when her baby became sick. She felt rushed in the pediatrician's office. She felt she couldn't go directly to an emergency room but had to call the hotline. In a moment of crisis, she had to speak with a nurse rather than a doctor. And then she was sent to a faraway hospital instead of a local one. In her eyes she had been ill served by a system that required members to deal with a remote gatekeeper when seeking treatment approval. As she fervently declared one evening at her home, "We don't need a gatekeeper if a child is in an emergency. We need all the doors to be wide open."

Such breakdowns in medical care are what this book will explore. A new health-care system known as managed care is taking hold in the United States, promising to make medicine more affordable, more efficient, and of higher quality. The best-known forms of managed care — tightly supervised medical plans known as health maintenance organizations (HMOs) — now claim 58 million members and are growing at a rate of 100,000 a week. In these health plans, doctors and patients no longer are left to themselves to seek whatever they consider necessary care. Instead new overseers have entered the picture via health-insurance plans, shaping treatment decisions from the start. These executives become medical commissars, deciding what doctors patients will see, what pills they take, and what hospitals they can use in a crisis. The architects of this system are supremely confident of their ability to make the right choices for millions of Americans; they believe they are creating such a decisive improvement over the fragmented, high-cost health care of prior years that it is only a matter of time before almost every American belongs to such a plan.

As we shall see, managed-care plans have the potential to do a great many things right. They can bring factorylike efficiency to the routine aspects of medicine. They can ensure that more babies get immunized on time, that more women in their 50s get regular mammograms to check for breast cancer, that diabetics get yearly eye exams. They can cut costs of health insurance 5 percent to 20 percent at the outset and then slow down further increases, chiefly by working with small groups of cost-effective doctors and hospitals and by taking away longstanding financial incentives for overtreatment. Most of all, managed care can redirect the priorities of American medicine so that good preventive care is no longer a stepchild in a world dominated by costly late-stage crisis care.

There is a dark side to managed care, however: the individuality of each patient doesn't matter much anymore. Planners have created a complex medical machine, full of channels and pathways designed to standardize most cases. The ascendancy of managed care may be correcting many misjudgments of unsupervised medicine. But managed-care planners are racing so fast to cover millions more people that they often lack the time — or the experience — to detect the potential blind spots of their system until tragedy strikes. That leads to a new class of blunder: the medical catastrophe that could have been prevented by overseers at several steps along the way, but wasn't. To wit:

- An elderly woman hoping to live out her last few months in dignity may find her health plan pushing for a transfer to a low-grade nursing home that is grossly unsuited to her needs.
- A middle-aged man needing heart surgery may find his HMO steering him to a hospital that has worse than average mortality statistics, in the interests of saving money.
- A young woman fighting breast cancer may find that her managed-care plan is badgering her doctors not to go ahead with a costly, long-shot treatment that has already been recommended as her best hope.
- A country doctor trying to stop an epidemic of a parasitic disease may find that the antibiotic he wants to prescribe has been declared off-limits by local managed-care plans for reasons of cost. While he appeals that decision, townspeople must cope with the epidemic by reverting to the public health norms of the 1940s: boiling clothes, washing hands incessantly, and closing schools.

To the planners trying to spread their new system throughout the United States, such reports of local failures hardly deserve attention. The champions of managed care focus on many thousands, even millions, of covered lives at once. At that level people's faces and individual experiences vanish. Only statistics remain. To be asked to focus on anything different is annoying. As the head of employee services at a major electric company put it in a mid-1995 speech: "Anytime health benefits are discussed — regardless of whether the group represents senior executives or workers from the line — it is difficult to keep the topic at a policy level. Conversation almost immediately deteriorates into personal preferences, concerns, and anecdotes. Will I have to give up my doctor? How far will I have to travel? Will I get the best quality care?"

What the planners forget is that health care only seems like a vast industry ready to be conquered by statistical methods. Ultimately medicine is intensely personal; it is a service delivered one patient at a time. The managed-care industry is dominated by people who see many statistics and few patients. They want to be judged by how they treat healthy populations overall. The crucial test of a health plan, however, is how it performs when anxious families are fighting medical disaster. After all, the main reason people seek health insurance is to have some medical security in a crisis. For that reason, any thorough assessment of managed care must concentrate on those moments when the risk of grave illness or devastating medical bills is palpable.

In Georgia, Kaiser and the Adamses never found a way to talk about such issues. The massive lawsuit drove the two sides apart; from mid-1993 onward, each viewed the other with great wariness. But one person on the Kaiser team did try to reach across the chasm between the health plan's policies and a mother's needs. It was Carol Herrmann, the pediatrician on call the night Lamona Adams phoned Kaiser for help. With sadness in her voice, Dr. Herrmann called Lamona at home shortly after the tragedy occurred. "We know about what happened to your son," Dr. Herrmann said. "I want to tell you how sorry I am to hear about it." The two women talked briefly about the telephonic relay system that night — and what had or hadn't been conveyed to Dr. Herrmann. At the end of the call, Dr. Herrmann told Lamona again how much the whole case concerned her.

"I have small children myself," the doctor explained.

2

Dismantling the Old System

Edward hennessy, the long-time chairman of Allied Signal Corporation, remembers the moment when soaring health costs finally prompted him to slam down his fist and declare, "Enough!" It was in early 1987, just after he learned that his company's expenses for employee health care were climbing 39 percent a year. Even though the big New Jersey conglomerate was doing well in its basic businesses — auto parts, aerospace, and chemicals — that sort of pell-mell growth in workers' health costs might ruin the company's prospects.

Determined to avert a crisis, Hennessy asked an aide to show him the most astronomical medical bills, in which care for corporate employees or their families topped $100,000. To Hennessy's astonishment, aides wheeled a metal cart into his office to deliver those documents. They were dealing with a mountain of manila folders nearly three feet high, a stack so huge that Hennessy initially refused to look at it. "Show me just the bills that are $250,000 or more," he told his staff. A short while later, a smaller mound of folders was delivered to his office. As Hennessy flipped through each binder, he encountered medical calamities from all over the United States, ranging from gravely premature infants to retirees with unending heart troubles. Each story involved desperate operations, unexpected complications, and an unending barrage of tests, exams, and therapies. Even when death was imminent, bills kept piling up, while the insurers hired by Allied Signal to administer this system did little to hold down costs. Ultimately, all these medical expenses were passed on to Allied Signal, either as premium increases or as direct costs.

From that moment on, Hennessy crusaded for change. "If we don't fix this ourselves, [corporate raider] Boone Pickens is going to fix it for us," he told subordinates in early 1987. At a top executives' budget meeting that spring, Hennessy angrily interrupted a presentation on health-care spending. The company's head of human resources, Ted Halkyard had been delicately explaining how he hoped to slow health care costs to a 15 percent increase in the coming year.

"That's unacceptable!" Hennessy snapped. "Come back and tell me how it's going to be zero."

Halkyard blanched. He couldn't imagine any strategy — short of canceling employee health insurance, thus inviting a workers' mutiny — that would slow costs that drastically. But Hennessy was serious. Struggling for a compromise, Halkyard suggested that Allied Signal begin wide-ranging talks with insurers about overhauling the company's health coverage. If those talks went well, Halkyard said, perhaps the rise in health costs could be slowed to the general inflation rate. "That's the most we can do," Halkyard explained. "And that's going to be a tremendous amount of work."

Over the next few days, Halkyard and his staff scrambled for a strategy to soothe what they dubbed "the Hennessy beast." Their solution: invite a dozen big insurers and health plans to compete for the chance to put most of Allied Signal's 76,000 workers, as well as their dependents, into managed care. Employees who chose not to use the cost-effective doctors and hospitals designated by this new system could still see their old physicians. But those workers would have to pay an uncomfortably large share of the costs themselves. Incentives to stay within the managed-care network would be so strong, Allied Signal and its consultants predicted, that 70 percent of employees' medical spending would be redirected into it. Because Hennessy wanted results in a hurry, Allied Signal decided not to phase in the new plan over several years. Instead, it would act as fast as possible, changing every worker's health coverage in early 1988.

What happened at Allied Signal in the late 1980s quickly became a model for the rest of corporate America. One after another, companies recoiled in horror at how much their open-ended health plans were costing them. Unwilling to bankroll this expensive system anymore, executives began dismantling the extravagant health plans that had allowed employees to draw upon the most that American medicine could offer, at hardly any direct personal cost. Instead, an austere new approach to medical care was put in place. Holding down expenses became the overriding goal, even if it meant telling employees that they couldn't see certain doctors; couldn't go to certain hospitals; couldn't have costly CAT scans and other tests performed.

This "businessman's revolt" was more than a money-saving issue; it had emotional and moral overtones as well. The companies that aggressively opted for managed care did so partly from a belief that doctors and hospitals, unsupervised, simply couldn't be trusted anymore. By the late 1980s the American medical establishment no longer occupied the revered position it had enjoyed a generation earlier. Images of greedy doctors abounded in popular culture, with some justification. Young doctors in training boasted about how much money they would make, often by relentlessly testing every patient they could, a practice known as "scoping for dollars." Health experts debated whether the huge American buildup in hospital-based medical technology — far beyond what existed in any other country — actually helped patients get better or simply helped providers get rich. As corporate payers began studying the health-care market in greater detail, they often convinced themselves that the savings offered by managed care not only benefited their own companies, but might actually be better for society at large.

The migration into managed care took place very suddenly at some companies, slowly and gently at others. From the late 1980s onward, however, the trend picked up speed until it became a juggernaut. Employers ranging from General Motors and Sears Roebuck to Hy-Vee Food Stores in Iowa overhauled their fundamental approach to employee health care. In the process they nudged at least 20 million Americans into HMOs and many millions more into preferred provider organizations (PPOs) or other, looser forms of managed care. As this migration happened, power flowed into the hands of the insurers who ran the tightfisted managed-care plans. Doctors and hospitals, even the best and most trusted ones, found their authority slipping away.

These transformations have proven intensely controversial. Workers at many companies have felt betrayed by the loss of their old all-encompassing health benefits. In some cases employees have sent petitions to corporate headquarters denouncing managed care. Secretaries have grumbled to their bosses about the injustice of the new system. Doctors and hospital managers have argued that managed care is a mistake — perhaps for patients and certainly for their own careers.

Allied Signal's boss bumped into an especially dramatic sign of this indignation in the late 1980s when an irate physician warned him, "Hennessy, you'd better not need to be operated on in New Jersey."

Yet the corporate executives who tore down the old health-care system insisted they were doing the right thing. "It was the only way we stood a chance of affecting our cost of health care," recalled Allied's Ted Halkyard. "We had tried asking for second opinions on costly procedures. We had tried switching to outpatient surgeries. We had tried everything else, and nothing was working." A hint of exasperation crept into his voice as he repeated, "Nothing was working."

All the subsequent upheaval associated with managed care must be understood against that backdrop of 25 years of business frustration with the mounting costs of medical care. After years of trying small, sensible steps that didn't work, corporate executives hardly worried about acting too boldly. Their overriding concern was whether *anything* could restrain the runaway health costs that were jeopardizing their businesses.

Men like Ed Hennessy and Ted Halkyard didn't ask to reshape America's medical system. In Britain, Germany, and most other industrialized countries, health insurance has been government-structured for decades. But the United States has taken a different path. Its health insurance markets evolved haphazardly and never came under central control. Corporate employers ended up in the curious position of being the leading providers of medical insurance.

In nineteenth-century America, doctors' bills were low and hospitals admitted many patients as charity cases. As a result, formal medical insurance was rare; individuals simply paid medical bills as best they could. In the 1920s private health insurance began as a cushion against unexpected hospital bills. Citizens generally bought coverage on their own, though a few companies, such as Montgomery Ward, offered health insurance as a fringe benefit. When World War II broke out, labor markets tightened and employers were subject to strict wage controls. Employer-organized health insurance caught on as a way to attract workers.

In the late 1940s, when medical services accounted for just 4 percent of gross national product, President Harry Truman tried to enact government-run health insurance for all. "We can afford to spend more on health," he told the country in 1945. His proposals bounced around Congress for several years but never won passage. Some of the most strident opposition came from doctors, who worried that their autonomy and their incomes would suffer. In a multimillion-dollar lobbying campaign, the American Medical Association repeatedly denounced the Democratic president's plan as socialized medicine. Legislators were cool to the Truman plan too, particularly after Republicans made heavy inroads in the 1946 elections. Most fundamentally, as author Paul Starr later noted, "growing confidence in American capitalism" led to dwindling public support for any big new government program.

As the postwar economy took off, corporations and unions filled the insurance gap. In 1940 just 12 million people enjoyed the luxury of private health insurance, less than one tenth of the population. Then labor leaders pressed for health coverage, provided either by unions themselves or by corporate employers. Companies generally obliged. The ranks of the insured swelled to 77 million in 1950 and kept climbing. In 1960 some 123 million people, or 60 percent of the population, had private health insurance. Every few years employers in the postwar boom further enriched health benefits, with the automobile industry leading the way. General Motors' original plan, enacted in 1941, covered only hospital costs and required employees to pay the full premium. In 1950 GM agreed to pick up half the cost of insurance and to extend coverage to doctors' services. In 1961 GM and other car companies agreed to pay the entire premium for employees and to cover half the costs for retirees and dependents. A few years later retirees and dependents were granted full coverage. Then prescription drugs and mental-health coverage were added to the menu.

Years later, directors and executives would rue their predecessors' generosity. "Chrysler opened its treasury door to doctors and hospitals," wrote Joseph Califano, a one-time secretary of Health, Education and Welfare who served as a Chrysler director in the early 1980s. "By agreeing to first-dollar coverage, Chrysler increasingly insulated its employees from any sense of what health care cost. . . . This gave the doctors the power to write their own checks on the Chrysler account." At the time, however, executives regarded all-inclusive health benefits for workers as both prudent and affordable.

The most profound implications of employers' generosity showed up in America's hospital bills. In 1946 a single night's stay in a U.S. hospital cost just $9.39 on average. Hospital equipment was spartan, and the nurses and aides who worked there were paid relatively low wages. Twenty years later hospitals' basic nightly rates had climbed to $45. By 1985 many community hospitals had turned into "medical centers" packed with expensive diagnostic equipment that could generate $2,000 a day or more in bills for patient testing. These hospitals bustled with nurses, X-ray technicians, and other skilled employees, all earning more than the median U.S. worker. Basic room rates alone often topped $600, even before tests and doctors' fees. Even something as simple as a hospital bed wasn't simple anymore. It was a high-tech medical marvel, packed with switches and controls to improve patients' safety and comfort. Top-of-the-line hospital beds cost $10,000 or more — at least as much as a new car. Someone had to absorb those costs, and corporate health-benefits plans or the federal government were the ultimate payers.

Medical schools and teaching hospitals fueled this technological buildup, encouraging thousands of young doctors to specialize in treating particular diseases. Physicians gravitated to the hardest, costliest cases, believing that they had not just the opportunity but the outright duty to spend many thousands of dollars in efforts to forestall the ravages of advanced disease. In the early 1970s physician Lewis Thomas warned against a growing national obsession with what he called "halfway technology" in medicine, which amounted to late-stage efforts to slow down disease without preventing or curing the underlying illness. "It is characteristic of this kind of technology that it costs an enormous amount of money and requires a continuing expansion of hospital facilities," Dr. Thomas wrote. "There is no end to the need for new, highly trained people to run the enterprise. And there is really no way out of this, at the present stage of knowledge."

In some cases doctors appeared simply to be pumping up their caseloads to make the most of each new facet of workers' medical coverage. When Chrysler put in a generous mental-health benefit, psychiatric treatment of its workers and their families jumped fivefold. There was no sign that the car company had begun hiring workers who were more disturbed, or that the new level of treatment was improving employees' peace of mind. Instead, the mere existence of the benefit was generating demand. As Chrysler director Califano later remarked, "Psychiatrists moved to southeastern Michigan the way prospectors went west for the Gold Rush."

By the late 1980s, America's immense medical machine was a

source of both national pride and national shame. The United States had 800 open-heart-surgery units, more than double the number in all of western Europe, even though the total U.S. population was significantly smaller than Europe's. The United States was the world leader, in fact, in almost every area of medical technology: three-dimensional scanners of internal organs; $2 million machines to crush kidney stones; new, minimally invasive ways to perform knee surgery. Individual success stories abounded of U.S. patients rescued by high-tech medicine. Yet American life expectancy wasn't any higher than that of most European nations. Americans actually died sooner, on average, than their Japanese counterparts, who spent a much smaller share of gross national product on health care. Meanwhile, the costs associated with this medical buildup were making comprehensive health insurance outright unaffordable for many businesses and for self-employed workers. The total number of Americans with private health insurance peaked at 188 million in 1982 and declined thereafter; in 1989 it had dropped to 182.5 million.

All the while, national medical spending kept climbing at double-digit annual percentage rates. By the end of the 1980s it totaled $604 billion, nearly 12 percent of gross national product. The one-year, 39 percent leap experienced by Allied Signal was an extreme example of how fast costs could escalate. But hundreds of corporations seethed at signs that employees' health-care costs were rising far faster than overall corporate sales. Even the federal government shared those concerns; it had become a major payer for health care as well, thanks to the creation of the Medicare program for the elderly and the Medicaid program for the poor in the mid-1960s.

Fixing this cost problem proved far harder than employers or the government originally expected. Workers had begun to regard health coverage as an unending free resource — an entitlement. They didn't want to give it up. Ultimately companies had only two basic choices: asking their own employees to pay more or putting greater controls on doctors and hospitals. Both routes were unpleasant.

Throughout the 1980s companies pressed workers to shoulder a bigger share of medical bills. Copayments and deductibles were introduced, then steadily boosted. Companies that once paid 100 percent of health-insurance premiums began asking workers to pay at least a token amount. Employees balked. Health benefits became one of the decade's most acrimonious labor-bargaining issues, playing a role in two thirds of all strikes in 1987. Even when companies got their way, cost sharing by itself was just a palliative. Employees might be liable for the first $250 of medical expenses, but that became essentially irrelevant when hospital bills often topped $10,000. And carefully designed copayment formulas, in which employees were expected to pay 20 percent of health bills, could be subverted if medical providers pressed hard for companies to pay their 80 percent share but treated employees' obligations leniently.

The hardest battle for employers involved challenging the medical establishment head-on. Corporate benefits managers generally shied from confronting anyone: they tended to be mild-mannered careerists, most comfortable in safe, orderly jobs. Besides, benefits managers shared the national attitude that *Fortune* magazine dubbed "MD-eification" — an almost obsequious deference to physicians' judgment. Medical experts had long encouraged this. As early as the 1950s, the head of the American Hospital Association told a meeting of Blue Cross insurers that they shouldn't meddle in medical decisions but should simply be "an agency for the prepayment of hospital care *as it is determined to be by the hospitals and doctors.*"

But the medical establishment in the 1980s began losing its aura of untouchability. Some of the first blows were struck by health-economics researchers, who pinpointed undeniable examples of medical excess. Dartmouth physician John Wennberg produced study after study showing astonishing regional variations in how often different doctors performed the same procedure. He found, for example, that pediatricians in Stowe, Vermont, performed tonsillectomies on 66 percent of local children, triple the rate in many nearby towns. There wasn't any evidence that children in Stowe were sicker — just that doctors in town were on a surgery binge.

In California, Rand Corporation researchers took the next step and began calculating how many inappropriate surgeries were being done each year. Rand was a think tank best known for its Vietnam-era military analysis. As its Pentagon contracts waned, Rand pushed into health-care research, led by Robert Brook, a Johns Hopkins–trained internist who believed that American medicine was riddled with waste. Brook and his colleagues won headlines from the mid-1980s on, with studies reporting that 14 percent of all coronary bypass surgeries in the United States were inappropriate; that 16 percent of hysterectomies were unnecessary and another 25 percent debatable. The Wennberg and Rand studies didn't lead to any immediate drops in surgery rates. Nonetheless, they became powerful ammunition for reformers who argued that American surgeons were operating far too often, treating patients as financial piñatas to be cut open for profit.

It took employers and their health insurance companies several years to find the most effective strategy for containing medical costs. Most early efforts in the mid-1980s concentrated on after-the-fact challenges to treatment costs. These early attempts didn't always work well; they irritated doctors and seldom produced lasting savings. Cost-control programs would work for a year or two, then lose their potency as doctors figured out how to maneuver around the insurance industry's barriers. Still, some of these initiatives — such as requiring doctors to get advance approval for routine hospitalizations, or requiring surgeons to get second opinions before performing some operations — showed that new ideas were seeping into the health insurance industry.

Gradually insurers became more adamant about their mission to hold down costs. Thanks to increasingly sophisticated computer programs, insurers could follow the money trail of individual doctors, hospitals, and medical-procedure codes much more closely. Alarming financial details emerged from this tracking. Stories circulated about doctors who performed hysterectomies that should have cost $2,000, but who billed for a $7,000 assortment of lesser procedures, including separate charges for opening up the patient, removing scar tissue, removing the uterus, and stitching up. "It's awful," an executive of Benefit Trust Life Insurance declared in 1990. "These unscrupulous doctors use any excuse to increase their revenues."

Equally repugnant in payers' eyes were doctors who owned their own diagnostic machines and found endless reasons to use them on patients. After studies showed rampant overuse of X-ray machines by some doctors who owned such equipment, Congress in 1989 barred physicians from getting Medicare payments on referrals to diagnostic centers that they owned. The California congressman most involved with that legislation, Pete Stark, vowed, "I'll be back with more legislation to weed out the greedy bastards."

As the case against high-cost medicine kept mounting, some employers wondered whether the basic design of America's health-care system was fatally flawed. From the 1920s onward, companies or their health insurers had paid doctors and hospitals for each service as it was provided. Employers and insurers also allowed the medical community wide latitude to decide what treatment each patient needed. Both practices had seemed logical. Corporations bought just about all their raw materials, from steel beams to envelopes, on a per-unit basis. And laymen originally had no intention of second-guessing their local MD-eities. By the late 1980s, however, many employers believed that those two practices invited wild overtreatment. The more tests, operations, and patient visits that doctors and hospitals conducted, the more money they collected. And who decided what level of care was appropriate? The doctors and hospitals themselves.

"We were the ones who created an out-of-control system," Allied Signal's Ted Halkyard later conceded. "A doctor could say, 'The more I treat, the more I get paid, and no one is watching me.' Or the doctor could decide: 'It's my responsibility to do everything I can for this patient.' All the incentives worked in the direction toward overtreatment. Doctors and hospitals were incapable, from an economic standpoint, of governing themselves." That message sunk home for Halkyard when he served for a few years on the board of a local New Jersey hospital, an experience that he dryly described as "very enlightening." Even as Allied Signal hoped that medical costs would moderate, executives at the local hospital rushed to create profit centers, such as an outpatient unit, that would capture more money from employers' budgets. Halkyard's conclusion: "They were acting rationally in a screwed-up system."

The only effective way to change the way medicine was practiced, some employers and insurers came to believe, was to intervene before doctors ever saw a patient. The name for such intervention was managed care.

Put bluntly, managed care amounted to a power grab by employers and the insurance industry. Its central tenet was that doctors, hospitals, and patients couldn't be given free rein any longer to choose whatever course of treatment they wanted. Outside supervision was needed — not only to hold down costs, but also to decide what constituted appropriate care. Managed-care experts would decide which doctors and hospitals to include in a treatment network. Outside supervisors then could monitor these medical providers according to standards of cost-effectiveness. Health plans would continue to cover the standard assortments of doctors' visits, tests, and hospital stays. But all the old incentives that encouraged abundant or excessive care would die. The new approach would reward thrift and punish overtreatment.

The all-purpose label of "managed care" applied to many varieties of reform. The most far-reaching versions were health maintenance organizations, or HMOs. Those health plans required patients to use only a preselected group of cost-efficient doctors and hospitals if they wanted any insurance coverage at all. Most HMOs also insisted on advance approval for specialist referrals, hospital stays, or other costly services. Some of these health plans, known as "staff-model" or "group-model" HMOs, delivered care at clinics they owned, using their own roster of physicians who worked full-time for that plan. Other HMOs, known as "independent practice" plans, sent members to nominally private doctors who had agreed to play by managed care's rules.

Whatever structure was used, most HMOs radically changed the way that physicians and hospitals were paid. No longer did each procedure generate extra income. Instead, many doctors were put on flat monthly rates — a system known as "capitation" — to cover all patient care, no matter how healthy or sick the plan member was. Hospitals were subject to similar payment schemes, most notably fixed-price "case rates" for treatment of specific illnesses. In this approach, medical providers thrived if they kept patients out of the intensive-care unit or the internist's office. No longer the big money-makers, sick patients became the heaviest drains on fixed capitation checks.

For employers or workers who found HMOs too severe, insurers offered more lenient versions of managed care. Members of PPOs were encouraged to use a preselected network of cost-effective doctors and hospitals, but weren't subject to advance-approval requirements for most care. In point-of-service (POS) networks, members essentially belonged to an HMO but had the option to go outside the network if they made steep personal copayments for that care, typically 30 percent of the charges. In general, looser forms of managed care put fewer constraints on doctors or made it easier for patients to see a wider range of physicians. But they typically involved higher premiums or members' paying of a greater share of the costs. As the managed-care movement evolved, new-products wizards at insurance companies fiddled with their basic formulas in much the way that a paint-store clerk might mix up different shades of tan or blue paint. Acronyms abounded as insurers marketed health plans with whatever blend of cost controls and flexibility that employers and their workers wanted.

On a small scale, many of the principles of managed care had been in use since 1929, when idealistic doctors in Elk City, Oklahoma, and Los Angeles separately set up tiny health plans to care for local workers. These "prepaid group practices" tried to make premiums as affordable as possible; during the Great Depression, members of the Community Hospital Association of Elk City paid just $12 a year. That single payment entitled members to full medical care without any extra charges, no matter what the ailment, as long as they dealt only with physicians in the group. Forced to operate within a fixed budget each year without knowing their caseloads, doctors in these groups tried to develop informal standards for good, low-cost care so that they wouldn't squander resources.

But these early versions of managed care were hardly a creation of the insurance industry or of employers angry about rising costs. They were frankly socialist in their approach, with just a few thousand members and no clear grasp of the potential for profit embedded in their way of doing business. There is irony in that beginning, considering managed care's later evolution.

In the 1940s more precursors to HMOs were started in other cities. The most successful by far was Kaiser Permanente, created by physician Sidney Garfield during World War II to serve workers in Henry Kaiser's shipyards, steel mills, and other enterprises. The Kaiser health plan started big and quickly grew bigger by covering workers from other companies up and down the West Coast. It built its own hospitals, ran its own clinics, and provided full-time work for hundreds of doctors. From a base of 30,000 members at the end of World War II, Kaiser Permanente grew to 250,000 in 1952 and more than one million in the 1960s. The Kaiser health plans became known as thrifty but reliable, appealing to labor unions that wanted to offer full health insurance to their workers without paying exorbitant rates. Similar group practices started by doctors in other cities evolved into Health Insurance Plan (HIP) in New York, Group Health Cooperative of Puget Sound in Seattle, and Group Health Association in Washington, D.C.

In those early decades HMO-type plans and their physicians were constantly attacked by mainstream doctors' groups. Social snubs were common, as were whispering campaigns about supposed flaws in the

HMO doctors' backgrounds. The AMA periodically debated whether prepaid group practices were unethical, chiefly on the grounds that they violated medical codes barring doctors from soliciting patients. Talk of expelling HMO doctors from medical societies arose at times. While few of these threats were carried out, the long battles over "ethics" issues took their toll. In his autobiography the founder of the Oklahoma plan, Michael Shadid, discussed his battles with organized medicine under the chapter heading "The Termites Attack."

Some early managed-care plans also developed a reputation for impersonal, clinic-style medicine, often delivered by doctors who couldn't succeed in traditional private practice. Officials at Kaiser and other major plans insisted that such stereotypes weren't true. Kaiser from the 1960s onward disclosed the percentage of its doctors who were board-certified in their specialty, confident that its percentages would exceed local averages in most communities. But the stereotype of cheap, second-rate care proved harder for other plans to overcome. As a result, managed-care plans were a sideshow to mainstream, fee-for-service medicine in the first three decades after World War II. In the mid-1960s barely 2 percent of the population belonged to HMOs.

Starting in 1970, the Nixon administration embraced HMOs as an alternative to Senator Edward Kennedy's proposals for national health insurance. Even that push didn't go far, however. Congress did pass the HMO Act of 1973, which required companies with more than 25 employees and a conventional health insurance plan to offer at least one HMO as an alternative. The act also authorized $375 million in grants and loans over a five-year period to speed up formation of more managed-care plans. Both those provisions proved quixotic. While employers did put HMOs on their benefits menu, they did so reluctantly, convinced that these new health plans were a bad choice for workers and employers alike. In one notorious case an HMO was told that it could market its services to one company's workers only on Monday, July 3 — a day when nearly all workers would be off for a four-day Independence Day weekend.

Start-up funding for HMOs, meanwhile, produced its own problems. Despite numerous $2 million awards of government aid, many of the new HMOs proved to have all the staying power of daisies in January. Some of the health plans failed quietly; others collapsed in scandals and bankruptcies. Nixon administration aides in 1971 had predicted that the United States would have 1,300 HMOs by the late

1970s, enrolling at least 65 million people. Those numbers proved far too optimistic. The national HMO roster stayed below 300 into the early 1980s. As late as 1985, HMOs covered just 18.9 million people, less than 10 percent of the population.

Then, step by step, the managed-care movement became stronger. The price savings that HMOs offered to employers began looking increasingly attractive. The industry no longer was run by amateurs; it became a multibillion-dollar business in its own right. Mainstream insurance companies such as Cigna, Prudential, Aetna, and the Blue Cross plans began moving aggressively into managed care. Independent HMOs grew into professionally managed enterprises themselves, with all the poise needed to win major corporate accounts. Scruffy no more, managed-care companies by the late 1980s could tell an appealing story about how they recruited capable doctors, put them on non-traditional pay schemes, and ran a medical system designed to be both cost-effective and reliable. That was exactly what employers wanted to hear.

Allied Signal's rapid conversion to managed care in the late 1980s — noticed by only a handful of business reporters at the time — turned out to be a trendsetter and a classic case study in its own right. The rapid dismantling of the company's traditional fee-for-service health plan in favor of managed care became a huge, frantic project. It involved some unpleasant tradeoffs, including a fraying of the basic trust that had made 50,000 workers across the country think Allied Signal was a good place to work. But the switchover undeniably saved a lot of money. It sounded good, at least as retold by Cigna, benefits consultants, and company executives. And because Allied Signal was such a bedrock American company (its stock is one of the 30 components of the Dow Jones Industrial Average), the company's willingness to adopt wholesale managed care legitimized the HMO movement in the eyes of many corporate executives.

To coax insurers to set up such a program, Allied Signal offered to let a single carrier handle all its health benefits for three years, a prize equal to nearly $1 billion in revenue. But the terms were tough. The managed-care vendor had to guarantee unusually slim rate increases through 1990. If costs jumped beyond projections, the insurer would have to cover every penny of the overruns. At first, groups ranging from Kaiser Permanente to a coalition of Blue Cross insurers said they might want to bid. But as Allied Signal's tough conditions became known, the field narrowed. By the deadline of June 1987, only two contestants remained: Cigna and Metropolitan Life. "We began to worry that we would come up empty-handed and look like fools," recalled Joseph Martingale of the benefits-consulting firm Towers Perrin, who helped run the selection for Allied Signal.

One Friday afternoon sealed bid documents arrived at Towers Perrin's New York offices. A scramble ensued to tear open the envelopes and see what terms the insurers were offering. "When we saw the Cigna bid," Martingale recalled, "we all breathed a huge sigh of relief." The big insurer was guaranteeing rate increases of just 6 percent a year on its managed-care business through 1990. Overall costs might be slightly higher if some employees still hadn't joined the managed-care network. But in aggregate Cigna said it could limit cost increases to single digits in each of the three contract years. Met Life, by contrast, offered higher rates and refused to provide the all-out guarantees against cost overruns that Hennessy and his aides wanted.

Allied Signal quickly cut a deal with Cigna, announcing that the great migration into managed care would take place January 1, 1988. Making that happen wouldn't be easy. The company's factories were scattered across the country, with major sites in Los Angeles, Phoenix, Kansas City, Baltimore, Massachusetts, and northern New Jersey. Unless Cigna could find enough dependable, convenient doctors in each location, the managed-care program would prove to be a mirage. Cigna executives at first assured Allied Signal that their network was so strong coast to coast that workers would move into it with hardly a hitch. At each location workers would be told to pick a primary-care doctor from Cigna's approved panel. That physician would see the employee and his or her family regularly and refer them to specialists if necessary. Trying to build enthusiasm for the new program, Ed Hennessy said he would forgo his own traditional doctor in favor of one in the managed-care network. Hennessy happened to be in robust health, with a cholesterol level so favorable that he boasted about it in magazine articles. Even if he didn't need much medical care, company officials thought his personal embrace of the system would make it seem more egalitarian.

In late 1987, just as the new arrangement was about to take hold, it became clear to insiders that Cigna's managed-care network wasn't nearly as good as promised. Employees' preferred internists and pediatricians weren't available in some Allied Signal locations, especially near the company's New Jersey headquarters. What's more, Cigna's pay scale for physicians was so stingy that even when the insurer tried to entice those physicians into its network, they wouldn't budge. Allied Signal delayed the launch two months, hoping that more doctors would join, and then nervously rolled out the program. Employees began haranguing Halkyard and even Hennessy about problems with the network. Halkyard couldn't sleep some nights for fear that he had made a dreadful mistake. "It was horrendous for a while," recalled Martingale, the benefits consultant. "New Jersey was the worst. Looking back on it, we hurried a little too much to put the network in place. We were reckless."

Despite such hidden problems, Allied Signal's jump into managed care soon was copied by big companies across the nation. Economists and benefits consultants suggested that HMOs could lower a company's health-care costs 10 percent or more, while also slowing down the future growth rate of those costs. The exact size of savings was intensely disputed; some HMO fans claimed gains as high as 20 percent, while skeptics held that most HMO "savings" were a mirage, reflecting no more than their ability to attract younger, healthier workers. But between those two extremes lay ample evidence suggesting that managed care could reduce the use of costly medical services and thus could save money for employers. That became an especially pressing goal when new rules on accounting for retirees' health benefits caused many big companies to take multibillion-dollar write-offs in 1989 or 1990. As a result, chief executives suddenly focused attention on the steep price of employee health care — making managed care's savings all the more alluring.

In another high-profile example, Southwestern Bell started offering managed-care plans to employees in 1987, gradually expanding them to cover the bulk of its 67,000 workers. Sears Roebuck began similar programs in Los Angeles and Houston in 1990, then rapidly expanded them to 47 other cities over the next three years. "It was emotional at first," said James Bronson, head of employee benefits at Sears. "But we felt we had to do this from a business survival standpoint." As workers settled into the new system, growth in Sears's health costs slowed to less than 4 percent a year, from well above 10 percent.

The table-pounding CEO became a familiar feature in benefits managers' lives in the early 1990s, goading them to take up managed care as fast as possible. In Detroit, General Motors chairman John

Smith personally lobbied the governor to block creation of Michigan's 29th open-heart-surgery facility, contending that it was wasteful and would only drive up costs. In Minneapolis, Kenneth Macke, chairman of the Dayton Hudson retailing chain, calculated that his company had to sell 39,000 Ninja Turtles just to pay for one appendectomy — a price he called intolerable. And in San Francisco, powerful banker Carl Reichardt, chairman of Wells Fargo, began a crusade against soaring maternity costs, focusing especially on what he perceived as overuse of costly cesarean sections. All three companies, not surprisingly, became regional leaders in the drive toward more managed care.

Sometimes a CEO's wrath could inspire subordinates to act in ways that changed a whole region's balance of power in medical-coverage negotiations. "I used to hate my meetings with Reichardt," recalls Steve Enna, the one-time head of human resources at Wells Fargo. "He kept pounding on me: 'What are we doing to contain this?' It was a killer." In 1989 Enna took a crucial first step by hosting a strategy breakfast for health managers from a dozen other Bay Area corporations, at which he enlisted them to develop a joint strategy for cutting health costs. That chat group soon evolved into the Pacific Business Group on Health, a renowned negotiator of low-priced managed-care contracts. By 1996 PBGH represented companies with more than 250,000 workers and dependents.

The crusade for managed care may have started in corporate CEOs' offices, but before long the trend was noticeable in many other places as well. The media played an important role, repeatedly declaring that a health crisis was at hand and that greater use of HMOs might be the only way out. In a 1991 cover story, *Time* magazine declared that America's medical bills "flow from a surreal world where science has lost connection with reality, where bureaucracy and paperwork have no limit, where a half-hour tonsillectomy costs what an average worker earns in three weeks. The prices, like the system that issues them, are out of control. . . . To control costs, care must be delivered through tightly managed private systems, such as a network of health maintenance organizations."

Consultants got into the game too. Benefits-consulting firms such as Towers Perrin, William Mercer, and Foster Higgins rapidly built up teams with "managed-care expertise." Then they went hunting for clients. Most consultants believed that the country truly would benefit from their ideas — but money, ego, and glory were important too.

Advisory fees for a wholesale conversion such as Allied Signal's could top $1 million. A consultant on such a high-status assignment was likely to be made a partner or win other promotions. Furthermore, once a basic managed-care program had been designed, consultants found it very tempting to travel around the country and install the same program elsewhere. "We'd like to think we played a large role and helped steer things," says John Erb, a veteran benefits consultant for Foster Higgins. "Consultants certainly stir the pot. And in some cases it becomes a competition between consultants and benefits managers. It almost doesn't matter if they reduce costs, as long as they get their names in the *Wall Street Journal* and get a reputation for being innovative."

Meanwhile state and local governments embraced managed care as the cure for their rapidly rising employee medical bills. California became the best-known example, holding a yearly contest from 1992 onward among nearly two dozen HMOs to see which could offer the best value on health insurance for nearly one million state employees and their dependents. Stanford University economist Alain Enthoven helped shape the rules for that contest, which he called "managed competition." It proved to be a huge cost saver for California, leading to several years of rate decreases in the mid-1990s. Other states, including Minnesota, New York, and Florida, rushed to make greater use of managed care as well. Like their corporate counterparts, top state officials acted out of a sense of fiscal urgency bordering on panic. "Health care costs have created an American state of siege," Florida's governor, Lawton Chiles, declared in 1991. "It's going to break us."

Unions continued to agitate for managed care as well. In contract talks in 1989, American Telephone & Telegraph proposed that workers share much more of the costs of the phone company's traditional indemnity health plan. That drew an angry reaction from leaders of the Communications Workers of America. "The union said, 'You've never done anything to manage these costs,'" one insider recalled. In its counterproposal the union urged AT&T to drop its cost-sharing ideas and try to make a major move toward managed care instead. Phone company officials resisted until just minutes before a strike deadline, then agreed to join the HMO parade.

Small employers joined the trend, too, thanks to business coalitions that sprung up in dozens of cities. By banding together and jointly negotiating health rates, even companies with just 25 employees could command the attention and the best prices of managed-care providers. In Denver the Colorado Health Care Purchasing Alliance began negotiating for 160 local employers, ranging from giant Coors Brewing to restaurants and tiny wildcat oil companies. Similar coalitions in cities such as Miami, Houston, and Des Moines helped concentrate bargaining power in the hands of business.

At Allied Signal some executives who initially pushed the hardest for managed care later conceded that the switchover had its painful side. "I don't think it ever will be embraced in the way that the old, solid-as-can-be indemnity system was," remarked Ted Halkyard, the company's benefits chief during the switchover, in a 1995 interview. Halkyard's long-time boss, Ed Hennessy, could testify to that personally. As CEO he found that the Cigna plan served him well. But when he retired in 1991 and began splitting his time between Florida and New Jersey, Hennessy discovered that he couldn't have regular doctors in both places. Under managed care he was required to pick one site as his home and then pay extra if he wanted care elsewhere. That was annoying. So were memories of rebukes from his employees. One time, Hennessy confided, his own secretary had lambasted him about her troubles with the new medical plan.

But the company's next generation of managers entertained no doubts. They goaded Cigna to expand its managed-care network and offered workers more HMO choices. In their eyes, Allied Signal's health-benefits package was steadily improving. Furthermore, managed care was saving money. As Russell Hawkins, the company's new benefits manager, observed, "Health care is our single largest outside purchase. It's $400 million a year — more than any raw material. It's at the top of our chairman's hit parade. His interest is ever-present. If we can keep our spending rate flat, that will be very good news for the company."

3

The New Mandarins

LIKE MOST OF THE FACULTY at Harvard Medical School, lung specialist Barry Levine and colon surgeon Paul Shellito thought of themselves as "star doctors." They weren't smug about it; they simply believed that their training and credentials qualified them for inclusion in America's medical elite. Both men had received federal research grants and had regularly published articles in leading medical journals. Both had staff privileges at Massachusetts General Hospital, regularly ranked among the five best medical centers in the United States. And both doctors had a nice way with patients. Dr. Levine brought a candid, upbeat style to the exam room. Dr. Shellito proved that even surgeons can be warm and caring, visiting patients frequently in the days after operations and doing all he could to improve their comfort as well as their healing.

Then curious letters arrived in the doctors' "in" baskets in the summer of 1993. The messages were from Tufts Associated Health Plans, an HMO that paid Drs. Levine and Shellito to treat some of its members. The two doctors were invited to three evening chat sessions, at which physicians and HMO managers would brainstorm about ways to manage hospital cases better. That easygoing request concealed a shrewd objective. Tufts had strong ideas about how to practice efficient medicine, and it knew which doctors had recently kept patients in hospitals for longer than the HMO felt was necessary. In its polite but iron-willed way, Tufts was singling out those physicians so it could bend them to its way of thinking.

When the evening conferences began, so did the reeducation of Drs. Levine and Shellito. Tufts officials offered the physicians a seat at a

cramped conference table and asked them to help review condensed
hospital records for nearly 20 HMO members. All the patients had
fared well; the main question was whether various attending physicians had kept the patients in the hospital for the appropriate length of
time. Dr. Levine, chatty as always, weighed in with his ideas. Then he
noticed that his hosts weren't exactly hanging on his every word.

The man in command was Joe Gerstein, a long-time community
doctor who now worked for Tufts full-time as a medical director. In
case after case Dr. Gerstein ticked off ways that he would have handled
things differently: discharging a heart attack patient a half-day earlier;
using a shorter-lived anesthetic in stomach surgery so that patients
could go home faster. Dr. Gerstein's tone was friendly, his medical
knowledge formidable and backed up with detailed statistics about
how Mass. General was handling Tufts patients. The star doctors
squirmed at times, yet they had no choice but to absorb this tutorial
on efficiency. Tufts was one of the hospital's biggest customers, sending
about 600 patients a year to Mass. General. All that business could go
elsewhere if the renowned hospital didn't please the HMO. As Dr.
Gerstein put it, "The flow of patients is clearly related to how well you
do at this."

Brilliant Harvard specialists weren't the only ones getting blunt
schooling in the ways of managed care. Almost every part of the
American medical establishment from 1990 on has been rocked by the
growing influence of HMOs. Primary-care doctors, specialists, and
hospitals all have been told to cut costs, improve efficiency, or simply
try harder to practice medicine in the orderly, disciplined fashion that
HMOs prize. Pharmaceutical companies have been lashed as well, as
managed-care plans snub their marketers and declare certain high-
priced drugs off-limits. The people delivering these messages have become some of the most powerful figures in American health care. They
all share a conviction that medicine has been an inefficient cottage
industry for too long and that their rules and statistical methods can
vastly improve the field.

Just a few years earlier, it would have been unthinkable for health-
plan officials to have such impact. Power in American medicine was
concentrated in the hands of highly regarded specialists at major medical centers. These doctors enjoyed free rein to order as many tests as
they wanted, to keep patients in the hospital for whatever period they
thought was appropriate, and to defy any attempts to standardize their

work. They were the top gods in America's pantheon of MD-eities, with immense reputations and even larger egos. If a nurse, hospital administrator, or insurance clerk questioned their methods, these doctors usually could overwhelm the opposition with a withering stare and a frosty rebuttal that typically began: "In my experience . . ."

With the advent of managed care, everything changed. Health plans could move huge blocks of patients away from doctors or hospitals that didn't practice cost-effective medicine. Fame, ego, and free-spending ways didn't count for much anymore. Managed-care plans wanted to do business with providers who shared their values and could keep a large panel of patients as healthy as possible for as cheaply as possible. Suddenly America's major health plans weren't just a collection of clerks paying bills or sour-tempered case reviewers challenging an occasional charge before yielding in the face of superior medical knowledge. Health plans were pumped full of medical-management expertise and power. Many HMOs believed they could teach even famous doctors a thing or two about how to practice more efficiently.

Within HMOs a new elite rose to power: doctors and statisticians who could wield computer-generated data in the battle for greater medical efficiency. These experts could pinpoint a medical issue — such as how long to hospitalize a heart attack patient or how best to care for asthmatic children — and then pick apart the problem with a computer-aided analysis of how 100,000 or more such patients were being treated. Many of these experts were former doctors who had mastered statistical methods; some were statisticians with a rough grasp of medicine. Either way, they zoomed to prominence as they spun out numbers that let them identify average performance, best practices, and subpar work. With that information in hand, HMO overseers could goad doctors to improve their scores. Some physicians fought this data brigade, claiming that their own medical practices were too distinctive to fit the standard mold. But in the world of managed care, people who relied on "In my experience . . ." seldom won an argument. Those holdout doctors were trumped, again and again, by the stern response: "According to our data . . ."

To keep their self-assuredness intact, HMO managers often shield themselves from any distracting information. They form their own professional societies and publish their own journals, promoting managed care and cost-effective medicine. They swap computer printouts and bar charts showing efficiency gains. And they try never to dwell on individual cases that have gone wrong.

One of the great clustering points for these medical mandarins is a suburban office park in Blue Bell, Pennsylvania. There 40 doctors in business suits work for the U.S. Healthcare division of Aetna Life & Casualty. Their mission: to nudge 30,000 or more practicing physicians into conformity with the HMO's notions of cost-effective quality care. These medical executives were internists or family practitioners themselves a few years ago. Vigorous and healthy, they could have stayed in private practice for decades before reaching normal retirement age. Instead they came to U.S. Healthcare, lured by high pay, generous stock options — and the chance to make the rules of managed care instead of following them.

Typical is Jay Rosan, a one-time family practice doctor who has worked full-time for U.S. Healthcare since 1984. One of his early projects was an initiative to get more doctors to perform annual mammograms on women age 50 and over. Such tests help detect possible breast cancer early, when treatment costs are cheapest and patients' prospects for long-term survival are best. Dr. Rosan started by mailing mammogram booklets to 1,200 doctors in U.S. Healthcare's network, but he didn't get much of a response. So he organized seminars on the importance of mammography, offering doctors $50 apiece if they attended the seminars and passed a simple quiz afterward. Compliance with the U.S. Healthcare program soared. "Most people work with incentives in most industries," Dr. Rosan later explained. "We decided, why not show physicians what we want and then let them drive toward it?"

Other medical executives at U.S. Healthcare have set up guidelines for immunizing babies, keeping asthmatic children out of the hospital, and reducing the rates of cesarean sections. Participating doctors who follow those guidelines get bonuses. Those who fall short are reprimanded. With 30,000 doctors to oversee — stretching from New Hampshire to Georgia — the HMO medical directors stay furiously busy. They collate data, pull together computer spreadsheets, and constantly go on the road to pitch their new objectives to doctors throughout the health plan's network. Their mission was tersely defined by company founder Leonard Abramson, who often declared, "It doesn't count if you can't count it."

In their marketing materials, HMOs such as U.S. Healthcare

claimed that they could monitor doctors' performance across the full range of sickness and treatment. But this supposed comprehensiveness was a mirage. The HMOs focused on a narrow cluster of treatments in which data were easy to gather and where cost savings did not compromise medical quality. Those criteria pointed almost exclusively to primary care doctors' records in carrying out simple screening tests. HMOs took much longer to get interested in systematic ways to improve care for sick patients. Even then, the plans concentrated on the cheapest, most mechanical aspects of care, such as whether patients with high blood pressure regularly weighed themselves.

If U.S. Healthcare's medical directors knew they were dodging the hard topics, they seldom let on. In a burst of self-importance in the early 1990s, they set up their own research institute, U.S. Quality Algorithms. They began a quarterly publication, grandly titled *USQA Quality Monitor: The Journal of Health Care Performance Measurement and Improvement.* Company physicians submitted footnoted articles; graphically, at least, the *Quality Monitor* closely resembled mainstream, peer-reviewed medical journals. But the articles weren't actually reviewed before publication by anyone outside U.S. Healthcare. Even so, the journal and the institute helped the HMO look rigorous in its work, winning admiration from employers and respect from many doctors.

As pure exercises in statistics, in fact, some of U.S. Healthcare's projects were magnificent. When the HMO decided that too many hysterectomies were being performed all along the East Coast, it gathered monthly practice data on 86 gynecologists in its network. That information turned into vivid charts full of red and orange dots, showing how often each gynecologist had performed a simple biopsy beforehand that could rule out the need for a hysterectomy. Those charts were mailed to each doctor, along with a little marker that identified one of the red dots as "Your office." The HMO hardly needed to do anything more. Gynecologists who were not doing enough biopsies before operating quickly changed their practice habits to conform with their peers. Over a four-year span biopsy rates for U.S. Healthcare members more than doubled, while hysterectomy rates dropped more than 30 percent. At the end of the project a U.S. Healthcare medical director proudly showed his graph of the change to a magazine reporter and declared, "It's beautiful. Especially where the lines meet in the middle."

Where did these analytic methods come from? They might have seemed fresh and startling to practicing physicians, but they were old news in the factories and service depots of industrial America. An entire discipline of quality engineering has sprung up since the 1930s, growing out of early work by Walter Shewhart, W. Edwards Deming, and Genichi Taguchi. By the 1980s the concept had been repackaged as Total Quality Management (TQM) or Continuous Quality Improvement (CQI) and was being hawked around the country by $5,000-a-day consultants. Devotees claim that these methods have done everything from helping Ford Motor cut the defect rate on its auto assembly lines to spurring the semiconductor industry to improve productivity.

In the eyes of many managed-care enthusiasts, medicine just wasn't that different from car making or computer-chip fabrication — no matter what doctors and patients thought. In a widely quoted speech to the Henry Ford Health System in 1990, physician and health-care consultant Donald Berwick observed, "The notion of controlling variation strikes fear into health care professionals. The objections come fast: 'This matter of quality control may be fine for manufacturing, but I am a physician. I don't make widgets.' Or: 'Medicine isn't like making cars. The product is not uniform. Every patient is different.'" Dr. Berwick acknowledged those anxieties but quickly dismissed them. As he put it, "It is essential that these connotations change if health care is going to benefit fully from modern total quality management."

To corporate employers, who were paying many Americans' health-care bills, the arrival of TQM on the medical scene was glorious news. Companies such as Xerox, GTE, and Digital Equipment had used these methods to improve quality in their own industries. TQM had raised the mean, reduced the variability, and lowered defect rates. Best of all, it had cut costs. These companies liked what quality-engineering principles had accomplished in the manufacturing of office copiers, phone equipment, and minicomputers. If health plans wanted to band together and promote standard measures of medical quality, employers were all for it. In fact, they offered to help. Throughout the early 1990s, a handful of employers and HMOs met to devise ways to gauge health-plan performance. They christened their benchmarks "HEDIS."* In 1993 individual HMOs began publishing their scores in

*The acronym stands for Health Plan Employer Data and Information Set.

this rating system, much as an air-conditioner manufacturer might report its energy-efficient rating.

These scorecards provided a skewed picture of medicine that played into HMOs' marketing strategies. Yet they attracted wide and generally positive media coverage. "HMO report cards . . . are starting to peel back the ignorance about who cures best," *Fortune* declared in October 1994. Clark Kerr, a BankAmerica vice president, told a health magazine that although it wouldn't be cheap to collect report card data, "we'll reap 10 times the cost in savings from increased quality care."

What outsiders didn't fully realize was how much the new medical quality reports were dominated by simple primary-care measures. Data abounded on how well the plans and their doctors did at checking cholesterol and providing routine cancer screenings. There was almost nothing on the hardest part of medicine: taking care of sick people. Xerox benefits manager Helen Darling later said she had pushed hard in 1992 for a basic measure of care for heart attack patients. But HMOs and cardiologists talked her out of it, saying the issues involved were too complicated. The result was a strangely lopsided picture of medical care, filled with healthy patients getting checkups but devoid of anyone fighting a serious illness. By the yardsticks of HEDIS, a health plan could achieve a fine score without having the least ability to deliver good care in a crisis.

Those omissions didn't happen by accident. Kathryn Coltin of Harvard Community Health Plan explained that her HMO's interest in HEDIS "grew out of an opportunity for us to establish a competitive edge. We said, 'Look, we can develop some measures that will show our value. If we can do that to purchasers' satisfaction, it will give us an advantage in the marketplace.'" Employers and their advisers couldn't do much to widen the choice of measures; they didn't know as much about medicine as did the HMO representatives at the drafting table. "If we needed expertise, we basically went to the health plans," conceded Janet Corrigan, who helped sketch out several early report cards while working for the group overseeing HEDIS, an HMO-employer coalition known as the National Committee for Quality Assurance.

In 1995 big employers belatedly began talking about monitoring HMOs' actual handling of illnesses. Working committees at NCQA started drafting new standards, known as HEDIS 3.0, that were to be launched in 1997. Those were meant, at last, to consider ongoing care of people with AIDS, diabetes, and other chronic illnesses. A different coalition of big employers, calling itself the Foundation for Account- ability, or FAcct, vowed to develop similar measures of treatment out- comes. Managed-care plans never opposed these steps outright; they simply kept pointing out complexities in the measurement of data that would have to be addressed. The net effect was that NCQA's most interesting new measures of HMO performance were put forward only as pilot projects to be "tested" for several years — a result that man- aged-care companies might not have minded at all.

When Harvard doctor Paul Shellito finished his tutorial on HMO-style efficiency, he emerged as an apparent convert to the new system. "It has changed the way I practice," he remarked in early 1994. "Tufts is very good at finding ways to get patients out of the hospital sooner with only a little inconvenience. Now I'm haggling with patients about going home the evening that I see them."

But Dr. Shellito's inner loyalties remained divided. "We know we have to do this, and Tufts is conscientious about the way they work with us," he said. "But this is all about cost, not improving patient care. Patient care was fine before." Enforcing the new rules, he found, sometimes left him with an unpleasant feeling. One touchy time oc- curred on a winter afternoon when he prepared to discharge a woman whose incision was still healing from major surgery. Ordinarily such a patient could expect a cheery welcome home from her spouse. But the woman's husband was in the hospital too, with a different ailment. She pleaded with her surgeon for an extra recovery day in the hospital, not because it was medically necessary but because she was afraid of going home to a lonely, empty house. Dr. Shellito's reluctant response, "I told her she had to go home."

Such everyday predicaments illustrate one of managed care's great- est challenges. Too much compassion and a health plan never saves any money. Too little compassion and the best aspects of American medical care are destroyed in favor of a grim medical assembly line that bounces patients along without any sensitivity to their unique con- cerns.

The architect of the Tufts/Mass. General relationship, the HMO's Dr. Gerstein, admitted in a series of 1994 interviews that he wor- ried about getting that balance right. "Physicians are resentful enough when colleagues look over their work," he observed. "When it's an insurance company, they go wild." His HMO did best when it could interest physicians themselves in analyzing their processes for handling common illnesses and making their own systems work better. When necessary, Dr. Gerstein was willing to play the tough cop in this process, pushing for lower-cost treatment. Still, he occasionally tore up his own drafts of letters to doctors and patients denying coverage after the fact for extended hospital stays — and left those letters unsent. "I had an attack of conscience," he later explained. "I thought there might be extenuating circumstances in a long hospital stay."

In many managed-care settings, such qualms seldom arise. Medical administrators stay at headquarters, where they are buffered from patients' individuality. Instead, cases are lumped together in computer printouts, making it almost inevitable that patients are treated as statistics. In this situation HMO executives usually let their wallets do their thinking. Dollar savings from managed-care guidelines are big. Minor inconveniences to patients don't matter; health-plan monitoring systems are set up to notice only more serious problems such as written complaints, hospital readmissions of prematurely discharged patients, or deaths. And if star doctors complain that managed care is cramping their practice style, the reaction within some HMOs is: good!

"There's been a history of 40 years of specialist contempt for primary-care doctors," observed Tom Rosenthal, a kidney-transplant specialist in Los Angeles. "Now it's payback time."

Sometimes the settling of old scores can be downright brutal. Edward Cadman, chief of staff at Yale–New Haven Hospital, was visited in the spring of 1995 by the chairman of one large HMO, who was furious about Yale's handling of a patient with unstable angina. The man had been in the hospital for 23 days — and for the first 10 days he did little but wait for doctors to get to his case. Only on the 11th day did cardiologists perform the essential test to learn more about his heart condition: inserting a fine tube into a vein, snaking it up toward his heart, releasing X-ray-sensitive dye, then capturing his heart function on film, a process known as angiography. That was soon followed by an artery-widening procedure known as an angioplasty, after which the patient recovered normally.

Dr. Cadman knew he had some apologizing to do about the extended delay. The patient's HMO, Health Systems International, had paid $3,000 a day for him to wait in the Yale intensive-care unit while the hospital's cardiologists completed other cases. The delay was wasteful, and it wasn't good medicine; an untreated patient with unstable angina is at risk of a heart attack. Dr. Cadman was quite prepared to extend Yale's regrets and to promise faster service in the future. What he didn't expect was the withering opening line from Health Systems' chairman, Malik Hasan, a one-time practicing physician himself.

"I wouldn't send my dog to your hospital!" Dr. Hasan declared. Shuffling through a stack of medical records on the case, Dr. Hasan pointed out delay after delay while his HMO was expected to absorb all of Yale's charges.

"All I could do was agree with him," Dr. Cadman later recalled. "I told him, 'I abhor inefficiency too.'" In an effort to make peace, Dr. Cadman added, "If you feel it's unnecessary to pay for the treatment, then don't." After that unconditional surrender the conversation became friendlier; by the end of the session Dr. Cadman could describe the two men's rapport as "nice." But it was nice on the HMO's terms, not Yale's.

On the West Coast as well, Dr. Hasan established himself as the scourge of famous medical centers that didn't meet his efficiency standards. In 1991 the Qual-Med subsidiary of Health Systems tried and failed to get a 30 percent rate cut from the most renowned hospital in Seattle, Swedish Medical Center. When talks broke down, Qual-Med simply stopped sending any patients to Swedish and began steering them to cheaper, less prominent suburban hospitals. The change generated plenty of protests from the HMO's members. The region's largest employer, Boeing, stopped offering Qual-Med to its employees because it regarded access to Swedish as an essential part of a decent local health plan. But the HMO didn't budge. "We weren't in the business of providing care that we couldn't afford," the HMO's regional medical director at the time, Raymond Austin, later explained.*

On a third occasion Dr. Hasan opened rate negotiations with the

---

*The HMO's chairman, Dr. Hasan, was even blunter. In a revealing interview with the *Wall Street Transcript* in 1992, he suggested that Boeing, not the HMO, was behaving strangely. Dr. Hasan said he was surprised that Boeing's "major priority was not to control costs but to keep their employees happy." He added, "I'm sure that when we talk with them again, their priorities will be different."

medical center at the University of California, Los Angeles, by arriving in a long white limousine and then telling shocked officials of the elite hospital, "It's a Darwinian world. We are not going to be subsidizing the University of California anymore." UCLA charged too much, he explained, and pulled out detailed analyses of Medicare data to prove his point. No matter how one examined the medical center — comparing it against other big centers in southern California or against other academic medical institutions in the western United States — it just didn't make economic sense to send patients to UCLA.

The hospital administrators were stunned. Dr. Hasan's health plans accounted for $10 million or more of annual business at UCLA; it would be hard to wave goodbye to all those patients. UCLA's director of managed care, Francine Chapman, patiently tried to explain that her hospital's costs couldn't help but exceed those at community hospitals because UCLA's doctors were researchers and teachers as well as practicing physicians. But Dr. Hasan wasn't buying it. In the early 1970s he had briefly been on the faculty of an academic medical center in Chicago, Rush-Presbyterian–St. Luke's, and he hadn't been impressed by the work habits he saw there. "When I was at Rush, I was the hardest-working professor," he told the UCLA administrators. "Most of the other doctors just worked three-hour days, three times a week. A lot of academic physicians are just plain lazy."

Such broadsides leave the men and women who run teaching hospitals aghast. For decades academic medical centers have enjoyed a special place in the national psyche and the national budget. Their high costs and inefficiencies have been excused because of the belief that those centers provide the country's best hope of future medical breakthroughs and the best possible care for the desperately sick. Insurance companies didn't fuss if patients went to a $2,000-a-day teaching hospital instead of an $800-a-day community hospital; it was considered part of a patient's right to seek the best care possible. No one questioned these hospitals' propensities to do more tests, regardless of whether the additional workups were vital for that patient or were simply providing good training for interns and residents. Liberal use of high-tech medical tests was considered part of the routine at a teaching hospital. Even the federal government blessed such practices, allowing academic centers to subsidize some of their medical research by collecting higher Medicare reimbursements.

HMOs shattered those arrangements. Price was the initial battleground, but managed-care companies didn't stop there. They adopted a highly skeptical, "show me" attitude toward teaching hospitals' claims of better-quality care. "Where are the data?" health plans asked. Teaching hospital's strong reputations among community physicians and accounts of dramatic single-case success stories didn't count for much anymore. Managed-care administrators wanted statistical reports — with means and standard deviations — showing that teaching hospitals really provided better care. Those sorts of data had already been gathered for primary-care doctors doing mammograms and immunizations, HMO negotiators crisply pointed out. Where were the comparable data for hospitals' treatment of patients with ovarian cancer or third-degree burns or spine injuries? And if high-priced teaching hospitals couldn't prove that they had better outcomes, why should they expect any business from managed-care companies?

Gamely, some renowned medical centers set out to enter the data race. But as they soon discovered, HMOs had set an almost impossible task. Much of the culture of the teaching hospitals involved a willingness to take the nearly hopeless cases on the belief that the best doctors in the United States might be able to pull off a miracle, or that at least the hospital's interns and residents would learn something. There was no way to explain those cases adequately to an audience dead certain that medicine could be reduced to a collection of orange and red dots above and below a median.

When teaching hospitals began collecting HMO-style data, more problems arose. Without some sort of adjustment for severity of illness, teaching hospitals' outcomes often looked *worse* than those at small community hospitals, simply because the people with the worst burns, the most advanced cancers, and the most devastating motorcycle injuries usually were sent to the major academic medical center in an area. Statisticians considered ways to adjust raw data on survival rates or other outcomes to reflect patients' varying conditions upon arrival. But doing those adjustments well was a hugely time-consuming and expensive project, which added to the top medical centers' already unattractive costs. If risk adjustments weren't done perfectly — as usually happened — arguments about the validity of the data broke out. When those squabbles were under way, HMOs had every right to say that nothing had been proven yet.

The teaching hospitals did have another alternative: to stop taking the hardest cases, to subsidize less research and teaching with clinical revenue — and to become more like lower-cost community hospitals with their relatively easy mix of cases. It was a repugnant choice for most of the men and women who ran world-famous medical centers. But as cost-minded health plans became an ever bigger part of the medical scene, the arguments for dismantling some of the special aspects of teaching hospitals became harder to ignore.

"Our core values are threatened by managed care," declared William Speck, the chief executive of Presbyterian Hospital in New York, in a June 1995 interview. "No one has dared use the rationing word. But this will drive it. We will see denial of expensive technology for elderly people. You survive in managed care by denying or limiting care. That's how you make money." As he reviewed what he regarded as managed care's assaults on his hospital, he likened his situation to President Franklin Roosevelt's position after the Japanese attack on Pearl Harbor in 1941. "It's not fascism, and we're not democracy," Dr. Speck noted. "But I have to mobilize people about this threat. Find allies. Hold this place together."

Even teaching-hospital executives who wanted to meet managed care halfway wondered sometimes if they could find a reasonable meeting ground. In Boston an earnest doctor with an MBA, Peter Slavin, became chief medical officer of Mass. General in 1994. There, he worked closely with Partners HealthCare, the umbrella company overseeing care at both Mass. General and another famous Harvard teaching hospital, Brigham and Women's. Dr. Slavin began as an ardent champion of greater hospital efficiency, contending that even the most famous hospitals needed to become better at simple things like making sure physical therapy sessions were scheduled promptly for patients recovering from knee surgery. He helped his hospitals develop more than 40 clinical pathways — flow charts that showed how patients with common illnesses should be routed through the system. Those programs often helped shorten the length of patients' stays by a day or more, eliminating bottlenecks and helping make the hospitals more cost-competitive.

But after several years of hunting for new efficiency steps, Dr. Slavin wondered if he had pushed as far as prudence would allow. "There are areas where length of stay is as low as anyone can get," he remarked in 1995. "We hear about other centers where complaints about patients being discharged prematurely are growing tremendously. I hope that the strategy we take relies on professional instincts and doing what's best by patients, instead of someone else's agenda."

In the pharmaceutical industry, the rise of managed care has created nearly as turbulent a shift in power as it has in hospitals. All through the 1970s and 1980s, drug companies not only participated in the great expansion of American medicine, they helped define it. Research labs devised new families of drugs: angiotensin-converting enzyme (ACE) inhibitors and calcium channel blockers to treat hypertension and heart disease; H2 antagonists to treat ulcers; nonsteroidal anti-inflammatory drugs to treat arthritis. The top-selling brands in these categories often generated $1 billion or more a year in revenue — allowing drug companies to build up huge sales forces, underwrite more research, and generate some of the richest returns to shareholders seen in any U.S. industry. Patients grumbled about skyrocketing pill prices. A few U.S. senators occasionally threatened "investigations" into the industry's pricing. For the most part, though, drug companies were free to develop, market, and price their drugs as they saw fit. Pharmaceutical executives depicted their medications as bargains, even at two dollars a tablet for common maintenance drugs that patients needed to take every day of their lives.

But if drug-company executives thought their position was secure, they badly misread both the political and the business climate. In February 1993, when President Bill Clinton tried to marshal public support for his ultimately doomed health reform package, his first target for attack was the pharmaceutical industry. Profit margins in the industry had reached "unconscionable" levels, he declared. Something ought to be done about it.

Waiting to pounce were the forces of managed care. In northern California, Kaiser Permanente had already established itself as a savvy buyer of prescription drugs for its members, using its size to negotiate discounts and its in-house pharmaceutical knowledge to steer doctors' prescribing habits toward cheaper drugs. Kaiser doctors treating ulcers, for example, prescribed far less Zantac than their peers did nationwide. At Kaiser the preferred choice was Tagamet, a very similar brand-name drug that was one half to two thirds the price of Zantac. As cost concerns intensified, and as Kaiser became more confident of its ability to make wise pharmaceutical decisions for its members without the advice of drug-company marketers, the HMO began squeezing manufacturers even more aggressively.

The obvious targets for Kaiser's axe were the squadrons of drug-company sales representatives, or detailers, who traveled throughout the United States with free samples, medical journals, pens, and sports tickets, making friends with doctors and encouraging them to prescribe that company's top brands. Kaiser regarded that entire marketing exercise — employing more than 50,000 people — as contemptible. "With very few exceptions, there is no legitimacy to drug detailing," declared Francis J. Crosson Jr., Kaiser's head of health policy for northern California. "It's not an objective educational process; it's selling. The costs are just being passed on to little old ladies who need their hypertension medicine. The whole process is offensive, and we have no interest in promoting it."

Because Kaiser owned its own hospitals and doctors' offices, it could shut down pharmaceutical marketing almost at will. Drug company sales representatives were occasionally allowed onto Kaiser premises, but they had to wear unsightly badges labeling them as "VENDOR." Distribution of scientific articles about the efficacy of various drugs was controlled almost entirely by Kaiser; drug detailers could not circulate reprints of academic studies without permission from the health plan. Slick marketing materials were banned from the HMO's premises, too, as were any efforts to promote a drug not on Kaiser's approved list. Salesmen called anyway, attracted by the plan's $700 million-a-year budget for pharmaceuticals. But their ability to influence the big HMO's prescribing patterns was minimal.

Such tactics moved great power into the hands of a few Kaiser pharmacists and doctors. These experts met regularly to decide which drugs passed the HMO's cost-effectiveness standards and could be used regularly — and which ones flunked. Most of the time Kaiser blackballed only drugs for which close, cheaper substitutes were available, thereby saving money while having a barely perceptible influence on care. Sometimes, though, the HMO waded into controversy. In 1993 it refused to pay for Cognex, which was touted as the first drug that could lessen symptoms of Alzheimer's disease. "We got ripped about that," recalled Bill Elliot, a Kaiser physician involved in the decision. "But we held our ground. Our neurologists felt it had poor safety, it wasn't effective, and it had high cost. We got a lot of sympathetic messages from doctors at UCLA and elsewhere, saying, 'That was a ballsy move. We applaud you. Everyone knows this drug is worthless.'" *

What Kaiser could do internally because its doctors worked only at its facilities, other health plans ended up doing externally. They hired specialized managed-care companies, known as pharmacy benefits managers (PBMs), to promote cost-effective choices of prescription drugs. Health-plan members simply presented to their pharmacy a plastic card, bearing the logo of PCS, National Rx, Caremark, or another drug-benefit plan. The pharmacy then charged a modest copayment (typically $5 to $10) for each prescription and handled the insurance paperwork themselves. The PBMs at the very least demanded discounts from pill makers. They also frequently phoned independent doctors in an attempt to guide the physicians' prescribing habits toward cheaper, older drugs in most major classes of medications. The newest, costliest drugs generally were designated as second- or third-line choices, to be used only if the cheaper medicines didn't work well. In some cases the costliest drugs were declared ineligible for health-plan coverage at all.

PBMs swept into the health-care marketplace in the early 1990s. Employers and their HMOs began using them because they promised to save money on health benefits. Workers tolerated or even welcomed the switch because the major PBMs made it much quicker and easier to get insurance coverage for a drug prescription. In getting prescription drugs, health-plan members no longer needed to deal with the bane of fee-for-service medicine: claims forms and a long wait to get reimbursed for up-front personal payment of bills. In 1995 national membership in PBMs topped 100 million people and was growing more than 10 percent a year. PBMs, in fact, reshaped the prescription drug business to such a profound degree that three major drug companies (Merck, Lilly, and SmithKline Beecham) in 1993 and 1994 spent a

---

*Three years later, medical experts regarded Kaiser as largely — but not entirely — right in its condemnation of that particular drug. Cognex turned out to be far less effective and far more encumbered with unwelcome side effects than its manufacturer, Warner-Lambert, originally had hoped. Even in the fee-for-service market, where doctors could prescribe any drug they wanted, sales of Cognex never took off. But some private neurologists continued to try it with patients, finding that in a handful of cases, the drug might slow the steady advance of dementia associated with Alzheimer's.

total of more than $12 billion to buy major drug-benefits companies themselves.

The true power of PBMs resided in something consumers seldom saw: paperback manuals, called formularies, packed with guidance for doctors about which drugs to prescribe and which to shun. A classic among those booklets — the *1993–1994 Formulary*, issued by PCS Health Systems through its Clinical Pharmacy Advantage unit — influenced prescription decisions for as many as 20 million Americans. On its cover the booklet promised "a focus on quality." Inside, however, cost-containment priorities were emphasized no less than the company's advice about wise medical choices.

A section on psychiatric medications, for example, declared: "All antidepressants are equally effective, but vary in side effects and cost." While technically true, that statement was stunningly muted. Treatment of depression has been radically changed since 1990 by the development of new medications virtually free of the debilitating side effects often associated with older drugs. The three leading such medications — Prozac, Zoloft, and Paxil — are more expensive than their predecessors but can be tolerated by far more patients. Major HMOs became some of the strongest supporters of these medications in the mid-1990s, finding that the extra cost of medication was easily recouped by the vast reduction in patients' need for therapy sessions and psychiatric hospitalization.

Those considerations barely registered in Clinical Pharmacy's charts. In a hard-to-read table the formulary noted different side-effect profiles for the various drugs, but didn't explicitly urge doctors to take those differences into account in making their prescription decisions. Its showcase table was a listing of 19 antidepressives, ranked in order of cost, with the cheapest medications listed first. A generic drug, amitriptyline, headed the list along with a rough indicator of its costs, the notation "$." Farther down, a seldom-used drug, Nardil, was rated "$$$." At the bottom of the list, Paxil, Zoloft, and Prozac all were tagged "$$$$$." In accompanying text Clinical Pharmacy told doctors: "Prozac is no more effective than other antidepressants and is much more expensive." Two years later — after Lilly acquired PCS — the drug-benefits company had a quite different view of Prozac. "Medications should be individualized to the patient in order to optimize treatment benefit and lower risk," PCS told doctors in its 1995–

96 formulary. "Factors to consider include: possibility of side effects." To make sure that this message wasn't overlooked, PCS referred to the cheaper antidepressants as "more toxic," while lauding Prozac, by name, for significantly fewer adverse effects. Those friendly words hadn't come cheaply; it had cost Lilly $4 billion to acquire PCS. But as the evolving language of the PCS formulary suggested, the takeover had helped convert a powerful opponent of Prozac into an ally.

When asked how their formularies are put together, the companies that produce them release only sketchy details. PCS officials say their data are compiled by an advisory board of eight outside doctors who meet periodically in Minneapolis. It refuses to divulge any of their names or backgrounds, saying that material is "confidential."

Most physicians who leave their own practices and go to work as HMO administrators make the switch for good. The rapid growth of managed care has meant plentiful job opportunities and generous salaries for these experts. Furthermore, most HMO medical directors genuinely believe that their statistics, oversight, and guidelines can improve American medicine. Every now and then, however, a practicing doctor takes a few steps into a managed-care career, encounters something deeply disturbing — and flees.

Linda Peeno was one of those doctors. A single mother who graduated from the University of Louisville Medical School in the early 1980s, she was delighted to get a job offer from Humana, a major HMO based in her hometown, soon after completing her training. For most of 1987 she worked alongside four other doctors as a medical reviewer for the health plan, helping it make coverage decisions in difficult cases. By her own account, it was stimulating work at first, with a chance to influence dozens of cases around the country each day. Most of the time wise medical judgments and smart business practices coincided nicely.

Then came a case that would haunt Dr. Peeno for years. A Nevada man in his mid-30s was near death, the victim of a viral illness that had attacked his heart. Doctors 1,500 miles away had put the man on a waiting list for a heart transplant. A matching donor had just been found. Now hospital officials needed to check the man's insurance status. He was a chef at a Las Vegas hotel; his health coverage was provided through Humana. A nurse working at Humana headquarters took down details of the case and passed the summary to Dr. Peeno.

The crucial question: would Humana authorize payment for a heart transplant?

Six years later, Dr. Peeno wrote a paper about the case for a graduate course in ethics, giving the following details:

> I sat at my desk, contemplating the paper given to me by the nurse, who had reminded me, in her dutiful way, that this was a "very expensive" case. I knew well by now what this euphemism meant: You better find a way to deny this. Medically the case was clear, with no grounds upon which I could issue a denial based on necessity. . . . I was left only with finding a loophole that would justify the denial of payment based on coverage limitations. A few quick calls to the benefit department about contracts in Nevada, and a review of the language in this man's own "certificate of coverage" gave me what I needed. I placed a call back to the hospital, rendered my judgment, supported it with convoluted rationale, and hung up the phone. That this man, who I would never know, would fail to get his heart was of less importance to me at that moment than the accolades I would get when word spread that I saved the company several hundred thousand dollars.

For nearly three more years, Dr. Peeno continued to work in medical management for HMOs. She switched to a different health plan in 1988 and collected a $156,000-a-year salary for a 35-hour work week: better pay and shorter hours than she would have had by practicing internal medicine in Kentucky. As she continued reviewing medical cases, though, she felt what she later described as "uneasiness" about her role in denying coverage. Before long she began approving expensive services out of compassion for patients' suffering, even if managed-care guidelines nudged her in the opposite direction. At her second HMO she approved a liver transplant for a desperately ill man who later died. She approved a speech-assist device for a paralyzed stroke patient — the first of many expenses necessary for aggressive rehabilitation. When colleagues and senior managers challenged her decisions, she regarded their criticism as signs that they weren't willing to put the full weight of the HMO into doing the best job possible for patients.

In 1990 Dr. Peeno quit her last managed-care job and became active in medical ethics issues. She went to Washington in 1993 to testify before a congressional committee about her glimpses of managed care, telling the panel, "There is no code of ethics. There is no oversight mechanism. . . . I was involved in the design and administration of many processes whose goals were explicitly to achieve fewer payments of claims and an increase in profitability."

Her testimony painted an unusually bleak picture of managed care — a picture heatedly disputed by HMO executives. Humana, for example, said it approved approximately 100 heart transplants from 1987 through the end of 1995, providing all medically appropriate care to those patients regardless of cost. But one of her criticisms was hard for HMO medical directors to refute. "The whole system is organized to keep you from thinking about the human dimensions of what you do," she said. "As a medical director, you are distanced from the consequence of your action. It's just numbers and claims that people talk about."

4

The Barons of Austerity

IN THE SKI VILLAGES OF central Colorado, many of America's richest movie stars, entertainers, and corporate bosses build $1 million vacation homes. They have transformed a gritty ranching and mining district into a place where tycoons can relax. Aspen's hillside chalets are home to celebrities such as Disney chief executive Michael Eisner, singer John Denver, and Hollywood superagent Michael Ovitz. Vail attracted takeover king Henry Kravis. The most exclusive town in the area, Beaver Creek, didn't even exist 20 years ago. In the past two decades, however, real-estate developers and their wealthy clientele have brought to life a glittering little resort, packed with shops that sell $800 cashmere sweaters and restaurants that brag about their Belgian chefs.

In November 1991 the HMO industry swept into Beaver Creek in grand style in the person of Malik Hasan, chairman of what is now Health Systems International.

Dr. Hasan shelled out $3.8 million to buy one of the town's most opulent homes: a 14-bedroom stone castle with a waterfall, a 100-foot-long Great Hall, and a 2,000-bottle wine cellar built into the side of a mountain. The previous owner had been a Mexican oil-industry millionaire whose extravagances were still talked about in Denver a decade later. When his fortune faded, the house was put on the market. Other people might have been awed by what oil money had purchased: enough china and gold-rimmed glassware to serve 50 people at once; a long driveway with heating coils underneath to melt the snow in winter. But Dr. Hasan and his wife, Seeme, didn't leave this luxury alone.

Instead, they made abundant changes to bring the house up to their standards.

Contractors ripped up and replaced the driveway when Dr. Hasan decided that the original heating coils didn't melt snow fast enough. The rough flagstones around the swimming pool were hauled away as well, in favor of sleek new marble. Inside, the couple built an elaborate home office so that Dr. Hasan could study individual medical reports for his HMO's 1.8 million members late at night, his favorite viewing time. They created a salon where Dr. Hasan could receive business guests as formally or informally as he wanted. Sometimes Dr. Hasan wore double-breasted suits to meet visitors; once he startled a prominent venture capitalist by wearing red silk pajamas to meet with him in the middle of the day.

Partway through the revamping, the Hasans invited the house's original architect to stop by. With a mixture of nervousness and pride, Charles Sink drove to Beaver Creek to see what was being done to his creation. It was a jarring encounter. As Sink discovered, all the airy features of his original design were being annihilated. The broad-plank wooden floors had been torn out in favor of marble and elaborate parquet. The house's vast windows were being masked by purple silk draperies. The new look was what Seeme Hasan wanted; she later told a ski-resort magazine that she and her husband had remade the house into a version of Sleeping Beauty's castle. Sink hardly said a word, fearful that he might offend his hosts.

The strangest moment came when the architect asked to see the kitchen, a large open room on which Sink and his partner Don Dethlefs had lavished more than $50,000 of equipment and labor. The kitchen was being abandoned. "They told me that Dr. Hasan's chef wouldn't cook in it," Sink recalled. "He said: 'You've got to build me another one.'" So the Hasans had paid for a new architect to gouge another subterranean room out of the mountainside. A 20-by-20-foot kitchen had been constructed deep below the garden and lawn, beyond the main wall of the house. It was packed with stainless-steel sinks and ranges and chopping tables, giving the chef as much culinary muscle as he might find in a big-city hotel. "Looking at the project," Sink recalled, "I just shuddered."

Every few years the U.S. economy offers a mouthwatering opportunity for people to get rich. The Texas oil boom of the late 1970s comes to mind. Or the dawn of the personal-computer industry in the early 1980s. Suddenly a fresh way of doing business roars into prominence, making millionaires of those associated with it. The biggest winners are the pioneers: the lucky or visionary people who enter a lonely little field before anyone else recognizes how lucrative it can be. When word of this new El Dorado circulates, a stampede ensues. Whoever can elbow their way into the action gets a chance to make big money. Such booms don't last forever, and their giddiest moments often come just before the collapse. When the money-making formula is working, however, everyone in the industry is filled with joy and cockiness and the certainty that they and their colleagues are brilliant.

Starting in 1990, the HMO industry emerged as one of those magical fields. People who once processed student loans, or practiced law, or taught college economics have flocked into managed care. They have been joined by former doctors, pharmaceutical salesmen, and nursing-home executives. Even a one-time governor of New Mexico, Garrey Carruthers, decided to get into the HMO business. "Managed care is where we're going," Carruthers explained in mid-1994, a few months after setting up Cimarron HMO. He added, "This is my third career. I don't know how long it will last, but I'll give it a try."

As corporate employers nudge millions of people into managed-care plans, the executives running HMOs have begun to swagger in their new prosperity. They have pampered themselves with corporate jets, sleek black limousines, and private chauffeurs. They have bought yachts, vacation homes, and expensive sports cars, unwittingly emulating the stereotypical "greedy doctors" that managed care was supposed to flush away. Given the chance to earn giant amounts of money, very few HMO executives have proven able to say no — or to reflect on how their social mission might change if they put corporate profit at the top of their priority list. Instead, executives have pushed their salaries and bonuses above $1 million a year and have splurged with the CEO's version of a four-scoop chocolate sundae for dessert: stock-option packages worth as much as $15 million.

These executives have reveled in what their money can buy. The chairman of Humana, David Jones, purchased his own plane, a Cessna 560 jet, and parked it in the HMO's hangar at the local airport in Louisville, Kentucky. Humana owned several corporate aircraft that Jones could use, but with his personal jet he could zip around on vacations without having to reimburse Humana for use of its planes. A stickler for details, Jones paid Humana $29,282 in 1994 for rental of the hangar and airplane maintenance. Those expenses were just a tiny nick in his checkbook; the HMO tycoon had become one of the richest men in Kentucky, with a fortune valued at well over $200 million, thanks to the soaring value of his Humana stock.

Retired HMO boss Richard Burke made headlines with an even grander display of wealth in 1995 — he bought control of a professional hockey team. Burke had grown up in North Carolina and never played much hockey himself. But during a decadelong stint as head of United HealthCare in Minneapolis, he had watched his teenage sons play countless hockey games at their prep school. Burke loved the sport and was sorry to see Minnesota lose its only major-league hockey team, the North Stars, in 1993. So when the Winnipeg Jets came up for sale, Burke put together a partnership to buy the team for $68 million. At first he talked about relocating the team to Minneapolis, which would have made him a local hero. But when he couldn't get enough subsidies from city officials to ensure that the move would be profitable, he pointed the team toward Phoenix instead. "This is not a social or other kind of lark," Burke explained during his negotiations. "If I didn't think this was going to work from a business standpoint, I wouldn't do it."

The wealthiest HMO tycoon of all has been Leonard Abramson, the founder of U.S. Healthcare, who appears each year on the Forbes 400 list of the richest people in America (estimated wealth: nearly $1 billion). The early stages of Abramson's career exemplify the self-made virtues of a Horatio Alger novel: driving a cab to pay his way through college, quitting a safe hospital-company job in 1976 to start a tiny HMO with $16,000 of his savings, and answering the switchboard himself on Saturdays when health-plan members called. As his company prospered, Abramson developed a taste for luxury that overshadowed his early commitment to thrift. He built a three-hole golf course next to his suburban Philadelphia home. He put two daughters and a son-in-law on the corporate payroll at various times, paying them salaries as high as $300,000 a year. In his biggest spree Abramson bought a 78-foot yacht for more than $1 million, naming it *Madlen* in an amalgam of his and his wife's names.

Are such achievements part of the way that healthy American capitalism works? Or is there something troubling about the piling up of wealth within the HMO industry?

Almost in unison, managed-care executives portray themselves as classic business success stories. As they see it, executives in any industry who do a good job of increasing sales, profits, and shareholder value deserve whatever rewards the market offers. To limit their pay or affluence would be almost un-American. Abramson, for example, bristled when asked how he justified his annual pay of $3.5 million and a further $11 million in dividend income. "This is a phenomenal company," he declared. "How do you measure what's the appropriate reward for someone who has created 5,000 jobs; someone who has devoted 25 years of very hard work. Is it $1 million? Or $2 million? Or some other number? If you want to regulate that, you take away what's great in this country: the free enterprise system."

What HMO executives can't bring themselves to admit is that their business priorities are fundamentally at odds with the workings of almost any other industry. Managed care is in large part a retrenchment tactic, a way to make medicine more efficient and bring costs under control. Successful HMOs do the exact opposite of most normal companies: they order *less* of everything. HMOs aren't like steel companies that try to sell record tonnage or restaurants that try to fill every table, so that everyone shares in the prosperity at the end of the year. A good year at an HMO is one in which doctors order fewer tests, patients are discharged faster from the hospital, and not every request for a specialist consultation is approved. That frugality is a tough message for an HMO's business partners to swallow. It becomes more palatable if those being asked to make sacrifices can see that even the rulemakers are being parsimonious.

Even more important, the moral justification for managed care is a belief that good health care can be achieved at lower cost if the American medical system is made to spend money more wisely. HMOs don't present themselves as the medical equivalent of a tawdry motel chain or a discount clothing store in a rundown part of town, blithely selling an inferior product in the name of having the cheapest possible price. Managed-care companies promise to uphold standards through their cost cutting, simply by targeting wasteful practices. Big corporate employers believed that assurance and gave these health plans tremendous leeway to decide what surgeries, X-rays, and home-care visits were "wasteful." But when people in the midst of a medical crisis discover that their supposedly thrifty HMO is spewing out enough wealth to allow the top executives to buy jets, yachts, and other extravagances, it raises bitter doubts about how wisely — or selfishly — HMOs decide what is "wasteful" and what is not.

Because managed care has caught on so fast, HMO executives seldom stop to think about what gives their industry its legitimacy. The economic forces pushing for medical austerity are intense. But that doesn't guarantee for-profit HMOs a permanent right to be national agents of change. For the American public to tolerate and accept a major role for these companies, people have to believe that the executives in charge sincerely want each health-care dollar to stretch as far as it can. When HMO executives adopt a different code of conduct — and decide that their mission is to make as much money as possible as medical middlemen — they invite scorn and distrust from the people most intimately involved with front-line care.

Tensions between rich HMOs and a disgruntled public haven't always existed. When the managed-care movement got started in the 1930s and '40s, it was run by doctors and health reformers who were filled with utopian ideas about delivering good care to the masses at a modest price. They weren't good businessmen and they didn't want to be. Their politics tended toward socialism; getting rich was seen as loathsome. Even in the 1960s and 1970s, most HMOs were nonprofit and proud of it. They paid administrators small salaries and plowed back 90 percent or more of premiums into direct patient care. HMOs in different parts of the country freely shared business ideas, seeing themselves as fellow evangelists trying to spread managed care rather than as rivals vying for market share. The heroes of the movement were men like Robert Biblo, a former auto worker who eventually became chief executive of two huge nonprofit plans, but who always personified the worker's interest in affordable medical coverage.

Those old-fashioned principles gradually eroded. In the early 1980s some ambitious HMO executives in California and on the East Coast wanted to expand rapidly but found themselves strapped for capital. Nonprofit companies couldn't issue stock and sometimes had trouble arranging bank loans. The remedy: switch the health plan to for-profit status, sell stock to the public, and voilà! — HMO executives could plunge their arms into $20 million, $50 million, or more of ready cash. That money could finance rapid internal growth or acquisition of other health plans. Being listed on the stock market had other allures too. Senior managers could become part owners of the business, building multimillion-dollar fortunes as the HMO's shares climbed. Many chief executives found these lures irresistible. As the former chairman of FHP International, California doctor Robert Gumbiner, said: "I never made much money practicing medicine. I made a lot through the greed and gullibility of Wall Street." His health plan went public in 1985, and it had plenty of company. By 1990 more than one third of the largest HMOs in the United States were for profit; by 1995, half the industry was for profit, according to researchers at InterStudy Publications, Minneapolis. New-listing parties became a regular occurrence at the New York Stock Exchange. Quotron terminals began showing up in HMO executives' offices, with little green lights that blinked out a company's stock price every few seconds.

Once managed-care companies entered the for-profit arena, the financial world's values started seeping in. Quarterly earnings mattered much more than before. Executives weren't likely any longer to know many patients or doctors by name. Instead, top managers hovered over computer printouts showing membership growth rates, hospital days per thousand members, and other favorite statistical benchmarks. Cost control became crucial. Securities analysts and big investors refused to support a health plan that spent "too much" on members and left too little for shareholders. Thanks to increasingly generous stock-option packages, executives' own fortunes became closely tied to the wiggles of their company's share price.

Before long, HMO bosses regarded boosting stock prices as a major priority, perhaps even their most important goal. Annual reports to investors talked about "providing the highest return on investment," about "enhancing the value of your investment," and about "our record-breaking financial performance." Of course, HMO executives usually insisted that financial gains at their companies went hand in hand with public service. Pictures of babies being immunized and doctors peering at X-rays were meant to suggest that an HMO's success was closely linked to enrolling more members and keeping them happy. In chief executives' eyes, their HMOs weren't just doing well, they were doing good.

The back pages of their annual reports told a darker story. During the early 1990s, publicly traded HMOs began spending ever smaller amounts of their premium dollars on patient care. That meant fewer doctors' visits, fewer lab tests, and shorter stays in the hospital for seriously ill patients. It also meant more money available for marketing, executive salaries, administrative overhead, and retained earnings — everything except patient care.

With the financial community, in fact, HMOs no longer talked about spending money on patients. Executives used a different term: the "medical-loss ratio," a phrase borrowed from the traditional indemnity insurance industry. Accountants used the term to describe the percentage of premium dollars used to pay out patients' medical claims, which an insurance company regarded as losses. But in the hands of managed-care companies, with their wide discretion to approve or disapprove treatments, the term took on a more sinister tone. The language of managed-care accounting now suggested that the very essence of medicine — spending money to fight illness — wasn't desirable. It would only increase the medical-loss ratio.

In the late 1970s leading nonprofit HMOs spent about 94 percent of premiums on members' medical treatment. Industry averages fluctuated greatly in the 1980s, because of a turbulent insurance market and some HMO bankruptcies. By the early 1990s, however, a two-tier trend had emerged. The handful of nonprofits still left in the business (such as Kaiser Permanente, Tufts, Harvard Community Health Plan, and Group Health Co-operative of Puget Sound) continued to spend 90 percent or more of premiums on direct patient care. But the largest publicly traded HMOs posted very different numbers. Their medical-loss ratio in 1993 dwindled to just 78 percent of premiums; in 1994 it fell further, to 76.6 percent. Some of the investment community's favorite HMOs pared spending even more. Oxford Health Plans constantly kept its medical-loss ratio below 75 percent in the early 1990s; U.S. Healthcare got its ratio as low as 68 percent in the fourth quarter of 1994.

In a blunt sign of Wall Street's priorities, U.S. Healthcare ran into a buzzsaw of hostile investor reaction when it announced in April 1995 that it would raise doctors' pay in an effort to upgrade the quality of its medical networks. Angry investors figured that the company's medical-loss ratio was going to rise. They sent the HMO's stock tumbling more than $8 a share over a two-day span in a selling spree that wiped out more than $1 billion of the company's shareholder value.

The less that HMOs spent on patient care, the more cash they could salt away. A survey of the 10 largest HMOs at the end of 1994 found that they were sitting on a combined $10.5 billion in liquid assets, enough money to buy every minute of advertising time on Super Bowl telecasts for the next 150 years. The richest HMO, United HealthCare of Minneapolis, basked in $2.6 billion of cash. Three other managed-care companies also topped the $1 billion mark: WellPoint Health Networks of California, Kaiser Permanente, and U.S. Healthcare. Some of those cash stockpiles were justified by the demands of ordinary business. HMOs needed liquid assets to meet state regulators' reserve requirements and to pay medical bills that hadn't yet been processed. Nonetheless, a leading securities analyst deemed the cash buildup "way, way beyond what HMOs need."

Money from members' premiums poured in so fast at Health Systems International that the head of treasury operations, Alan Bond, was briefly flummoxed. At one point, he told a newspaper reporter, he had $475 million to invest, with a further $500,000 coming in each day. Membership growth, and the resulting premium income, was simply outstripping the company's spending on medical care. As Bond sheepishly put it, "Our problem is what to do with the money that comes in, not whether we have enough cash."

If HMOs weren't spending every dollar of premiums on patient care, other uses beckoned. Companies such as U.S. Healthcare, Foundation Health, and Oxford Health built splendid suburban headquarters with landscaped grounds, waterfalls, and big, bright work areas. Their offices weren't necessarily any more lavish than those of comparable Fortune 500 companies that made cigarettes, missiles, or motorcycles. But HMOs no longer regarded it as a point of honor to house themselves in spartan quarters. Monklike thrift was an anachronism from the early days. In 1948 Kaiser Permanente had a policy that employees could get new pencils only if they brought in a used stub less than three inches long. Such penny-pinching had long since stopped. HMOs in the 1990s were among America's biggest dispensers of free pens, coffee mugs, and T-shirts, in an effort to get their names known.

Other administrative costs ballooned too. Rather than leave doctors and hospitals lightly supervised, managed-care plans hired thousands of case managers and other reviewers to peer over the shoulders of caregivers. HMO executives portrayed these employees as patients' hidden allies, making sure that sick people got to the right specialist at the right time and were properly guided through hospital stays and subsequent recovery. Doctors, therapists, and practicing nurses, however, were caustic, grumbling about the influx of "utilization-review clerks from hell" and "1-800-DENIAL" services that were intruding on their lives. Shareholders and Wall Street analysts didn't seem to care much which version was right, as long as the case managers helped keep spending down. As HMO analyst Douglas Sherlock put it, "Money spent on administration yields declines in medical costs."

A small but intensely controversial part of HMOs' budgets was the compensation set aside for top management. When HMOs were small and nonprofit, even the chief executives didn't earn much more than a typical physician, corporate lawyer, or division chief at a manufacturing company. Robert Gumbiner, the long-time head of FHP, earned about $60,000 a year in the mid-1970s. Leonard Abramson earned $126,000 in 1982, just before U.S. Healthcare went public. As HMOs grew bigger — and as management pay throughout the United States began soaring much faster than worker pay, corporate profits, or any other yardstick — the men and women who ran HMOs started drawing paychecks that would make movie stars and professional athletes jealous.

Dan Crowley, the chief executive of Foundation Health, became the industry's king of compensation in 1994, with a $19 million pay package. It consisted of $558,288 in base salary, a $2.7 million bonus, $342,172 in deferred pay, $43,482 in reimbursements for taxes on his income — and stock options valued at $15 million. Foundation hadn't even had an especially good year; it had temporarily lost a military contract that accounted for more than one third of its earnings. But the HMO's directors said they voted to award the bonus and options package anyway, "in view of Mr. Crowley's continuing role in determining the future success of the company."

Among the outraged observers was Tom Elkin, health-benefits chief for 400,000 California state employees, one of Crowley's biggest customers. In a face-to-face showdown, Elkin demanded justification for such a big pay package. When Crowley began explaining how poorly paid he had been in previous years, Elkin, a career civil servant, shot back, "Dan, there are an awful lot of us who are working very hard and making a hell of a lot less than $19 million." A year later Crowley accepted a much smaller pay package, with a 50 percent pay cut and only one fifth as many stock options. Crowley also came close to apologizing for his previous takings. In a speech to a northern California doctors' group, he conceded, "In this environment, it's doggone piggy to put your face that far in the trough when other people are hurting."

On the East Coast the lure of big money captivated two young executives who always insisted that they had gone into the HMO business for the most idealistic of reasons. One was Steve Wiggins, the founder and chairman of Oxford Health Plans. A boyishly handsome manager with a down-home style, Wiggins was known for wearing rumpled khakis to high-level meetings and for driving a beat-up 1976 Saab to negotiating sessions with doctors, when he could easily have afforded a better car. When asked how he got into health care, Wiggins explained that a close high school friend had broken his neck in a diving accident. That tragedy had led Wiggins in his early 20s to set up a small nonprofit company to provide rehabilitative services. From that base, moving into HMOs was a small step. Beneath his rumpled charm, though, Wiggins quickly figured out how the for-profit health-care industry worked. He collected options on 500,000 Oxford shares between 1992 and 1994 — a package subsequently valued at more than $35 million.

Just as financially savvy was Norman Payson, a Dartmouth-trained physician who helped found HealthSource in 1985. Dr. Payson's résumé included idealistic deeds, such as a brief stint working on an Indian reservation after becoming an MD. His financial disclosures, however, showed a keen eye for money. In 1994 he collected a $385,000 salary from HealthSource and options on one million shares — valued at $11.4 million. The HMO's compensation committee used the quaintest language in justifying the options award, saying that it "will provide a significant incentive for Dr. Payson to increase the value of the company's stock over the next several years and will totally align Dr. Payson's interests with those of the shareholders." Eight months later the options had done their magic; HealthSource's stock had jumped more than 50 percent. Even so, the financial chiropractors on the compensation committee decided that Dr. Payson's interests needed to be realigned some more. So he was awarded options on a further 100,000 shares, valued at $1.7 million.

White-collar HMO employees weren't paid nearly as well, but they also found managed care generous. Clerical workers, computer programmers, and marketing specialists all flocked to an industry with above-average pay scales and a constant demand for more workers.

Some of the best prospects were in sales, particularly in the lucrative business of pitching Medicare HMOs to elderly Americans. In south Florida, Humana in early 1996 was paying $9,400 a month — an annual rate of $112,800 — for marketers who could sign up seven or eight elderly people a week. Some rivals paid even more. Foundation Health ran ads in the *Miami Herald* offering new sales representatives a car allowance, a monthly bonus, dental and health coverage, and a chance to earn as much as $190,000 a year if they could sign up 50 elderly members a month. Those big checks meant that sales commissions would chew up more than half of the first month's premium for each new Medicare HMO member. That might seem like an extravagant use of money that is meant to cover medical care, but HMOs made no apologies. They simply tried to hire the best marketers they could and to keep the competition from poaching them.

From 1992 onward HMOs used much of their excess cash on acquisition binges. Companies such as HealthSource, Foundation Health, and Humana routinely snapped up at least one — and sometimes three or four — smaller health plans in the course of a year. Outlays of $100 million became routine; megadeals of $1 billion or larger weren't unknown. Power was increasingly consolidated in the hands of a few dominant HMOs in each region, which was exactly what the managed-care industry wanted. Big HMOs could mount the marketing campaigns necessary to make themselves seem like the best choice in town. Big HMOs could put in state-of-the-art computer systems to track members' status and manage costs better. And big HMOs could dictate contract terms to doctors and hospitals, for both sides knew that a provider who didn't agree to those terms could instantly lose access to thousands of patients.

The HMOs' takeover spree made onlookers nervous. "We're losing competition," complained Jim Foreman, a benefits consultant who helped companies pick health plans for their employees. "That's potentially bad." Doctors' groups echoed his concerns. "We at the AMA have real problems with the for-profit mentality of some health plans," said James Todd, executive vice president of the American Medical Association. "Whatever money is paid out for investors or acquisitions is money removed from the health-care system. We would like to see it recirculated and used for patient care." But employers and doctors couldn't do much more than grumble; HMOs were calling the shots.

In the Darwinian world of stock-market investing, in fact, any evidence that doctors and employers were squirming was seen as good news for HMOs. Securities analysts applauded United HealthCare in mid-1995 when it agreed to spend roughly $2 billion to buy a traditional health insurer, MetraHealth. "It will be a very successful strategy that blankets the eastern half of the U.S. with health plans," analyst Tom Hodapp told the *Wall Street Journal*. The combined company started out with 4.5 million HMO members and millions more subscribers in conventional health insurance. United executives said the acquisition would give them "critical mass," a coded way of saying that the combined HMOs would be so dominant that employers and doctors would have no choice but to do business with them.

Similar arguments surfaced in April 1996, when Aetna Life agreed to buy U.S. Healthcare for $8.3 billion. Analysts enthusiastically spoke about the combined company's clout — with 14 million subscribers spread through all 50 states. Executives of the two companies predicted that they would "redefine the way health care is provided."

Whenever an industry expands as fast as the HMO business has, historians debate whether the boom was shaped by economic events in the background or by a handful of entrepreneurs who made the trends happen. Both points of view generally contain considerable truth. It could be argued, for example, that corporate demand for cheaper health care, the nationwide surplus of hospitals and medical specialists in the early 1990s, and the rip-roaring stock market of modern times made the emergence of a rich, rapacious managed-care industry almost inevitable. Still, it is hard to imagine that HMOs would have caught on so fast — or would have pushed the marriage of capitalism and medical cost control so audaciously — if it weren't for a handful of trailblazers.

The boldest and most controversial barons of austerity are the doctors who decided to stop seeing patients and start managing populations. Those MDs brought an intensity, a stubbornness, and a knowledge base to the HMO business that nonmedically trained executives often lacked. Many of the physician/executives, though they originally seemed unlikely recruits, became the most zealous champions of managed-care principles. Some of these doctors in pinstripes also displayed a raw hunger for wealth that shocked competitors. In all those respects, the front-runner has been Malik Hasan, a stocky Pakistani immigrant in his late 50s.

Born into a rich family, Dr. Hasan came to the United States in 1971 after completing training in neurology in England. He spent a few years as an assistant professor at Rush-Presbyterian–St. Luke's medical school in Chicago, then started his own private practice in Pueblo, Colorado. Pueblo, a steel town 110 miles south of Denver, was a medical backwater. But that was fine. "I wanted to go to an area that was neurologically underdeveloped," Dr. Hasan later recalled. "I felt it was somewhere that I could make my mark. That was what appealed to me. There was nothing there!"

The unwritten rule of private practice in the mid-1970s was "bill a lot," and colleagues at the time believe that Dr. Hasan quickly mastered it. When he learned that local hospitals lacked the high-tech equipment that a good neurologist needed, he set up investment vehicles so he could acquire the machines himself. One Hasan partnership bought a CAT scanner, a $500,000 machine that provides three-dimensional X-ray images of internal structures, including the brain, neck, and spine. Another Hasan partnership bought a magnetic resonance imaging (MRI) machine, a $1 million device capable of even better soft-tissue scans. When patients with seizures or headaches needed sophisticated tests, Dr. Hasan referred them for examination with his machines.* He soon became known as one of the hardest-working doctors in southern Colorado, putting in long hours in Pueblo, then driving into ranching towns 100 miles away to conduct once-a-month clinics for people with neurologic problems. Those visits improved care in rural areas that otherwise would never see such a learned specialist. They also improved Dr. Hasan's income. Some of his rural patients were told to travel to Pueblo for a brain scan on his machines. "Malik always knew how to maximize the system," a Pueblo hospital administrator cheerfully recalled. "Anybody that got referred to him got a CT scan."

Then the unwritten rules changed. HMOs in the early 1980s began making inroads in Colorado. It became clear that the only people who would thrive in this new system were those who got managed-care contracts, made sure that frugal medicine was practiced — and pocketed the difference. That was such an alien idea at first that when a small HMO tried to enter Pueblo in 1982, Dr. Hasan led local doctors in a successful attempt to repel the intruder. A few years later he was

---

*Such self-referral was legal at the time and tolerated by professional societies. In recent years it has been labeled a conflict of interest and has been sharply curtailed.

ready to switch sides. Managed care wasn't so bad after all, he told colleagues. In fact, it was inevitable. "We could see the writing on the wall," Dr. Hasan later recalled. "There was a feeling that this thing was going to be unstoppable. We, the specialists, were going to be run out of town if we didn't do something."

In 1985 Dr. Hasan helped form Qual-Med, a tiny HMO with 7,000 members in southern Colorado. He didn't get much backing from fellow doctors; he asked 100 physicians to invest with him, and 94 turned him down. But the few doctors who did pitch in were wowed by Dr. Hasan's conviction that he was about to start a great business. Pueblo physician Robert Dingle put up a few thousand dollars, mostly on the strength of Dr. Hasan's personality. "He promised us investors that we would realize more than we could dream," Dr. Dingle warmly recalled.

When Qual-Med's growth in Colorado proved slower than Dr. Hasan had expected, he started acquiring other HMOs. First he snapped up a New Mexico health plan that appeared to be in such bad financial shape that the seller *paid* Dr. Hasan's company $2.5 million to take the business off its hands. Then he acquired medium-sized HMOs in Washington, Oregon, and California. Pretty soon he was running a 200,000-member health plan that was earning more than $1 million a month.

People who watched him in action say that Dr. Hasan embraced dealmaking with even more passion than he showed for his first professional love, neurology. Sometimes he got his way through sheer stamina, turning a two-hour afternoon meeting into an eight-hour haggling binge that broke up late at night only when the other participants were too sleepy to resist. On other occasions, elaborate politeness worked in his favor. One hospital administrator kept a secret tally of the number of times Dr. Hasan referred to him as "my very good friend" — in the midst of a high-pressure attempt to cut the hospital's prices by 20 percent. And in acquisition negotiations Dr. Hasan could adopt the classic good cop/bad cop strategy all by himself. One moment he would praise a seller's business and talk about how well they could work together if a deal were completed. The next moment he would protest that the seller's terms were "very steep," even if Dr. Hasan knew he was being offered a bargain.

One of the most potent tributes to Dr. Hasan's skills came from Boston venture capitalist Robert Daly, who served for several years on

Qual-Med's board of directors. Their friendship had its rocky moments; Daly's firm at one point sued Dr. Hasan over a contract dispute, which was eventually settled out of court. In the end, though, Daly's firm made more than five times its original investment in Qual-Med. And Daly referred to Dr. Hasan as "the most brilliant HMO executive I've ever met."

After acquiring an HMO, Dr. Hasan would install an aggressive medical director and tell him or her to shrink the medical-loss ratio. The results offended some patients and doctors, but the approach was a financial success for Qual-Med. One executive, emergency physician James Riopelle, took a 50 percent pay cut to work for Qual-Med in New Mexico, but got stock and options that a few years later were worth $5 million. With such compensation packages, medical directors naturally did what was best for Qual-Med shareholders. If an obstetrician wanted to keep a new mother in the hospital for a second or third day after delivery, Qual-Med's medical directors would say no on the grounds that it wasn't medically necessary. If an orthopedist wanted to order a second MRI, he was told no as well, on the same grounds. Even neurologists were told to stop practicing in their old, extravagant ways. Physicians and patients sometimes squawked about Qual-Med's rules, but the HMO's managers shrugged it off. Qual-Med insiders believed that their system was providing good, cost-effective care. Besides, it was making a fortune for those who were lucky enough to own stock.

In June 1991 Qual-Med went public in a massively oversubscribed stock sale. The transaction created 13 instant millionaires, all physicians who had invested modest amounts in the company early on and then had watched the value of their holdings soar. The supreme winner was Dr. Hasan, whose modest investments had skyrocketed to a market value of $67 million. As a practicing physician, Dr. Hasan's biggest indulgence had been the purchase of a Rolls-Royce. Now, as a successful inventor and an HMO executive, he could afford something 40 times more expensive than a Rolls: the mansion in Beaver Creek.

Many entrepreneurs might have slowed down for a year or two to savor those new riches. But that wasn't Dr. Hasan's style. In mid-1991 he began stalking Health Net, a major nonprofit HMO in California. Qual-Med already operated a 100,000-member HMO in that state, and Dr. Hasan feared that the 900,000-member Health Net might soon become strong enough to crush his local health plan. His solution: a hostile $300 million bid to acquire the bigger rival. When Health Net executives resisted, Qual-Med sued.

In that suit Dr. Hasan zeroed in on Health Net's weakest point. Health Net executives in 1991 were feverishly trying to convert their HMO to for-profit status, a move that would clear the way for top managers to make millions in the company's stock. But under California law, such switches can be carried out only if the converting HMO properly compensates the "public interest" that it previously served as a not-for-profit company. That compensation usually involves creating a public interest foundation, bankrolled with stock or cash equal to the appraised value of the HMO at the time of conversion. Hoping to get state approval of the conversion, Health Net initially proposed to put $127 million into a new foundation that would promote the use of seat belts, campaign against smoking, and pursue other wellness initiatives. When state regulators deemed that amount too small, Health Net in early 1992 raised the foundation's funding to $300 million. But Qual-Med in its suit protested that even $300 million was not a full valuation for the company. Californians deserved more for having allowed Health Net to thrive for years as a nonprofit company that didn't pay taxes, it argued. Until that time few people had expected a for-profit HMO to show a deep interest in such issues. In mid-1992, however, Qual-Med proposed to direct $325 million or more into a "Wellness Foundation" if its own higher bid prevailed.

The suit was a masterstroke. Consumer activists unwittingly helped Dr. Hasan's cause by labeling Health Net's original and revised plans an asset grab by management. Lawyers at Consumers Union said the state would be better served if Health Net were sold at open auction. Eventually Health Net chief executive Roger Greaves realized that his hopes for a management-led conversion to for-profit were doomed. In a series of talks in 1992 and 1993, Greaves did the unthinkable: he flew to Denver, shook hands with Dr. Hasan, and agreed to merge their companies into a new entity, Health Systems International. In August 1993, the two men finally settled on a merger value of $725 million, reflecting the steady improvement in both companies' prospects during the two-year takeover battle. In an apparent sign that they were making peace as equals, Greaves and Dr. Hasan decided to be joint chief executives of the combined company.

Within 18 months Greaves was out of a job and Dr. Hasan held sole command of a 1.8 million–member HMO. The power play left

Greaves, a cheerful man who believed he was the better strategist and marketer of the two, bewildered. But Dr. Hasan had quickly seized the two most important levers of power within Health Systems. He installed his own medical directors in crucial jobs and took the steps needed to reduce Health Net's medical-loss ratio. And Dr. Hasan put himself in charge of the hunt for more acquisitions. His most ambitious project, an attempted $3 billion merger with WellPoint Health Networks, proved impossible to complete. But when the deal looked imminent, negotiators envisioned such a tiny future role for Greaves that the long-time Health Net executive decided to quit.

Partway through 1995, Dr. Hasan rang up two smaller deals in Pennsylvania and Connecticut, giving his HMO a coast-to-coast presence. With outright glee Dr. Hasan later told how he had convinced executives of the Pennsylvania plan to accept his $100 million bid, even though another suitor wanted to offer $115 million. "Anyone can pay top dollar," he explained. "But that's not what my shareholders are paying me to do. They're paying me to get a better deal done for better terms than anyone else." As Dr. Hasan bluntly put it, "I'm not representing the other party's shareholders."

Because of his aggressive negotiating, Dr. Hasan became a symbol of HMO power and strong-mindedness. But that didn't bother him, and at times he even played to the image. After one especially bruising round of negotiating lower prices with groups of physicians, Dr. Hasan accepted an invitation from the California Medical Society to talk about his philosophy of managed care. It was a hostile audience, but the HMO boss enjoyed the chance to match wits. After his talk a plastic surgeon rose to berate him for profiting at physicians' expense. Without missing a beat, Dr. Hasan shot back, "There's nothing I can do to help you. I'm a neurologist by training. You need a psychiatrist."

From 1991 onward Dr. Hasan was far too busy with HMO duties to treat individual patients. Nonetheless, he remained intimately involved in treatment decisions, thanks to an unusual two-shift workday that he developed. From late morning till 6 P.M. or 7 P.M., he worked in a conventional office at Health Systems headquarters in Colorado or California. Then he went home and began a second shift, combing through computer printouts of patient care and calling up aides at home if he saw something he didn't like. His workday continued well past midnight, and he made no apologies for phoning subordinates after hours. "If you don't want a phone call from me at 3 A.M., you'd better get everything right," Dr. Hasan once remarked.

For his troubles Dr. Hasan collected $3.6 million in salary and bonus in 1994, along with stock options initially valued at $5 million. It was a pay package that incensed his critics, yet most of the time Dr. Hasan breezily dismissed their concerns. "I get people asking me: 'How do you justify your compensation? Aren't you denying care so you can have a larger salary?'" he volunteered. "But I tell them most of the amount isn't cash, it's stock options. The cash that I got doesn't amount to two cents per member per month. To say that I deny care to have a high salary is sophistry. The link isn't there." At times Dr. Hasan even worried that he wasn't being paid well enough. "We are being innovative, and we are helping to solve some very difficult and knotty problems," he told one interviewer. "If we are successful, then I think we deserve not only this, but more."

Every now and then, however, a trace of regret slipped into Dr. Hasan's world-view. In Pueblo he had been a popular, even loved, physician. Patients not only hurried to pay their bills, he remembered, they brought him small presents and thanked him for his care and devotion. In his new career things had changed. He did have national impact on the American health system, along with more than $150 million in stock and options and a yearly pay package eight times higher than what he had made in his best year as a practicing doctor. But he had forfeited the public trust he once enjoyed.

"When you're a doctor, people constantly tell you that you're wonderful," Dr. Hasan wryly remarked. "Now I sit here all day long, paying people. And I have nothing but hassles."

5

Turning Doctors
into Gatekeepers

IT WAS A CLASSIC MOMENT in a young doctor's education.
Third-year medical student Brian Greenberg was completing back-to-
back evening and night shifts at the pediatric ward of a Florida hospital. A night nurse woke him from a catnap at 2:40 A.M. and asked him
to draw blood from a patient down the hall who was fighting an
infection. Irritated at the interruption, Greenberg walked over to the
bedside — and found a humbling sight: a 13-year-old blind boy, suffering from terminal cancer. "He had every reason in the world to
be angry," Greenberg later recalled. "Much more than I did. But he
wasn't angry at all. He was calm and friendly, and told me which vein
would be the easiest for me to draw blood. I felt this incredible sorrow
and love for him right there. I wished there was more I could do to help
him. And I knew right then that I wanted to be a pediatrician."

Such dramatic personal encounters become career turning points.
They can occur at any point in a medical education: in a maternity
ward as a newborn safely enters the world, in a psychiatry rotation
helping a mentally ill person battle schizophrenia, in an operating
room as a veteran surgeon explains the intricacies of the craft. Whatever the setting, the moment marks the occasion when a young doctor
suddenly knows what specialty to choose and what types of patients to
help. Medical school instructors deliberately kindle that passion, telling students and doctors in training, "Do the most that you can for
every single patient."

For more than a decade, Brian Greenberg has pushed himself to be
the best pediatrician he can be. After graduating from medical school

in 1986, he moved to California for advanced pediatric training at UCLA, concentrating on children with asthma and allergies. Today he sees nearly 150 children a week, as a pediatrician in private practice in Tarzana, a northwestern suburb of Los Angeles. He is a popular doctor, with a gentle voice and a bouncy sense of humor that makes most children regard him as an oversized playmate in corduroys. All day long he ministers to earaches, broken fingers, and asthma attacks, providing the essential primary care that has been a backbone of American medicine for more than a century. The abstract ideas of managed care seem incredibly remote in his offices, where giggles and yelps ring through the halls, where little boys and girls with stuffy noses say "Aaah," where mothers gently struggle to hold a baby still for a vaccination.

But when the children and their parents go home, Dr. Greenberg pours out a litany of frustrations with managed care. Half his patients now come via HMO contracts, something he never expected. Every day, he says, he must put up with ways that the managed-care system malfunctions, humbles him, or subverts his expertise. When he needs a blood sample drawn, managed-care plans tell him to bypass his own carefully trained nurses in favor of a cheaper site off premises — which has unfriendly technicians that leave children howling. When he wants to prescribe costly but powerful medicines, faraway HMO clerks second-guess his drug choices. And when very sick children need a specialist, managed-care rules can make it difficult or impossible to get a referral to the right one. "None of this helps me be a better doctor," the pediatrician says. "Much of it doesn't even save money in the long run. It just makes everything harder."

Dr. Greenberg's predicament points out the great paradox of managed care. It is a system that appears to work well overall from the panoramic vantage point of an HMO's head office, but that is often callous and clumsy in its dealings with individual patients. In the noisy commotion of a doctor's office, patients come in one at a time, with distinctive names, faces, and symptoms. Some of them truly need extra attention. All of them would like to believe that their doctor is committed to doing the most that he or she can to promote their well-being. Under the old medical model, that one-patient-at-a-time approach was regarded as the right way to practice. Yet managed care, with its emphasis on the aggregate, tugs doctors in a different direction. It makes physicians think like economists, causing them to pull back from individual cases and focus more on the allocation of resources across the whole patient population.

It is easy to see why managed-care companies want this sort of industrial logic brought to the primary-care doctor's office. Routine office visits are a major piece of overall medical spending, accounting for an estimated $50 billion a year, or 5 percent of total national health outlays. Not all that money is spent wisely or well; some patients in fee-for-service care get too much treatment while others get too little. Furthermore, most complex cases begin with an office visit to a person's regular doctor. As a result, managed-care companies tend to regard doctors' offices as facilities to be supervised with the same attention to cost-effectiveness that General Electric would apply to a light bulb factory or American Airlines would devote to a downtown ticket office.

Most HMOs start this efficiency campaign by assigning each member to a primary-care physician such as Dr. Greenberg, who is designated as the member's "gatekeeper." Health plans like to portray the gatekeeper as a patient's friendly personal physician, an image that is partly true. But the gatekeeper also is meant to keep a close eye on costs. Patients cannot see a specialist or have most medical tests performed without the explicit approval of either the primary-care physician or the managed-care company itself. A typical gatekeeper may handle 1,500 to 2,000 patients, with individual HMOs contributing a minimum of 100 and a maximum of the entire practice. To keep doctors efficient, HMOs every few months tally up how frequently their physicians are providing desirable, low-cost forms of care, such as immunizations, cholesterol checks, and cancer screenings. Other computer printouts keep tabs on doctors' use of costlier services such as X-rays, specialist referrals, and hospital days. Once health plans have such data at their fingertips, they can use a variety of incentives, penalties, and TQM techniques to encourage all doctors to practice in the manner that the managed-care plan has deemed "efficient."

From a patient's perspective the gatekeeper system is part of a whole family of controls built into managed care — affecting everything from a baby's birth to an elderly person's stroke or terminal illness. In theory, managed-care rules should steer patients to the right doctor at the right time. Often HMOs succeed in this. But as will become clear in the following chapters, managed care's guidelines can hamper vital care. Specifically:

- When patients need heart surgery, HMOs have strong ideas about what hospitals to use. In several prominent instances HMOs have chosen to steer patients to centers that offer deep discounts, even if survival rates are far from the best available.
- When a person is diagnosed with cancer, getting an oncologist's candid advice about treatment choices is crucial. But one major HMO had its own ideas about what the cancer specialists should favor; it repeatedly lobbied doctors not to request a costly investigational treatment that the health plan didn't want to pay for.
- When an unexpected crisis strikes, HMO members must decide whether to call their managed-care plan for permission to go to the emergency room or simply dash ahead and call later. Patients who didn't ask for clearance have been stuck with medical bills as high as $26,000. Several patients who played by the rules suffered tragic delays and died.
- Mental-health spending is a favorite cost-cutting target of managed-care plans. Many have cut overall spending in half, which may leave schizophrenic and manic-depressive patients without the care that their doctors or family members believe they need.
- Millions of older Americans have found HMOs an attractive alternative to the conventional Medicare program. But a senior who suffers a stroke is likely to be discharged from the hospital while she still is having trouble moving her arms and legs, walking, or seeing clearly.

Fortunately, most Americans don't need a lot of medical care in any given year. Most people require only routine treatment, such as flu shots or ulcer medication, and for them the channels of managed care tend to work smoothly. Healthy members also are likely to appreciate HMOs' low copayments — $10 or less — and minimal paperwork. Surveys regularly show that 80 percent or more of HMO members say they are satisfied with their plans, a rating every bit as high as that of traditional insurance plans. Even in many cases of severe illness, the orderly paths sketched out by managed-care planners actually have helped patients get appropriate treatment.

Yet in a disturbing number of cases, the constraints of managed care, starting with the gatekeeper system, can lead to a breakdown of trust. Patients and their families no longer feel certain that their physician is making an all-out effort to help them. They are beginning to ask questions that never would have arisen 20 years ago: "Are you doing everything possible to treat my condition?" "What more could you be doing?" Persuading the new system to provide full medical care can become a negotiation, much like getting a plumber or car dealer to honor a service contract. Rather than the patient's friend and guardian, the doctor is simply a provider to bargain with.

In Orlando, Florida, internist Barbara Beeler felt so hemmed in by bureaucracy that she quit her staff-physician job at a Cigna HMO in the late 1980s to return to private practice. "It was all 'Spend less, do fewer tests,'" Dr. Beeler recalled. If a patient complained about blood in the urine, she found, Cigna's system required her to check with a referral coordinator and then the director of the local HMO center before getting clearance to order an intravenous pyelogram, the standard test to determine whether bleeding might be a sign of kidney cancer. Such tests cost more than $100 and usually don't find anything. But in a small percentage of cases the test indicates serious trouble. In a private-office setting, Dr. Beeler could order whatever tests she wanted right away; at the HMO it could take an extra day of paperwork to get her treatment approach approved. At Cigna, she said, "it became exceedingly difficult to feel good about what I was doing."

One of the most contentious issues for both patients and doctors involves managed-care protocol for referral to a specialist. HMOs argue, with some justification, that unmanaged care sends too many ailments directly into specialists' hands. As the health plans see it, cost-effective medicine means making greater use of a primary-care doctor rather than sending every rash to a dermatologist, every stomach ailment to a gastroenterologist. Academic researchers have found that some ailments, such as stomach disorders, often can be treated just as well by primary-care doctors and at lower cost.

As a result, managed-care plans deliberately make it hard to get specialist referrals. At the very least, plans require gatekeepers or the HMO itself to approve a visit to a specialist. Many health plans set up financial incentives for primary-care doctors; those who don't send many cases to specialists get bonuses, while frequent referrers may suffer penalties. Bonuses vary by plan, but in the course of a year, they can amount to several thousand dollars for a practice that relies heavily on HMO patients. Without such constraints, HMO executives contend, patients would be preyed upon by specialists eager to jack up their bills by using costly probes, scopes, and imaging machines as much as possible.

By tilting economic incentives in the other direction — and paying gatekeepers to withhold care — HMOs create a different set of potential problems. Those issues were spotlighted by Jerome Kassirer, editor of the *New England Journal of Medicine,* in a 1995 essay entitled "The Morality of Managed Care." He observed:

> On the one hand, doctors are expected to provide a wide range of services, recommend the best treatments and improve patients' quality of life. On the other, to keep expenses to a minimum, they must limit the use of services, increase efficiency, shorten the time spent with each patient and use specialists sparingly. Although many see this as an abstract dilemma, I believe that increasingly the struggle will be more concrete and stark: physicians will be forced to choose between the best interests of their patients and their own economic survival.

To guard against neglect of patients, HMOs periodically look for signs that their gatekeepers are not providing sufficient care. Extremely low rates of specialist referrals — less than half the norm — will set off warning bells at some plans. Numerous member complaints also may prompt action. And many HMO officials say that doctors who ignore their patients' needs ultimately will suffer financially, because manageable ailments will become much more serious and generate big medical bills that will be charged against the doctor's earnings. That safeguard only works, however, if patients stay with one plan for many years.

In any event, HMOs and their gatekeepers are hardly flawless in their efforts to deny needless referrals while allowing the essential ones to go through. A mid-1995 survey by Robert Blendon, a professor at the Harvard School of Public Health, found that 21 percent of HMO members in poor health said they hadn't been able to see a specialist when they needed to in the past year. Only 15 percent of comparable fee-for-service patients made the same complaint. Lawsuits across the United States allege that HMO gatekeepers have restricted access to specialists so tightly that medical tragedies have occurred. In an extreme case, computer programmer William Bacigalupo alleged in a 1992 lawsuit filed in New York state court for Dutchess County that he incurred temporary kidney failure at least in part because of his HMO's unwillingness to refer him to the appropriate specialist. Bacigalupo sufferd from cryoglobulinemia, a blood-plasma disorder that can damage internal organs. Prior to joining Healthshield, a New York HMO, he had been seeing a rheumatologist for his condition. In his suit, Bacigalupo alleged that the HMO and his primary-care doctor had stymied his requests for referrals to a specialist, causing his condition to deteriorate. A New York State jury in May 1995 awarded the 40-year-old patient more than $1 million in damages. The HMO appealed the verdict.

Even when HMOs do allow referrals, their choice of available specialists can be problematic. Allan Schwartz, a New York cardiologist, observed, "When I used to encounter an aneurysm, I would send the patient to the best aneurysm surgeon I knew. It would be where you'd want your mother to go. Now I have to look at a list of surgeons who are in an HMO's network. I do my best to identify someone in the network who is OK. But it isn't someone of the caliber that I could get otherwise."

Aware that some doctors reluctantly join HMO networks but never fully welcome managed-care tactics, several major HMOs explicitly bar their participating doctors from making any negative comments about the health plan. Breaking this code of silence can be grounds for expulsion from the network. That provision was tested in late 1995 when David Himmelstein, a Massachusetts internist participating in U.S. Healthcare's HMOs, spoke out against the health plan on the *Donahue* television show. Two weeks later Dr. Himmelstein was told that U.S. Healthcare wouldn't need his services anymore. The HMO said only that it was realigning its network in Massachusetts, but Dr. Himmelstein interpreted the ouster as punishment for his comments. The Massachusetts legislature subsequently passed a law banning such HMO "gag clauses." Dr. Himmelstein eventually was reinstated into the U.S. Healthcare network.

Many physicians take a warmer view of managed care, contending that the benefits — more affordable care for the public, better data on how each doctor is performing — outweigh the flaws. The doctors who really thrive in HMO settings simply don't see limited access to tests and specialists as a major problem. "I want first crack at treating a disease," says New York internist Steven Tamarin, rather than sending everything from acne to yeast infections on to a specialist. Even more assertive is Richard Morrow, a Bronx family practitioner. Everywhere he turns he sees examples of specialists overdoing it. In his view, otolaryngologists put middle-ear tubes into far too many children who don't need them; cardiologists order batteries of tests that aren't always necessary; and back surgeons collect huge fees for operating on bulging disks that may not be the cause of patients' pain. "When you go in for all these treatments, you're just helping put those doctors' kids through school," Dr. Morrow snips. From that point of view HMO guidelines are the best way to rein in specialists.

One of the most intense battlegrounds over managed care has been southern California. Nearly half of all workers in the area belong to HMOs, one of the highest rates of managed care in the United States. Since the early 1990s big employers have been especially aggressive in negotiating cheaper rates for health insurance. That has led HMOs to cut their payments to doctors and hospitals and to tighten the rules on what services will be paid for. Doctors have banded together into large negotiating groups in efforts to increase their clout. Health-care consultants frequently cite the southern California market as a bellwether for the rest of the country, predicting that changes occurring in the Los Angeles area will play out in similar form throughout the United States in the next three to five years.

The promise and pitfalls of the rush toward managed care come to life in the day-to-day practice of pediatrician Brian Greenberg in Tarzana.

An easygoing man in his late 30s, Dr. Greenberg became an HMO gatekeeper by accident. When he finished his training at UCLA in 1991, Dr. Greenberg toyed with the idea of practicing full-time as a pediatric allergist, but decided he preferred the variety of general pediatrics. Rather than set up a solo practice, he joined a small medical group run by a veteran pediatrician, Robert Barnhard, whom he already knew and liked from his UCLA years. Dr. Greenberg agreed to share a patient population of nearly 8,000 with Dr. Barnhard and two other younger doctors, Victoria Millet and Elaine Rosen. Dr. Barnhard divided up the income from the partnership, paying Dr. Greenberg a flat salary slightly above $100,000.

Until the end of 1992 the four doctors catered only to patients with traditional fee-for-service insurance. But then parents began mentioning that changes in their health insurance might force them to look for different pediatricians. One of the biggest local employers, the Los Angeles County Unified School District, decided in late 1992 to move all its employees into HMOs. Parents began scouring for new pediatricians. The threatened exodus was especially unsettling for Dr. Barnhard, who had been in practice for more than 25 years. In that time very few of his patients had quit, and when one did leave, he wondered whether he had disappointed them in some way. Now parents were telling Drs. Barnhard and Greenberg that everything about their practice was fine, except that the doctors weren't signed up with their HMOs.

Eager to keep their doors open to long-time patients, the doctors decided to affiliate with as many HMOs as they could. To do so, they were required to use a middleman, an independent physicians' association, or IPA, that negotiated pay rates and contracts for hundreds of doctors with managed-care leaders such as Aetna, CaliforniaCare, Cigna, and Health Net. Doctors at the local hospital sponsored one such association: Tarzana IPA. Physicians a few miles away had formed two other such groups. Drs. Greenberg, Barnhard, Millet, and Rosen promptly joined all three IPAs to be sure of keeping almost all of their patients.

The managed-care package looked soothing at first. Dr. Greenberg and his colleagues could stay in private practice and take patients with all kinds of insurance. The physicians simply needed to agree to treat HMO patients according to managed-care rules. Pay rates would change; instead of being reimbursed for each visit or test, the doctors would be paid through capitation, the system of flat monthly rates per patient. But Dr. Greenberg and his colleagues didn't foresee the enormous consequences of these changes. The physicians briefly scanned their 40-page contracts with the IPAs, then signed them.

Three years later Dr. Greenberg musters a thin smile when recalling his early optimism. HMOs now provide half his patients, and the percentage continues to climb. Managed-care companies "have taken over our practice," he says. The values that he learned in medical school no longer are universally admired — or even taken seriously. As Dr. Greenberg observes, "I think my patients like me. I believe I practice good medicine. It used to be that if you did those two things, you were in good shape. But now none of that may matter. It all comes down to contracting decisions. Which HMO do you sign up with?

Which IPA? How many patients can they send you? And will they decide to keep you or not?"

Some of the most wrenching situations involve the managed-care rules for pediatric and maternal care right after a child is born. Medical experts, notably the American College of Obstetricians and Gynecologists, recommend that mothers with no complications be discharged 48 hours after a vaginal delivery and 96 hours after a cesarean. That allows time to detect any abnormal postpartum bleeding and to check that the newborn doesn't have jaundice, infections, congenital heart problems, or other complications. But the decision about when to send a mother and baby home no longer is left up to the obstetrician and the pediatrician. Power has moved over to the health plans that pay the bills, and they often put patients on a different clock. Many HMOs pay only for shorter stays: 24 hours or less after vaginal deliveries; 72 hours after cesareans.

For HMOs the monetary rewards from shorter maternity stays are immense. Whittling away one hospital day from every birth can translate each year into 5 million fewer hospital days nationwide, or roughly $6 billion in savings. But such financial gains may carry hidden costs. Pediatric journals carry accounts of life-threatening infections and congenital heart problems in newborns that were spotted only in the second day of a maternity stay. Rapid medical treatment or surgery can save such children; delays may prove fatal. Such cases are rare. As Dr. Greenberg puts it, "The overwhelming majority of babies are fine, no matter what you do." Even so, the notion of losing even one rescuable newborn appalls him.

So, like many physicians, Dr. Greenberg now feels pressured to practice two-tier medicine. Patients with generous insurance can remain in the hospital for the full maternity stay recommended by medical panels. Patients with skimpier HMO coverage must settle for the shorter stay unless the family wants to pay for extra care themselves or Dr. Greenberg can outwit the managed-care guidelines. He has a few favorite ruses that can win his patients a few extra hours in the hospital, such as the sudden "meeting" that prevents him from signing discharge papers right away. By and large, though, he has ended up doing what managed-care companies want — and he is not proud of it. "I don't want to live in a world where insurance companies have decided to sacrifice a few patients to save a buck," he says.

On this life-and-death issue, doctors and patients have mobilized fast against HMOs' cost-saving guidelines. In the 1995–96 legislative cycle, more than a dozen states passed laws requiring insurance companies to pay for 48-hour maternity stays. A similar bill was introduced in the U.S. Congress and won support from President Clinton. HMOs generally opposed such bills as unnecessary meddling in medical issues. Health plans contended that some publicized deaths of quickly discharged newborns didn't constitute a trend, noting that a study of 30,000 deliveries at Kaiser Permanente showed no connection between short stays and higher complication or mortality rates for newborns. But HMOs' statistics couldn't allay public concern about the well-being of mothers and babies sent home barely one day after birth. Besides, other researchers found evidence that short-stay babies might be at greater risk, particularly for conditions such as jaundice.

Rapid discharge of seemingly normal babies occasionally has upsetting consequences for parents too. Consider the standard test of a newborn's thyroid gland. If thyroid output is abnormally low, the baby is at risk for mental retardation unless synthetic thyroid is taken for years. Normally, thyroid tests are done on a baby's second day, with results available 48 hours later. When the baby leaves the hospital after one day, however, the test must be done a few hours after birth, when the thyroid gland may not yet be working properly. The test's error rate, usually less than 0.1 percent, can be appreciably higher. False alarms can be caught by a retest a few days later, but in the meantime parents must endure a needless scare until accurate results come in.

Managed-care rules can create more mischief in a baby's first year of life, typically the pediatrician's busiest time. Infants receive a battery of immunizations against mumps, diphtheria, and a half-dozen other diseases. They are supposed to have a well-baby checkup every two or three months. Inevitably, most infants also see the doctor at least once or twice for fevers and other ailments. Those repeated brief visits allow pediatricians to do a great deal of preventive care, something that HMOs play up in their marketing brochures. But when it comes to paying the pediatrician, managed-care pay scales vary tremendously. Some companies pay as much as $600 for a year's worth of infant care; others' rates may be less than $50 for the same work. Such pay scales leave doctors seething; they also raise the risk that physicians will skimp on care.

Curiously, the managed-care system starts with enough money that it could pay its front-line soldiers — the primary-care doctors — quite well. But each premium dollar travels a long path, from a corporate employer through an HMO and other intermediaries, before reaching physicians. At each stage middlemen who never see patients skim off their share. By the time Dr. Greenberg presses a stethoscope to a baby's chest or asks a mother if her child is eating properly, only a sliver of the original premium dollar is left.

On his Macintosh computer at home one evening, Dr. Greenberg called up a summary of his managed-care contracts, and brooded. Employers in southern California typically were paying about $120 a month, or $1,440 a year, for each worker's or dependent's health insurance. Of that amount, 15 percent to 20 percent went to marketing, administration, management salaries, and profit. Another 35 percent or so was set aside for members' hospital expenses. The rest usually was routed to the IPAs, which divided up money for primary-care doctors, specialists, lab work, and tests. These IPAs, naturally, kept some money for their own administration. In the end pediatricians and other primary-care doctors seldom got more than 20 percent of the premium dollar, and sometimes ended up with 5 percent or less.

Some of the skimpiest paychecks in 1994 and early 1995 came from Southern California IPA, known as SCIPA. At that time, the IPA paid Dr. Greenberg $108 a year for children between ages two and 18. For children under two, he got $266.40 a year. But that apparent pay boost for infants was deceptive. The pediatrician himself had to pay for vaccines, which cost $222 in an infant's first year. The money left over, $44, was meant to cover managed care's contributions to doctors' incomes, overhead, and supplies. It barely matched what parents might pay for a single oil change and tune-up at the local gas station.

"How can you do decent care on $44 a year?" Dr. Greenberg asked. When he chose pediatrics, he knew he was going into one of the lowest-paying areas of medicine. His yearly income is far higher than that of most Americans, but barely half what his medical-school classmates who went into radiology, pathology, or other specialties can command. And his income is largely at the mercy of plans such as SCIPA, which links doctors with most of southern California's dominant HMOs: Cigna, Aetna, FHP, PruCare, and nearly a dozen more. SCIPA in late 1995 boosted its pay rates considerably after being acquired by a larger IPA, Huntington Provider Group. But for several years the managed-care plan valued Dr. Greenberg's work at less than 50 percent of what he charged fee-for-service patients. Inevitably, he speeded up his rate of seeing patients, to about six an hour, trying to cover expenses by shuttling more patients through the office in a day.

Such pay gripes are part of a fundamental worry among some physicians: that HMOs regard the fine points of doctoring with disdain if they think about them at all. Managed-care companies can track several dozen aspects of a doctor's practice, including such essentials as a pediatrician's immunization rate for all children assigned to that doctor. Over the past decade, many HMOs have nudged doctors to do better in most of those categories, often surpassing the rates of preventive-care measures in fee-for-service medicine. Physicians applaud those gains. But they contend that their best work is in subtle, impossible-to-quantify areas that won't ever show up on HMO spreadsheets.

At least a half-dozen times a day, for example, Dr. Greenberg carries out a 10-minute well-baby visit. Such a session may seem like merely a friendly chat with the baby's mother or father, but it is packed with rapid, careful probes for potential problems. Are the infant's feet and hands cold? Maybe there is a circulation problem. How does the heart sound? Maybe there is a congenital problem that can be caught early. Is the baby rolling over? Starting to crawl? Making different sounds? This is where development problems can be spotted early and treated if necessary. How is the child sleeping? Eating? Such questions check that the parents are caring for the child correctly. If there are problems, they can be discussed before the child's well-being suffers. "I think that's important," Dr. Greenberg says. "But all the HMO wants to know is: did I do the immunizations on time?"

Managed care is at its best in the treatment of routine illnesses. The capitation system ensures that doctors get their flat monthly payment even if they provide only a few minutes of phone advice for a nervous parent. A meaningful part of primary care consists of brief oral advice: the equivalent of "Put ice on it" or "Take two aspirin and call me in the morning." For basically healthy children, Dr. Greenberg finds, the capitation system lets him treat simple ailments simply, without feeling any financial incentive to insist on an office visit.

HMOs also try to make sure that doctors follow managed-care formularies — and don't prescribe costly drugs when cheaper alternatives will do. Among antibiotics, for example, generic amoxicillin is a favorite, costing $10 or less for a multiweek prescription. Stronger new antibiotics that can cost $50 or more are off-limits unless a doctor can make an overpowering case for using them. Nationwide cost savings from following formularies may total $1 billion a year or more, money that can go toward other types of care or lower insurance premiums.

Yet almost every doctor can cite cases where overly strict HMO formularies led to mean-spirited or wrong decisions. Dr. Greenberg, for example, sees a fair number of children under age six who have minor eye infections. He can prescribe several different antibiotics that are generally effective. His top choice, Polytrim, can be administered painlessly. But on several occasions HMOs vetoed that prescription and told him to switch to a cheaper substitute, sodium Sulamyd, which must be applied four times a day and can sometimes sting a child's eyes. Boxed in, he had no choice but to rewrite the prescription or tell parents to pay for the better drug out of their own pockets. "To me it matters a lot whether a four-year-old is in pain," Dr. Greenberg says. "But to the HMO it's just money. They don't see the child, and they don't care."

Managed-care reviewers frequently relent if a doctor insists that good medical judgment requires an exception to the drug formulary. But the review process can be draining. That may be no accident; a favorite cost-saving technique at some HMOs is known as "management by inconvenience." Even if a persistent doctor or patient can win special treatment, the thinking goes, most applicants will become discouraged and give up. It may take two or three phone calls — and a journey up the hierarchy of a managed-care company's utilization-review department — before a doctor can win an appeal. That takes away 20 minutes from other patients, Dr. Greenberg observes, a diversion that he can't always afford.

Such skirmishes also are a humbling reminder to doctors that they no longer have total control of their practice. Managed-care pharmacists and review nurses can second-guess their decisions by telephone from hundreds of miles away. Dr. Greenberg likes to recount how he won a minor tussle over his attempt to prescribe Lorabid, a costly nonformulary antibiotic, for a child allergic to the cheaper drugs. A series of managed-care reviewers questioned the doctor's judgment, but capitulated when he convinced them that the allergy was serious. Offsetting that small victory, however, Dr. Greenberg admits to losing other squabbles, including an attempt to stray from the formulary when he felt that a standard drug came in pill sizes too big for a six-year-old to swallow comfortably. A Utah-based HMO clerk pulled up the child's medical records and declared during a phone review, "He was able to swallow an even larger pill last week." Stunned by the amount of detail in the HMO's records, Dr. Greenberg caved in and agreed to use the formulary drug.

Similar tradeoffs of cost versus comfort arise with medical lab contracts. Managed-care negotiators get rock-bottom prices on blood testing, X-rays, and other ancillary services by signing exclusive contracts with a few suppliers willing to give sizable discounts. In southern California some managed-care plans have trimmed lab costs by 40 percent or more, saving millions of dollars for their members. But as different bargain hunters cut different deals, doctors can end up with a crazy-quilt assortment of service contracts.

Patients needing X-rays, for example, may end up on a long zigzag because of bargain shopping by an HMO or an IPA. Children who see Dr. Greenberg through Tarzana IPA can get their X-rays done across the street at the radiology department of Encino-Tarzana Regional Medical Center. But Southern California IPA negotiated a different cut-price contract with a radiology group six miles north. So SCIPA patients must bypass the nearby X-ray facility and drive to Northridge. The rules are ironclad; if a SCIPA patient mistakenly goes to the nearby facility, the IPA will refuse to pay for the resulting X-rays.

This bargain-hunting approach faces its toughest test in managed-care coverage of the seriously ill. It is a health insurance truism that the sickest 3 percent of policyholders account for 40 percent of all medical spending. Those are the cases that an HMO most avidly wants to avoid — or at least "manage." Managed-care executives like to portray themselves as watchful shepherds of sick members, lining up the best possible care while occasionally saving a few nickels. But primary-care physicians such as Dr. Greenberg see a different picture.

Tensions start when Dr. Greenberg wants to refer an ailing child to a specialist, which happens several times a day. Dr. Greenberg's general skills let him treat 90 percent or more of the children who walk in his door, but when a young boy's bladder disorder doesn't respond to the first two programs of treatment, or a teenager's mood swings alarm a parent, it is time to call in an expert. Under traditional indemnity insurance, such referrals are a snap. Pediatricians simply tell parents whom to see next and let the insurer pick up the bill. Parents can even hunt for a specialist on their own if they disagree with their pediatrician's suggestions. But in managed care Dr. Greenberg must fill out a referral form, send it over to his IPA, and wait for approval. Patients may wait a week or two — sometimes more — before they see the specialist, unless a dire emergency exists. And the choice of specialists is a far cry from the medical all-star team to which Dr. Greenberg can steer his fee-for-service patients.

On a bookshelf next to Dr. Greenberg's examination rooms are two thin folders listing all the specialists to whom he can send his managed-care patients. The 32-page SCIPA list is in a blue folder; the 28-page TIPA list is in red. As the last patients leave his office one evening, Dr. Greenberg flips through the list and marvels at his lack of choices. In the TIPA folder there are only two dermatologists, neither of whom specializes in children. The list of general surgeons has shrunk to two. Originally there were five, but three pulled out because they were not getting paid on time. Only two oncologists are listed, and one of them isn't really available. Next to the cancer specialist's name, Dr. Greenberg's office manager, Vernalie Dermajian, has written "No new patients!"

That skimpy roster of experts vexes Dr. Greenberg. "I don't expect to be able to use the best in the world every time," he says. "But I do expect conscientious care." Some doctors on the approved lists were chosen, he suspects, mostly because they agreed to discount their fees 45 percent or more, accept outside review of how often they order tests, and otherwise play by managed care's rules. Top specialists won't agree to such terms, Dr. Greenberg notes. His most trusted dermatologist, in fact, briefly was part of the TIPA network, but dropped out when the managed-care plan tried to cut her fees further.

Sometimes Dr. Greenberg and his colleagues can persuade a managed-care plan to bend its rules and allow a patient to see a nonnetwork specialist. Such a request, however, almost always is a struggle. One such case involved a young girl with eosinophilic leukemia, a rare blood cancer. After five weeks of haggling with IPAs and HMOs, one of Dr. Greenberg's colleagues, Dr. Millet, won the right for the girl to be treated by a top pediatric oncologist at Children's Hospital in Los Angeles. During that time, though, the girl's treatment was delayed because the managed-care companies tried to steer her to an in-network adult oncologist who had limited experience treating the child's condition. By eventually getting the girl to the appropriate specialist, Dr. Millet believed she put her on the road to remission and perhaps outright cure. But she remained troubled by the lost five weeks and the narrowly avoided outcome of sending a very sick child to the wrong expert.

When specialists agree to work under managed-care rules, they surrender their long-standing freedom to bill insurers for whatever tests and equipment they think are needed. Dr. Greenberg, for example, continues to practice part-time as an allergist, treating children with asthma. He would like health insurance to cover whatever he prescribes, but his HMO patients sometimes run into nasty surprises. In one case he prescribed six inhalers, a three-month supply, for a boy. The parents' HMO approved only five. To a managed-care company that cut represents a 17 percent saving. To Dr. Greenberg such cutbacks squeeze out a margin of safety and make it more likely that the child will run out of medicine before his refill date. If that happens, the boy could succumb to an uncontrolled asthma attack — a scary outcome for him and a potential trigger for a $1,000 emergency-room visit that would wipe out the HMO's earlier cost savings.

In another case, Dr. Greenberg wanted to prescribe two inhalers for a boy with exercise-induced asthma, one for home use, the other for school. Managed-care reviewers vetoed that plan, saying they would pay for only one. HMO accountants may call that step a 50 percent cost saving, but to Dr. Greenberg, it once again compromises the margin of safety. Unless the boy proves scrupulous about taking his inhaler back and forth from school to home — something that many adults sometimes forget — the HMO's approach increases the risk of an asthma attack with no medicine at hand.

In the worst predicament of all are children with major chronic diseases struggling to fit into the capitated, gatekeeper system of managed care. Such children may need a raft of specialist referrals every month, and never-ending tests and office visits. Those needs don't square well with a system that pays doctors a flat monthly rate for each patient. Dr. Greenberg, for example, gets $8 to $12 a month for children older than two, without any extra cash for patients who need the most care. Easy and hard cases are supposed to average out. But his monthly capitation checks don't begin to cover the costs of seeing a child with muscular dystrophy, Down's syndrome, or juvenile rheumatoid arthritis.

As a result some doctors with HMO contracts are quietly closing their doors to high-risk patients. The standard excuse among such physicians: "I don't know if I'm skilled enough to take care of such a child. Try someone else." The dodging of high-risk patients has long been an unpleasant aspect of the health insurance industry. Now, as HMOs push the financial responsibility for patients onto doctors' shoulders, some physicians are starting to behave like insurance companies themselves — redlining the patients that could annihilate their capitation budgets. "I think it's unethical," says Dr. Greenberg, who takes in some of these economically orphaned children. "But if you get only $96 a year to take care of these children, they will be a financial drag on your practice. I know I'm going to see them every month, and every visit will mean five referrals."

At 6 P.M. one autumn day, Drs. Greenberg and Barnhard sit at their small desks in the back room of their Tarzana office suite and debate a tantalizing question. What would happen if they shed all their HMO contracts and went back to a pure fee-for-service practice? Both doctors can cite what they believe are deep flaws with managed care and its gatekeeper system: underpayment for important preventive treatment, undue meddling in the doctors' choice of labs and pharmaceuticals, and limited access to good specialists who can help the sickest children. Yet after a few minutes of discussion, the two doctors realize that the idea of breaking away from managed care is only a pipe dream.

"Overnight, we'd lose 15 percent to 40 percent of our revenue," Dr. Greenberg says. "Maybe some of our HMO patients would switch insurance so they could keep seeing us. But a large percentage would just drop us and go to another doctor. Either we've never established a relationship with them, or they just don't want to pay more."

Dr. Barnhard is even blunter. "We could say 'We don't like managed care, and we'd like to go back to what was.' But the truth is, the old practice doesn't exist anymore."

6

Heart Trouble

IN EARLY SEPTEMBER 1995, top executives of the Health Insurance Plan of Greater New York gathered for a weekend retreat at the Montauk Yacht Club on the eastern tip of Long Island. Away from the hubbub of their Manhattan offices, surrounded by golf courses and ocean breezes, the HIP executives decided to cut a clever strategic deal with a big suburban hospital. A week later HIP president Anthony Watson announced a far-reaching alliance with North Shore University Hospital in the Long Island town of Manhasset. HIP promised to steer many of its members to North Shore. In return the hospital agreed to "maximize" discounts for 375,000 HIP members throughout Long Island and the neighboring New York City borough of Queens. And North Shore agreed to buy two small hospitals that were HIP-owned and hard to manage.

Crowning this alliance was a new heart-surgery contract. For 10 years HIP had sent all its heart-procedure candidates in Queens to be treated in Manhattan at New York Hospital–Cornell Medical Center. As of October 1, 1995, however, the relationship with New York Hospital was over. All HIP's Queens members would be pointed toward North Shore instead. For North Shore's administrators and heart surgeons the new contract was a tremendous boon. It would mean an extra 200 or more surgery cases a year, establishing North Shore as a truly high-volume heart center. It would generate at least $1 million a year in new revenue for surgeons, cardiologists, and anesthesiologists, and perhaps $4 million a year more for the hospital.

The only losers were HIP members with heart disease.

The facility that HIP dropped, New York Hospital, was widely regarded as one of the best heart-surgery centers in the United States. One of its young surgeons, Jeffrey Gold, had the lowest mortality rate among all 220 active heart surgeons in New York State. His boss, cardiac surgery chief O. Wayne Isom, was the surgeon of choice for many celebrities, such as talk-show host Larry King, who could pick any doctor they wanted. The hospital's ultimate seal of approval came in March 1995 from the state Department of Health. State officials found that patients undergoing bypass surgery — the most common type of heart operation — had some of the best risk-adjusted survival rates if they were treated at New York Hospital. Even HIP, just before switching contracts, had bragged about its affiliation with New York Hospital. Throughout the summer of 1995 the health plan aired television ads showing the hospital's doctors in action. The message: if viewers joined HIP, the elite medical center was at their disposal.

North Shore, by contrast, was an adequate but hardly inspired choice for heart surgery. The Long Island hospital had stumbled in the late 1980s, posting one of the worst heart-surgery mortality rates in New York, according to state health department data. In 1989–90, 5.15 percent of patients having bypass operations died in the operating room or soon afterward. Deaths became less common in the early 1990s, in part because the hospital promised state regulators that it would stop taking some high-risk cases. In 1993 North Shore had a risk-adjusted mortality rate of 2.65 percent, according to state data. That ranked the hospital in the middle of the pack: 14th best out of 31 hospitals performing open-heart surgery. New York Hospital's rate, in contrast, was just 1.70 percent.

Even at North Shore there was little belief that HIP's choice of this hospital was made for clinical reasons alone. "I think we've got a good reputation, but New York Hospital did have some of the very best mortality numbers in the state," observed Anthony Tortolani, chief of cardiothoracic surgery at North Shore. He added, "When managed-care companies look at things, I think quality is an issue, but the three most important things are cost, cost, and cost. The business side is probably an important factor in why HIP decided to be with us."

That line of thinking frightened some HIP members. In mid-September 1995 a middle-aged HIP patient arrived at New York Hospital for a consultation with Dr. Isom and pleaded with the surgeon to schedule his heart surgery quickly. The request startled Dr. Isom, who believed that the man's condition could be managed with less drastic measures for some time. "I asked him, 'Why do you want surgery now?'" Dr. Isom recalled. The answer: the patient's cardiologist had informed him that after October 1, heart-surgery patients would not be sent to New York Hospital. They would have to go to North Shore instead. Rather than gamble on another hospital, the patient wanted accelerated surgery with the doctor he trusted.

HIP's own approach to hospital selection was more detached. "It's our job to get the best terms for our members, and that includes financial terms," said Jesse Jampol, a long-time HIP medical director. State officials had spent years trying to distinguish the best heart-surgery centers from ones that weren't as good, but HIP officials didn't seem nearly as interested in such distinctions. As Dr. Jampol put it, "New York is blessed with a large number of first-class institutions. I don't know that you can tell the difference in any realistic way among a half-dozen institutions. We haven't compromised on quality to any degree."

It would be some comfort if HIP's decision to save money by dropping a top-flight hospital were an aberration. Unfortunately it is not. In the past few years managed-care executives have brought an aggressive business focus to the most expensive aspect of American medicine: the treatment of heart disease. In public the HMO directors have said all the right things: they would preserve and even improve quality, while looking only for ways to trim waste. A close look at contracting practices, however, suggests something very different. When it comes to caring for people with heart disease, especially the very sick, managed-care companies have repeatedly opted for what is cheap instead of what is best.

Of all the subspecialties of medicine, the stakes are highest in treating heart disease. Each year more than 900,000 American men and women die of cardiovascular disease, making it the leading killer for both sexes. Over the past 50 years, advances in medicine and surgery have greatly improved patients' chances of delaying, stalling, or even reversing heart disease. As author Sherwin Nuland points out, a man having a heart attack in the early 1950s was likely to die on the spot, even if he was in a hospital with a physician beside him. Treatments at the time were "few and too often inadequate." Today such a patient is likely to walk out of the hospital within a week or two, often with a stronger heart than before. New clot-dissolving drugs, vastly improved cardiology techniques, and the ability to do open-heart surgery quickly and with reasonable safety have given doctors and patients tremendous hope.

Such progress has not been cheap. A free-spending mentality took hold in the 1970s and 1980s, and the treatment of heart disease was seen not just as an urgent medical priority but also as an economic bonanza. Drug companies, medical-equipment makers, cardiologists, and heart surgeons all kept widening the circle of patients they treated, sometimes leading to unnecessary procedures and inflated "demand" for their services. Providers also learned that their lifesaving work could fetch stunning prices, far in excess of the direct costs. As a result, ostensibly not-for-profit hospitals salted away millions in earnings from highly profitable cardiac units. Heart surgeons earning $1 million or more a year began collecting Jaguars and fine art. Pharmaceutical companies posted giant profits and bathed their executives in luxury. Meanwhile, patients muttered in disbelief at $100-a-month prescription drugs and $1,500 tests of heart function. But they or their insurance carriers kept paying. Total spending on treatments for heart disease has surged to the point that it is currently more than $117 billion a year, equivalent to the gross national product of Sweden.

For managed-care companies the remedy has been clear: do whatever it takes to get costs for heart care under control. Most HMOs have taken a three-step approach. First, they have stressed diet changes, exercise programs, and smoking cessation, on the sound theory that such low-cost preventive care is the most cost-effective way to protect members from heart ailments. Second, they have clamped down aggressively on tests and surgeries for people already suffering from heart disease, trying to avoid overuse of costly services. Some leading managed-care plans perform heart surgery just half as often as the national average. And in a third, controversial initiative, HMOs have used their purchasing clout to pick the cheapest surgeons and hospitals. Within managed-care plans, MBA-trained contracting executives run an exercise that has been dubbed "buying hearts." Their goal: to negotiate rock-bottom hospital contracts with the same price-focused discipline that the HMO would use in buying paper towels or office supplies.

Such bargain hunting need not hurt patients if it is done with a close eye on medical quality. Some widely admired heart-surgery teams, including those at the Cleveland Clinic, have cut prices to win managed-care contracts. Heart care, in fact, provides some uniquely good opportunities to identify the best doctors and hospitals. If HMOs wanted, they could work predominantly with these quality leaders, helping them expand capacity. Then HMOs could try to negotiate the best possible prices with universally recognized "centers of excellence." Mediocre hospitals wouldn't be driven out of business, but they would see fewer patients unless they improved their results — and the overall level of national care would improve.

In fact, many HMOs do use the "centers of excellence" approach in one small corner of their business: treating patients who need organ transplants. Successful heart, lung, or liver transplants carry tremendous prestige for both hospitals and managed-care plans, and often are cited in HMO marketing material. Even though transplants and associated care can cost $100,000 or more per case, their extreme rarity makes them a trifling part of a typical HMO's annual budget.* Thus managed-care plans can afford to make clinical quality their highest priority on the few occasions that they shop for transplants. Business generally is directed to renowned centers such as Johns Hopkins, the Mayo Clinic, or Stanford University.

More typically, though, managed-care plans fail to sign up such centers of excellence. In easily standardized, high-volume aspects of heart care, HMOs repeatedly fail to compile rigorous data on surgical outcomes, and they ignore publicly available quality reports. Price is what matters most. As a result, managed care's record in treating advanced heart disease is sprinkled with missed chances and patient-unfriendly decisions. Those failings can be seen in areas ranging from the formularies that determine which pills are prescribed to something as complex as the quality of surgeons available to treat rare congenital disorders. This chapter will examine all those issues, starting with the main event in heart surgery: coronary-artery bypass operations.

Each year about 600,000 Americans have their hearts mended on the operating table. Valves are replaced, pacemakers are installed, occasionally even an entire heart is transplanted. The most common operation is coronary-artery bypass graft surgery, known as CABG (familiarly pronounced "cabbage"). This operation attaches new lifelines for

---

*All told, about 9,000 Americans receive a heart, lung, or liver transplant in any given year. Many of those recipients have indemnity insurance or qualify for Medicare, Medicaid, or other federal insurance. HMOs are unlikely to set aside more than 0.1 percent of their total premiums to cover transplant costs.

freshly oxygenated blood to the heart muscle itself. Done properly, CABG surgery can give patients a second chance at a healthy life, correcting the damage that smoking, obesity, a fatty diet, or unlucky genetics has done to the heart's own arteries. In CABG surgery doctors open up the chest wall, briefly stop the heart, and typically stitch short stretches of vein taken from the patient's legs onto the surface of the heart. These grafts take on a new role as replacement coronary arteries, transmitting blood that will keep the heart muscle alive and healthy. While surgeons perform this delicate reassembly, medical technicians redirect the patient's blood through an external heart-lung machine for half an hour or longer. Once the grafting is complete, surgeons restart the heart, close up the chest, and send the patient to the hospital's intensive-care unit to begin an in-hospital recovery of at least four to six days.

First carried out in 1964, bypass surgery initially evoked the same feelings of awe, enthusiasm, and national pride that attached to NASA's space program. Pioneering heart surgeons such as Michael DeBakey, Denton Cooley, Norman Shumway, and John Kirklin became national heroes. In an admiring cover story in 1965, *Time* magazine lionized Dr. DeBakey as "the Texas Tornado," praising everything from his skill with a scalpel to his humble beginnings and his boundless energy. Two U.S. presidents, John F. Kennedy and Lyndon Johnson, championed heart surgery for the nation, setting up presidential commissions that called for rapid dissemination of these new techniques to hospitals throughout the country.

By the time managed-care companies rose to prominence, America's gee-whiz attitude toward CABG surgery had changed. What once was a rare, heroic operation had become common: 100,000 CABGs in 1979; 200,000 in 1983; 400,000 in 1990. The field had become far more competitive too. In 1990 some 900 hospitals could boast of having their own heart-surgery unit. Hospitals throughout the 1980s jockeyed for market share mostly by advertising, by befriending cardiologists who might refer patients, and by trying to build a reputation for convenient, good-quality care. Price competition didn't exist yet; most hospitals and surgeons thought it would be unseemly (and bad for business). But that was about to change.

One of the first big price cutters was Gerald Kay, a charismatic California heart surgeon. In the early 1980s, well before most people had become concerned about medical efficiency, Dr. Kay began arguing that hospitals weren't doing nearly enough to save costs in the operating room, rehabilitate patients quickly, and discharge them swiftly. In 1986 he was recruited to head up the heart-surgery team at the Hospital of the Good Samaritan, a midsize Los Angeles facility with big ambitions. Before Dr. Kay's arrival, Good Samaritan hadn't been a major factor in the CABG business. Its inner-city location was unappealing; it lacked the prestige of an academic medical center; and its list prices weren't cheap enough to attract California's quickly growing managed-care plans. When heart-surgery patients did arrive, Good Samaritan charged the region's going rate: $50,000 or so for hospital fees, plus $10,000 or so for surgeons and anesthesiologists. But where others saw problems, Dr. Kay saw opportunity. If Good Samaritan could become the region's "low-cost producer" in heart surgery, he believed, it could slash prices, attract big new managed-care contracts, and use the extra volume to become even more efficient.

Hospital executives embraced his ideas. They ripped out half a floor of surgery and recovery units and rebuilt them to Dr. Kay's liking. That let him create a heart-surgery "assembly line" that could handle more than 1,000 cases a year. Then Good Samaritan offered eye-popping discounts to managed-care plans in return for promises of numerous patients. On some contracts, hospital fees plunged to $18,000; surgeons' fees were halved to about $5,000, for an all-inclusive charge of $23,000. "We wanted to put through as many patients as we could, seven days a week," recalled John Westerman, president of Good Samaritan in the mid-1980s. Two-tier pricing took hold, in which Good Samaritan still charged its old rates to non-HMO customers, but wooed managed-care plans with much better terms. The gamble paid off; big medical groups and HMOs responded by steering hundreds of patients a year to the deepest discounter in town. Good Samaritan's cardiac-surgery caseload rose to a peak of about 1,300 cases a year in 1989 and 1990, up from just 250 in 1985.

To Good Samaritan's chagrin, its competitors didn't sit still. Other hospitals overhauled their heart units, cut costs, and dropped their managed-care prices. A price war broke out in southern California, and the all-inclusive rates for CABG surgery and hospital stays sank below $20,000. Before long, rates had dropped even further, to $16,500, and weren't done falling. In 1990 the greater Los Angeles area turned into a spectacular buyer's market for heart surgery. HMOs could pick and choose among 71 hospitals in the region that provided heart surgery — twice the number as in all of New York State. With price established as the main competitive yardstick, hospitals wanting extra business embarked on an almost suicidal race to be the cheapest. At one point, when Dr. Kay tried to snatch away CABG business from another hospital with an all-inclusive bid of just $13,000 per case, he was rebuked by Charles Munger, the hospital's chairman, for bidding below Good Samaritan's marginal cost. (Munger was known for his business savvy as a partner of legendary investor Warren Buffett.) After that Good Samaritan's contract prices inched up slightly, but the hospital found that it couldn't dictate prices any longer. Its HMO customers now controlled the market.

If managed-care plans had picked hospitals on the basis of patient survival rates instead of price, Good Samaritan might not have become nearly so popular. Each year the federal Health Care Financing Administration (HCFA) compiles hospital-by-hospital data on CABG mortality rates for Medicare patients. In states, such as California, that don't compile mortality rates for all heart-surgery patients, Medicare data are the next-best gauge of a hospital's outcomes. They track all patients age 65 and over, who account for half of all CABG surgeries. The frailness of many elderly patients makes them risky candidates for surgery; a hospital with a 3 percent overall death rate from heart surgery may have a 5 percent rate for its Medicare patients. Medicare mortality rates tend to be higher than those for the general population; they also provide an especially sensitive gauge of a hospital's ability to handle tough cases.

At the apex of Good Samaritan's business success, the hospital had a markedly worse than average death rate for coronary bypass surgery on Medicare patients. In fiscal 1989, HCFA found, 6.7 percent of the hospital's Medicare CABG patients died on site or within 30 days of discharge. That figure climbed to 8.2 percent in fiscal 1990 and remained high, at 7.2 percent, in fiscal 1991. Each of those figures was at least a full percentage point above HCFA's predicted rate, given the ages and complications of the hospital's Medicare patient mix.

For the 1991–1993 interval, Good Samaritan's 30-day mortality rate for Medicare patients climbed to 10.4 percent, one of the highest among high-volume heart centers in its region. Kaiser Permanente's main Los Angeles hospital, by contrast, had a Medicare mortality rate of just 2.2 percent. Defending its record, Good Samaritan pointed out that the 1991–1993 mortality data weren't adjusted for the hospital's unique mix of easy and hard cases, including second surgeries on patients whose initial bypass grafts had stopped working well. Such "re-do" surgeries are generally regarded as riskier than first-time cases. "We operate on sicker people as a group," declared Gerald Kay's son, Gregory, who took over as chief of heart surgery at Good Samaritan in the early 1990s. "Fully 30 percent of our patients are age 75 or older, and 20 percent of our cases are re-dos." Nonetheless, two other Los Angeles hospitals that also handle many unusually sick patients, UCLA and Cedars-Sinai Medical Center, had lower death rates on Medicare CABG surgery during the 1991–93 period. Their mortality rates were 7.9 percent and 5.6 percent, respectively, according to Healthcare Data Source, an Aurora, Colorado, company that analyzed HCFA data.

Despite Good Samaritan's lackluster record in the early 1990s, the hospital continued to win contracts from managed-care plans. Among the hospital's patrons were the two California HMOs with the largest number of Medicare members, PacifiCare and FHP International. Federal authorities in the early 1990s stopped announcing hospital-specific mortality rates, but surgeons at Good Samaritan say their own data show a marked improvement in heart-surgery mortality rates in 1994 and 1995. According to Gregory Kay, 30-day death rates for CABG patients aged 65 and over totaled 3.6 percent in 1994 and 3.9 percent in 1995.

Hospital consultants have not been shy about emphasizing the importance of cost containment in winning heart-surgery contracts. A major hospital consulting firm, APM Incorporated, in San Francisco, told its clients about an unidentified HMO chief executive who declared, "For a 2 to 3 percent difference in mortality I'm not willing to spend an extra $40,000 per case." The implication, APM told its clients, was that even hospitals with better-than-average survival rates couldn't expect to win much HMO business if they didn't have competitive prices.

The scramble for cut-rate heart surgery can degrade patient care in subtle and not-so-subtle ways. Hospitals trying to win managed-care contracts have committed themselves to extensive reengineering of their cardiac-care units, looking for ways to lower costs whenever possible. Postsurgical tests have been scaled back. Nursing staff levels have been reduced. Patients are being zipped through various recovery units faster, often spending less time in the most expensive area, the intensive-care unit, and being moved quickly into lightly staffed general recovery units. In the vast majority of cases, such cutbacks can lower costs without producing a rise in the death rate or a surge in "red flag" complications such as infections or hospital readmissions after discharge, which would be widely regarded as signs of bad care. Sometimes, in fact, efficiency campaigns have eliminated needless delays or outdated practices, thereby actually improving patient care. Nonetheless, nurses and doctors who work closely with heart-surgery patients ask themselves if the cost cutting induced by managed-care contracts may be going too far.

"Hospitals are cutting their budgets to the point that one nurse is managing 10 patients," observes a worried David Perkowski, a Laguna Hills, California, heart surgeon. "That's nothing but crowd control. It used to be one nurse for every three patients. We haven't seen any disasters yet, but the trend is worrisome." Dr. Perkowski got a blunt lesson in the hazards of having fewer nurses on duty when his brother-in-law, a hospital efficiency consultant, went into the hospital for an angioplasty. During his hospital recovery, the brother-in-law bled into his sheets for 12 hours before a nurse noticed. The mishap didn't prevent a full recovery, but it unnerved family members. Dr. Perkowski says he warned his brother-in-law, "That's what happens when you have these kinds of cutbacks."

Rapid discharges of heart-surgery patients also can be cause for alarm. In southern California, many hospitals now send bypass patients home just four days after surgery, down from the 10-day stays that were common a decade ago. Experts say that medical advances, such as anesthesia agents that leave the system faster, and brisker forms of in-hospital rehabilitation, justify much of that shrinkage. Yet new financial incentives also play a role. In particular, the switch to all-inclusive case rates — instead of the older system of per-day charges — can lead hospitals to discharge patients "quicker and sicker." That shifts much of the care burden to patients and their families.

One of the hospitals that has done well by managed care is St. Francis Medical Center in Lynwood, California. In the early 1990s it won a major contract to handle heart-surgery patients who belong to MedPartners/Mullikin Medical Group. But its case price of just $16,500 doesn't provide much of a cushion to finance long hospital stays for patients recovering from surgery. As a result Anne Billingsley, chief of cardiothoracic surgery at the hospital, often is in the awkward position of nudging elderly patients out the door just a few days after she has operated on them.

"Most of them are scared to go home after four days," Dr. Billingsley confides. "You have to get them out with a shoe horn. I come around and say, 'All right. It's time.' It's really bad. These poor old guys look at you. They're terrified. But they end up doing fine when they go home. There's nothing else we really do for them at that stage of the recovery. It's just babysitting and helping them walk up and down the hall a few times. Their wives can do that for them at home."

Some surgeons, cardiologists, and hospitals take a warier approach toward cost cutting in pursuit of managed-care contracts. But those providers admit they are losing business by doing so. In Los Angeles, UCLA once had the busiest heart-surgery program in the region. Now it ranks well behind Good Samaritan, St. Vincent, and other hospitals in the yearly tally of heart-surgery cases. UCLA officials say their changes for CABG rates remain several thousand dollars above those of competitors, in part because of the extra costs associated with being a research and teaching hospital. "If we were as aggressive as Good Sam, we'd be a lot busier," says Lawrence Yeatman, a UCLA cardiologist. "But our name and reputation still attract the dwindling number of people who can choose us. We see people who were unhappy elsewhere. We see horror stories, cases that were mismanaged."

Those schisms among hospitals can be found in many other parts of the United States as well. In Philadelphia in 1993 the lowest CABG mortality rate occurred at Temple University Hospital, according to data compiled by the Pennsylvania Health Care Cost Containment Council. That year just 1.4 percent of bypass-surgery patients died at Temple, markedly better than the state's expected range. But Temple has relatively high posted charges, compared with a peer group of Philadelphia hospitals, and it hasn't been an aggressive discounter to managed-care plans. So while local HMOs use Temple for some rare, complex heart cases, such as transplants, they send most routine CABG cases elsewhere.

One of the HMOs' favorite picks in Philadelphia is Hahnemann University Hospital. Its death rate on bypass surgery was 3.6 percent in 1993, more than double the rate at Temple for that year. Even so, the two biggest managed-care plans in Philadelphia — U.S. Healthcare and the Blue Cross–affiliated Keystone Health Plan East — together send more than 100 heart cases a year to the hospital, making it one of their top referral centers. Hahnemann was one of the earliest hospitals in Pennsylvania to agree to discounted pricing for HMOs, and its negotiated prices for bypass surgery are said to be among the most competitive. That is what the HMOs like. "Mortality data alone is a pretty small factor in determining physician referrals" for heart surgery, says Gary Owens, a Keystone medical director.

Even Philadelphia's Episcopal Hospital, with a 5.0 percent mortality rate in 1993, attracts some CABG cases from U.S. Healthcare. State officials identified Episcopal as a hospital with a greater number of deaths than expected. But Joseph Carver, a U.S. Healthcare medical director, contends that his HMO's more sophisticated system of assessing hospital outcomes allows U.S. Healthcare to use centers like Episcopal for routine, easy cases and still achieve a better-than-expected overall mortality rate on heart surgery.

In Rochester, New York, the choice for top-quality heart surgery should be easy. The city's largest heart-surgery program, at Rochester General Hospital, has a risk-adjusted CABG mortality rate of 2.96 percent, according to state data for 1993. Its main competition, Strong Memorial Hospital, has a far higher risk-adjusted death rate: 4.90 percent. Strong's fatality rate is "significantly higher than [the] statewide average," according to New York State's Department of Health. Nevertheless, some managed-care plans continue to contract with Strong, which has been willing to discount its services.

In New York State public information on different hospitals' heart-surgery programs is especially plentiful, thanks to the efforts of Marc Chassin. A physician by training, Dr. Chassin began gathering mortality data in the early 1990s when he was state commissioner of health, then refined the data with a sophisticated risk-adjustment system, so that hospitals handling many tough cases could be compared with those whose cases were easier. Dr. Chassin says he is heartened that some hospitals and surgeons use the findings to identify problem areas and improve their performance. He is less impressed, however, with the response among HMOs. As he puts it, "There is no evidence — and in fact some evidence to the contrary — that managed-care plans are using this data in New York State."

Janet Monroe has learned about HMOs' indifference the hard way. She negotiates managed-care contracts for New York University Medical Center, another standout hospital in the state's heart-surgery rankings. Its risk-adjusted CABG mortality rate was just 2.14 percent in 1993; its death rate in the 1991–93 period was significantly below the state average. She likes to present such data, hoping to persuade HMOs to pay extra for her hospital's results. But she reports, "They give lip service to quality. Unless there's just a huge, gaping difference between hospitals, though, the decision is based on price, price, price."

When surgical plans change, HMOs' procurement plans may take precedence over continuity of care. Eric Rose, chief of cardiothoracic surgery at Columbia Presbyterian in New York, recalls a 1993 case involving a U.S. Healthcare member sent to him for a heart transplant. On examining the patient, Dr. Rose determined that a simpler operation, replacing an aortic valve, would suffice. The HMO at that point proposed moving the patient to Boston or Philadelphia, where it could get a cheaper rate on valve surgery. "Columbia Presbyterian is a very expensive institution," U.S. Healthcare medical director Hyman Kahn later explained. "If there's nothing urgent about the case, and it can be done elsewhere, equally as well, then why pay that premium? That's the whole idea of managed care."

Both the patient and Dr. Rose balked. U.S. Healthcare countered that it would approve the surgery at Columbia only if the hospital cut its price 40 percent and if Dr. Rose agreed to do the surgery for $2,000 — less than one third his usual fee. Outraged at the proposal, Dr. Rose and Columbia held firm and finally received approval to do the surgery on their standard terms. Nonetheless, Dr. Rose came away shaken at the HMO's apparent willingness to shuttle a very sick patient up and down the East Coast for a cheaper surgery rate.

In the early stages of cardiovascular illness, when symptoms may not extend beyond high blood pressure or elevated cholesterol, managed-care plans perform well. Surveys have shown that HMOs generally do a good job of monitoring members' cholesterol and encouraging them to make dietary changes that can reduce the risk of a heart attack. A detailed study of 1,296 patients with high blood pressure, published in November 1995, found little difference between HMO and fee-for-service participants over a seven-year period in death rates and in quality of life. Sheldon Greenfield, a researcher at New England Medical Center who ran the study, said it suggested that HMOs were saving costs without skimping on necessary care for those patients.

As heart disease worsens, the cost-cutting side of managed care bites more deeply. One frequent target has been angioplasty, the artery-widening procedure that many cardiologists perform as an alternative to bypass surgery. Many managed-care strategists contend that 30 percent or more of all angioplasties are unnecessary — and could safely be skipped in favor of much cheaper regimens of diet, exercise, and prescription drugs. In some markets HMOs have stopped paying cardiologists on a per-case basis for angioplasties and instead have put in capitation contracts that pay a flat rate per member per month, regardless of the number of angioplasties performed. Those contracts are meant to take away incentives for overtreatment. Like any capitation system, however, the contracts create new incentives for undertreatment. The cardiologist who decides that hardly any of his or her patients need angioplasties can pocket the monthly capitation check without doing much work; the cardiologist who takes many patients into the hospital for artery-opening procedures loses financially. Whether HMOs can safeguard members against underuse of a potentially lifesaving procedure is an open question.

As researchers develop better ways to treat heart disease, managed-care plans often lag behind other insurers in authorizing payment for new treatments. A major case in point involves the Palmaz-Schatz stent, a half-inch-long stainless-steel sleeve that props open coronary arteries narrowed by a buildup of plaque. Many cardiologists regard the stent as a powerful enhancement for angioplasty, improving the chances that an artery will stay open for years rather than clogging up again, as often happens after conventional angioplasty. But HMOs have been reluctant to reimburse doctors and hospitals for the full $1,600 cost of the stent itself. Some managed-care plans have openly said that in the interest of cost control, they will cover only about $350 of the new stent's price — the price of the surgical balloon used in conventional angioplasty. That puts doctors and hospitals in the uncomfortable position of either taking a financial loss every time they use the stent on an HMO patient or forgoing an advanced device in the face of budgetary pressure from a managed-care company. Alan Johnson, a top cardiologist at Scripps Memorial Hospital in La Jolla, California, says he regards HMOs' limited reimbursement policies on stents as "a horrific thing to do, let alone publicize."

Other controversies arise concerning on-the-spot treatment of heart attacks. Since the mid-1980s, hospitals have been able to save many thousands of patients by prompt administration of clot-dissolving drugs. These powerful medications can unclog coronary arteries and allow normal circulation to resume before major parts of the heart muscle die from oxygen insufficiency. The best such drugs are extremely expensive, though, and managed-care plans haven't always been willing to pay.

In particular, some HMOs have been stingy in allowing the use of recombinant tissue plasminogen activator, or t-PA, an enzyme produced through biotechnology at a cost of $2,200 per dose. A major 1993 study showed that patient survival rates with t-PA were two percentage points higher than with an older clot-busting agent, streptokinase. But researchers D. S. Lessler and A. L. Alvins reported in 1994 that patients being treated in HMO-owned hospitals were only 51 percent as likely to get t-PA as were patients treated in a fee-for-service setting. HMOs justify that lower level by saying that t-PA doesn't benefit all patients equally. Nonetheless, cost considerations in the managed-care environment may loom larger than the benefit to patients.

After heart patients leave the hospital, doctors often prescribe extensive physical therapy. When fee-for-service medicine prevailed, insurers suspected that the medical industry profited from overlong rehabilitation programs. Employers and managed-care companies insisted on severe cutbacks, despite claims that patients' recoveries might be jeopardized. One such controversy arose in Phoenix, Arizona, in 1994. Cardiac-care nurses were accustomed to putting patients through an 18-session program. That wasn't how Cigna wanted to do things; it offered nine-session coverage to some managed-care participants and left nurses with the impression that it might prefer just three sessions. "We tried to reconcile the idea of taking our complete program and compressing it into three sessions," says Joan Ming, a cardiac nurse who worked in Phoenix at the time. "We couldn't do it. It seemed like a window-dressing rehab program — and nothing more."

One of the most vexing shortcomings of some managed-care plans is their treatment of children born with heart defects. From the high-altitude vantage point of an HMO budget director, these rare cases are regarded as "outliers" — statistical flukes that don't fit into the central concentration of business. An HMO with 100,000 members may have just seven pediatric heart-surgery cases per year. For the affected children and their families, however, these are life-and-death dramas, in which surgical success can win many decades of full, normal life, while an operating-room failure will doom a child to endless medical attention and an early death.

In fixing a child's heart, the choices of hospital and surgeon are even more crucial than in adult cardiac surgery. "These are extremely dangerous, complex operations," explains James Lock, head of cardiology at Boston's Children's Hospital. "To do them well, you need a lot of resources, talent, and supervision." Mortality rates vary enormously among pediatric heart centers, he finds. On certain benchmark operations the top pediatric centers keep all but 3 to 4 percent of their patients alive after surgery; the laggards post death rates as high as 25 percent. Historically, corporate benefits managers have not asked HMOs to justify their choice of pediatric heart-surgery centers, leaving the decision up to HMO executives' consciences . . . and their wallets. "If something bad is going to happen in managed care," Dr. Lock contends, "you're probably going to find it here first."

Indeed, a 1995 study of pediatric heart-surgery outcomes found disturbing variations in death rates, depending on patients' sources of insurance. Kathy Jenkins, a Boston cardiologist, studied 7,000 heart surgeries performed in 1992. She found that after adjusting for the riskiness of the surgery, patients with regular commercial insurance were less likely to die than those with HMO coverage. The difference was especially pronounced in the largest HMO market, California. In many states, results for HMO patients were no better than for children covered by the government's Medicaid program for the poor — and in Illinois, the HMO outcomes tended to be worse. The most likely explanation for the difference, she suggested, was that HMOs were less willing to send patients to preeminent, high-cost hospitals.

What Dr. Jenkins found in her statistics, pediatric cardiologist Stuart Kaufman encounters repeatedly in his own practice. Based in Morristown, New Jersey, Dr. Kaufman sees hundreds of children each year with congenital heart defects. "I tell my patients: if there's any way to get to the best hospital, do it," Dr. Kaufman says. "But it's a daily battle. The managed-care companies think that any one place is equivalent to all the others. They just go on the basis of what is cheapest."

A handful of those cases still haunt Dr. Kaufman, years after managed-care companies overruled his choice of surgeon and sent children elsewhere. In one instance Dr. Kaufman wanted to send a child with a small hole in an interior heart wall to Columbia Presbyterian in New York for corrective surgery. The child's managed-care plan balked, saying it would pay only if the child went to a cheaper hospital in New Jersey. Dr. Kaufman protested, to no avail. The New Jersey hospital handled the case, which ended up with profound complications. After being hospitalized for three months, the child emerged disfigured with skin grafts, necessary to patch up unexpected wounds. At Columbia, Dr. Kaufman believes, those complications never would have occurred and the child would have been home within five days.

The surgeon that Dr. Kaufman most frequently wants to use is Jan Quaegebeur, a brilliant, irascible Belgian in his mid-50s who heads Columbia Presbyterian's pediatric heart-surgery team. No one picks Dr. Quaegebeur for his personality; he tosses off one barbed remark after another in his office and in the operating room, including the famous complaint "I've managed to do half of this operation in the amount of time it is taking them to get my next patient ready. What is wrong with these people?" And no one picks Dr. Quaegebeur because he is cheap; his annual earnings at Columbia Presbyterian routinely top $1 million, making him one of the nation's highest-paid doctors in academic medicine. But as Dr. Kaufman says, "You pick him for what he can do with his hands."

One of the hardest operations for most pediatric surgeons is the repair of a condition known as transposition of the great arteries, a congenital defect that is fatal if not corrected within a few weeks of birth. Typical death rates for this surgery average 7 percent or higher. In the 150 such surgeries he has performed since coming to the United States in 1990, Dr. Quaegebeur has had just two deaths — a mortality rate of 1.3 percent.

Yet Dr. Kaufman, like many pediatric cardiologists in the New York area, finds that his favorite surgeon frequently is off-limits because of price if a child belongs to an HMO. That's not just bad medicine on the HMOs' part, Dr. Kaufman argues, it is bad business. He contends that well-done pediatric surgery ought to be viewed as a bargain, even if the initial cost is high, because it greatly reduces the expense of follow-up care. Yet he has made little headway with that argument in his battles with managed-care plans. As one HMO executive told him, "If you pay for a Chevrolet, don't expect a Cadillac."

The hobbling nature of managed-care rules is especially stark when one takes a look at the contrasting sagas of Bryan Jones and Trey

McPherson. Both boys were born in the New York City area in the mid-1990s with hypoplastic left heart syndrome, in which half the heart is shrunken and almost useless. Without a heart transplant, most doctors believe, such children will die in infancy. In the past decade, however, a handful of surgeons have developed a radical way to redirect blood through the functioning half of the heart and allow it to be oxygenated during an unusual detour past the lungs. This method, known as a Norwood procedure, requires a series of three operations over a span of several years. Long-term survival rates can approach 80 percent in the best circumstances. The first surgery must be done just days after birth if the rescue plan is to have any serious hope of success.

In both the Jones and the McPherson case, doctors diagnosed the problem within a few days of birth and urged the parents to get their babies to Dr. Quaegebeur for surgery as quickly as possible. At that point their stories diverged sharply.

Trey McPherson was the lucky one. Soon after his condition was diagnosed at a New Jersey hospital, the infant was helicoptered to Columbia Presbyterian and prepared for surgery. Dr. Quaegebeur in March 1995 began the process of redirecting the boy's blood flow in a four-hour operation that went perfectly. Ten months later the boy returned to Columbia Presbyterian for the second round of surgery. A week later his parents were thrilled to see their son climbing out of his crib at the hospital, full of vigor and ready to be discharged. Except for a bandage across his tiny chest, it was hard to tell that the boy had recently undergone open-heart surgery.

"I thank God every day for what the doctors have done," said the boy's father, Bruce McPherson, as he watched his son cavort around. "They've given us back something very precious that almost slipped away from us." One more round of surgery lay ahead for the boy in another year or two. But doctors said the child's long-term prognosis was very encouraging.

Bryan Jones wasn't so fortunate. In April 1994 the boy was readmitted to Winthrop-University Hospital in Mineola, New York, just two days after birth. His breathing was labored, his skin was bluish gray, two obvious signs of severe heart problems. As the extent of his plight became clear, a cardiologist recommended that the family pursue a Norwood procedure at Columbia Presbyterian. But the Joneses didn't have free rein in choosing where their son could go for treatment. The baby's medical coverage was provided in part by U.S. Healthcare, through his mother's job as a kindergarten teacher. The HMO didn't have a contract with Columbia Presbyterian. And so, as Susan Jones later told the *New York Post,* the HMO refused to approve the New York City hospital. Instead, U.S. Healthcare suggested that she take the boy to Philadelphia Children's Hospital, which was much farther from home than she wanted, or to Long Island Jewish Hospital, which was nearby but lacked extensive experience with such advanced surgery. In a hurried scramble, the family pressed U.S. Healthcare to relent; the family also took steps to rely more on the boy's other insurance carrier, Blue Cross–Blue Shield, available through the father's job at a family-owned construction company. Those maneuvers allowed the Joneses to get to the hospital they wanted.

The delay amounted to only a day or two, but the boy's parents believe it made a difference. During the wait, his condition deteriorated further. Dr. Quaegebeur carried out the first stage of the Norwood surgery when the boy was 10 days old, to little avail. Bryan remained in the hospital for another 31 days before being discharged. Throughout that time he was heavily medicated and barely able to eat. Late that summer, at age four and a half months, he died.

Ironically, the boy who made it to Dr. Quaegebeur in time, Trey McPherson, lacked employer-funded health insurance of any kind, either managed care or fee-for-service. Bruce McPherson worked as a handyman at an apartment complex, a job that provided no medical coverage at all. From the time he was born, Trey McPherson qualified for Medicaid, the free government health program for poor people. Traditionally, Medicaid has been viewed as second-class health insurance: better than nothing but spartan. Nonetheless, New Jersey's Medicaid program allowed gravely ill children such as Trey McPherson to see whatever doctor and hospital would take them. That privilege was denied to the Joneses because of their HMO coverage.

Cases like those two leave Dr. Quaegebeur very uneasy about the workings of American managed care. He practiced in Holland, Italy, France, and Germany for much of his career before coming to the United States in 1990. He says he left Europe because of frustrations with the ways that national health insurance plans limited patients' access to top specialists in the name of saving money. In the United States he expected freedom to build a large practice and attract all the patients that he could help. Instead, he finds that many health plans block him and his hospital from treating desperately sick children, in favor of community hospitals that are cheaper but don't have nearly as good surgical-survival rates.

"I'm not denying that financial aspects are very important," Dr. Quaegebeur says. "But there's something even more essential that you should keep in mind. If you don't do some of these operations in the first few weeks of life, kids will die. There's no time to shop for the best price on surgery. And some of the HMOs are playing off hospitals against each other as if they were buying a car."

7

The Breast Cancer Battles

For MOST OF HER CAREER at Health Net, Janice Bosworth liked and admired the California HMO. She was one of the company's most successful sales managers, calling on corporations with more than 1,000 employees and trying to convince them to offer the health plan to their workers. The trunk of her car invariably was filled with Health Net brochures. She drank coffee at home from a Health Net mug. Her own medical coverage was with Health Net; she talked up the virtues of managed care not just on her job, but at parties, picnics, and family reunions.

Then, in a single afternoon, her faith in the HMO was shattered.

In August 1991 Bosworth paid a surprise visit to the office of one of Health Net's administrators to discuss her own medical crisis. She was 31 years old at the time and fighting breast cancer. The latest report from her oncologist, Gary Davidson, was grim. The disease had spread to her liver, he told her. Standard chemotherapy was unlikely to keep her alive much longer. Her best chance of survival, Dr. Davidson said, might be a risky new technique: high-dose chemotherapy followed by a bone marrow transplant. Bosworth didn't yet know the cost of this procedure — which at the time could be $150,000 or more — or even whether she wanted it. But she had arranged for a preliminary consultation at Duke University, a renowned cancer center. Before she traveled to Duke, she wanted to know how much of the transplant cost her HMO would cover.

The man with the answers was R. Clifford Ossorio. A chatty, self-assured medical director at Health Net, Dr. Ossorio reviewed many of the HMO's cancer cases. In trial testimony two years later, Bosworth recalled her meeting with Dr. Ossorio as follows. When she arrived at his cubicle, she found him talking on the phone, his back to her. He sounded annoyed. As she waited for him to finish the conversation, the source of his peevishness gradually became clear: a cancer patient was causing trouble. Then, with a start, Bosworth realized whose case he was analyzing: her own.

"How did she find out about Duke?" she heard him ask. "I'm going to have to call them. Maybe Gary told her. I'm going to have to call him, too."

Bosworth was stunned. Something about the tone of his voice was deeply unnerving, she later said. The fact that her own doctor had told her about a potentially lifesaving therapy wasn't seen as good news; it was being viewed with disapproval. Even more ominous was the implication that the HMO executive was about to intervene in her case. After Dr. Ossorio's next few calls, would Dr. Davidson still encourage her to think about a bone marrow transplant? Would Duke even want to see her?

A few minutes later, as Bosworth recalled in her testimony, she and Dr. Ossorio met face to face. His apology for the overheard critique of her case was brief. "I'm really sorry you had to hear that," he told her. "It's hard with these open cubicles. No doors." Then he began to share his views of bone marrow transplants for breast cancer. He was deeply skeptical. He told Bosworth that many women who have the transplant die from the procedure itself, citing mortality statistics that she later regarded as overstated. He said that Health Net officials were very concerned about her welfare and wanted her to "be around for Christmas" with her son and husband. He didn't spell out the cost of the transplant or forbid her to get a simple consultation at Duke. He simply held to his central theme: a bone marrow transplant wasn't appropriate in her situation.

Years later executives at Health Net couldn't understand what was so alarming about their policy, whether applied to Bosworth or a series of other breast cancer patients. The California HMO was simply doing its job. After all, managed care works only if administrators say no to some forms of care that patients or doctors request. Some health-plan executives have even claimed that bone marrow transplants — with their sky-high cost and erratic results for breast cancer patients — represent a particularly valid occasion to say no.

To many people outside the managed-care industry, however,

Health Net's conduct was alarming. In clear life-and-death situations the HMO was prepared to override patients' wishes, their doctors' judgments, or even the apparently pro-coverage language in its own contracts. Instead, the company applied its usual cost-control doctrines with even greater zeal. Members such as Janice Bosworth came away angry and bitter, convinced that the HMO was trying to wiggle out of expensive contract obligations and simply didn't want to spend enough to let them live. Doctors felt bullied by a health plan that not only turned down their proposed cancer treatments, but also tried to change the fundamental way that they dealt with patients. In perhaps the most jarring reaction of all, some breast cancer patients with Health Net coverage began showing up at major teaching hospitals saying they had *no* insurance and would pay cash themselves. The reason for that ruse was fear that doctors might withhold their best advice if the HMO's shadow touched the case file.

Because of a series of court cases, the public record now includes more than 5,000 pages of previously confidential material about Health Net's treatment of breast cancer patients in the early 1990s. Those papers provide a remarkable six-year portrait of how a major HMO wielded power, interpreting coverage rules to its advantage and making its decisions stick. Those cases aren't necessarily typical of how HMOs treat patients in a crisis; by their very nature, as evidence in a court case, they represent some of managed care's most extreme conduct. Nonetheless, the breast cancer cases show how an HMO can deny care, save money, and attempt to impose its version of medical truth on patients and doctors.

All those issues were simmering in Janice Bosworth's case in late 1991, when Health Net abruptly backed down and paid for a bone marrow transplant. Bosworth's long-time boss, Rita Duarte, one of the top five officers of the company, confronted Dr. Ossorio, the main opponent of the transplant, and reminded him he was dealing with a valued employee. Health Net should support whatever Bosworth's physicians wanted to do, she added. Dr. Ossorio continued to tell people that he regarded a bone marrow transplant in Bosworth's case as futile. But Health Net in early 1992 paid for the therapy at Bosworth's chosen facility: City of Hope National Medical Center, just outside Los Angeles. Nearly two years later she was disease-free and telling people, "If I had not had a bone marrow transplant, I would not be alive today."

Other Health Net subscribers weren't so lucky. From 1991 to 1993 the HMO rejected at least a dozen other requests similar to Bosworth's. Each time the HMO asserted that the costly procedure had not been proven effective and thus did not have to be covered. Patients and doctors fumed to no avail. Health Net ignored threatened suits, actual suits, and a protest rally outside its headquarters. It also disregarded a raft of pleas from practicing oncologists, who defended the procedure, saying their patients needed it to stay alive.

Appeals to executives' compassion fared worst of all. The mother of one breast cancer patient wrote the chairman of Health Net, imploring him to approve a transplant for her 33-year-old daughter. "Dear Mr. Greaves," the letter from Joyce Nesmith began. "I do not know if you have children, but you have no idea how agonizing it can be for the patient as well as the mother when you are offered realistic hope to beat this dreadful disease, and yet it is impossible to pay." Health Net chairman Roger Greaves never answered. A subordinate wrote Nesmith a terse letter 19 days later to say that coverage would be denied.

Until late 1993 Health Net's hard-line strategy appeared unstoppable. But in December of that year a California jury awarded $89.1 million in damages to the family of Nelene Fox, a Health Net member who had tried unsuccessfully to get the HMO to cover her bone marrow transplant. Health Net ultimately paid a much smaller out-of-court settlement, in return for forgoing its right to try to overturn the verdict on appeal. Even so, the giant jury award was seen as a warning signal to other health plans.

One of the key witnesses at the Fox trial was Janice Bosworth, testifying against the HMO where she once worked. Asked why she was appearing on the witness stand, Bosworth explained, "They hadn't learned anything by going through it with me."

Breast cancer cases generally are divided into four stages. In the most easily treatable form, Stage I, the cancer is localized in breast tissue. Champions of preventive medicine — including most managed-care executives — argue that the single best strategy in fighting breast cancer is to catch it early and treat it quickly. As a result, HMOs' main initiative in breast cancer is to encourage women to do regular self-exams and visit their doctors for periodic mammograms. When Stage I cancers are found this way, a lumpectomy or a series of radiation treatments often can eradicate all traces of cancer at modest cost to both health plan and patient. Patients' 10-year survival rates can be 90 percent or higher.

For thousands of women each year, however, routine self-exams and mammograms aren't enough. Some breast cancers elude early detection and some, even if caught, continue to spread despite medical or surgical treatment. In the most severe cases, known as Stage IV, breast cancer metastasizes to other parts of the body, such as the liver, bones, or bone marrow. In those cases standard treatments are almost powerless. Chemotherapy can slow the disease slightly, but patients typically survive for less than a year and a half once Stage IV cancer is diagnosed. The chances of becoming disease-free under conventional treatment are just 8 percent.

In the early 1980s medical researchers at Duke University, the Dana-Farber Cancer Center in Boston, and other centers began an audacious new assault on Stage IV breast cancer. They stepped up the dosage of chemotherapy as much as tenfold in an attempt to annihilate cancer cells. Ordinarily such high doses would be fatal because the drugs would wipe out the patient's bone marrow, crippling the immune system and the production of blood cells. But the Duke and Dana-Farber doctors quickly followed the massive chemotherapy with a reinfusion of bone marrow, generally using marrow harvested from the patient shortly before treatment. Those transplants rescued patients from the worst consequences of intense chemotherapy, allowing them to tolerate a much greater chemical attack on their cancer. Doctors in the mid-1970s had established that this regimen of high-dose chemotherapy followed by a bone marrow transplant could fight other cancers, notably leukemias. That spurred interest in extending this technique to one of the most common malignancies of all: breast cancer.

Progress was fitful. Early transplant attempts for breast cancer patients had 30-day mortality rates as high as 20 percent. The procedure involved a monthlong hospital stay and bills of $200,000 or more. For many patients, even the massive chemotherapy didn't significantly improve their long-term survival. But researchers saw enough promise that they kept refining their techniques. A major breakthrough came around 1990, when doctors found that they could revive blood-cell production faster, more safely, and more cheaply if they transplanted stem cells — the fast-growing, undifferentiated "baby" cells that soon turn into red or white blood cells — rather than whole bone marrow.* In the early 1990s, many researchers reported that immediate mortality rates for their transplants had fallen to 5 percent. Hospital stays in some cases shortened to as little as a week. Costs per patient kept dropping, to as low as $60,000 in 1995. The new regimen fell far short of being a reliable cure; one study found that only 43 percent of patients survived for two years or longer. Still, the treatment did leave many patients disease-free for at least a few months afterward, and improved their quality of life. In the brightest successes, a few of the earliest transplant recipients remained alive more than 10 years after getting bone marrow transplants. Encouraged by such gains, transplant specialists have come to regard their procedure, known informally as BMT, as the best hope for some patients.

For HMOs and traditional insurers, this new therapy was problematic at best, and in some circles downright unwelcome. It was extremely expensive, and it often didn't work. Many health plans in the late 1980s and early 1990s tried to deny BMT coverage for Stage IV breast cancer patients, arguing that the new therapy was unproven and not necessarily effective. Health plans believed they had legal grounds for doing so; most insurance contracts explicitly said that "experimental" and "investigational" treatments wouldn't be covered. But those terms seldom were clearly defined. When coverage disputes went to court, as they often did, the internal workings of a health plan looked cold and ugly, especially when juxtaposed against the drama of a young mother fighting for a potentially lifesaving treatment. As a result, many health plans capitulated if breast cancer patients threatened to sue over denial of coverage. Rather than go before a jury, the plans agreed to pay.

At Health Net questions about breast cancer coverage in the late 1980s went straight to the desk of Leonard Knapp, the firm's chief medical director. Dr. Knapp was not a cancer expert; he had been a general practitioner for 27 years before moving into medical administration. But he thrived at Health Net, in part because of his ability to round up expert advice in a hurry. The first few BMT advisers on Dr. Knapp's list said they regarded the treatment as experimental or inves-

---

*By the early 1990s most "bone marrow transplants" for breast cancer patients actually involved stem-cell infusions instead. But in everyday usage, doctors, patients, and insurers still referred to the procedures as bone marrow transplants.

tigational and thus exempt from coverage. That was the message he got from the national Blue Cross–Blue Shield association in 1988; it also was the recommendation of an informal circle of seven California oncologists that he consulted soon afterward.

In late 1990 Dr. Knapp decided he needed more advice. The BMT issue wasn't playing out as health plans had wanted; some East Coast insurers were being ordered, in court, to pay for members' transplants. So Dr. Knapp hired a San Francisco consulting firm, Technology Assessment Group, to provide a systematic overview of BMT. The consultants reviewed 15 years of medical literature from the United States and Europe; they surveyed dozens of California hospitals, oncologists, and insurers, asking each group what was regarded as standard care. The consultants' conclusion: BMT wasn't yet viewed as a standard protocol, but it could well become one within a year, particularly if ongoing clinical trials continued to show improving survival rates.

That forecast was good news for patients — but it wasn't what Dr. Knapp wanted. He dismissed the consultants' optimism about BMT as an "egregious" mistake and told other people that his hired experts had "exceeded their charter." He refused to contract with Technology Assessment Group for any updates or additional work on BMT. And in a telephone call to one of the consultants, Jannalee Smithey, Dr. Knapp lashed out at the advisory firm he had signed up just a few months earlier. He accused the consultants of severely compromising their credibility and again asserted that their findings "did not warrant a prediction such as this." As Dr. Knapp later put it, "I raised a little hell."

A few months later Dr. Knapp found the expert he wanted: Cliff Ossorio.

Dr. Ossorio had all the right traits to help Health Net hold the line on breast cancer care. He was a star doctor in his own right, a part-time UCLA faculty member in oncology who had helped set up a BMT unit for leukemia patients at Cedars-Sinai Medical Center in Los Angeles. He could examine a cancer patient's medical records and rigorously challenge a community doctor's treatment plans, an impossibility for a typical HMO medical director who lacked special training in cancer care. And unlike many of his peers, Dr. Ossorio scorned the use of BMT for advanced breast cancer. He saw no evidence of improved survival rates. In his view it was associated with longer hospital stays, 11 to 12 percent immediate mortality rates, and possible damage to other organs. BMT was useful in fighting leukemia, Dr. Ossorio later explained, but he never used it for his own breast cancer patients. Asked in 1993 for his views on whether BMT should be tried for Stage IV breast cancer, he declared, "It would never be appropriate."

After some casual chats, Dr. Knapp decided that he wanted Dr. Ossorio not just as an adviser, but as a fellow medical director within Health Net. The HMO couldn't quite match Dr. Ossorio's earnings in private practice, but it offered a base salary of well above $100,000 a year, a bonus if he did good work, the prospect of a quick promotion, and more money if the company sold stock to the public. Attractive as those rewards were, Dr. Ossorio seemed most excited about getting a chance to change the way medicine was practiced throughout southern California. When he began work at Health Net in July 1991, his colleagues saw a great future for him. Asked some years later what he liked about Dr. Ossorio, Dr. Knapp explained, "He is a very persuasive individual and has a good grasp of managed care. He is able to modify physicians' behavior in directions we would like."

Health Net dealt Dr. Ossorio a tough hand, though. The HMO didn't tell its members that BMT was not a covered treatment for breast cancer. In fact, it left many of them with exactly the opposite impression. Each new member got a pamphlet entitled *Evidence of Coverage,* which spelled out covered benefits. On page 40 of the pamphlet, Health Net listed some ultrasophisticated procedures that it covered, including heart transplants, liver transplants . . . and bone marrow transplants. Only in a different clause, 19 pages away, did Health Net say that its coverage excluded experimental or investigative procedures. That contract ambiguity helped Health Net's package look attractive to employers and workers; the HMO at the time had blanketed southern California with billboards declaring, "When you've got your Health Net, you've got everything." But the murky contract, which appeared to promise BMT coverage for all relevant diseases, put tremendous pressure on its in-house medical experts. The only way that Health Net could deny coverage for breast cancer patients — and expect to withstand challenges from angry patients and their doctors — would be if the HMO could unleash a highly convincing argument that BMT was medically ineffective in fighting Stage IV breast cancer.

The decisive case reached Dr. Ossorio's desk in early June 1992. It involved Nelene Fox, a 39-year-old mother of three, who received Health Net coverage through her husband's teaching job. She had been diagnosed with breast cancer a year earlier. By the time Dr. Ossorio became involved in her case, her disease was quite advanced. So were her medical preferences for fighting it.

For 12 horrifying months Fox's doctors had been powerless to stop the spread of her disease. They started with mastectomies and moderate chemotherapy in the summer of 1991, only to discover a few months later that her cancer had metastasized to her bone marrow. In early 1992 she began a regimen of Adriamycin, a grisly chemotherapy agent that Fox took each Monday, only to spend the next few days in her room, vomiting. She couldn't eat with her children until Thursdays; she couldn't go outside until Saturdays — at which point it was almost time to start the cycle again. In spite of all that anguish, doctors didn't expect Adriamycin to help much. One of her oncologists, Elber Camacho, told her in December 1991 that her disease was terminal. With the best available conventional chemotherapy, he told her husband, she might have one more year to live.

Nelene Fox wanted a better shot at life. Even as Dr. Camacho relayed the bad news to her and her husband that December, he suggested she consider a bone marrow transplant. A few months later another oncologist, Stanley Schinke, urged them on, telling Nelene's husband, Jim, at one point, "If it was my wife, I would try to get her to transplantation as soon as possible." Dr. Schinke helped her line up appointments at the University of Southern California's Norris Cancer Institute for evaluation as a candidate for BMT. In May 1992 one of USC's transplant specialists, Aziz Khan, pronounced her a "good candidate." For Nelene Fox that was a joyous, even giddy moment. It was the first piece of good news about her health she had received in nearly a year.

Ordinarily the HMO's gatekeeper system would have tightly limited Fox's ability to see specialists and thus to explore costly treatment choices without the HMO's permission. But in her situation the gatekeepers had lost control of the case. Rather than wait for each HMO referral form to be filled out before proceeding, Nelene and her husband used the initial referral to a cancer specialist as a jumping-off point to start a regular dialogue with these oncologists and to seek the best care possible. The couple figured that managed-care rules could catch up later. In May 1991 Nelene Fox's primary-care gatekeepers at Rancho Canyon Medical Group told her they believed Health Net would refuse to pay for BMT on the grounds that it was an unproven, experimental treatment. But Nelene Fox's oncologists, the doctors she trusted most, disagreed with the gatekeepers' assessments and appeared ready to battle Health Net for coverage. In late May and early June 1992, Drs. Camacho, Schinke, and Khan submitted letters to her managed-care plan, saying that they believed BMT was appropriate and essential for her.

A showdown was imminent. An old-line insurer might have yielded to the combined tuggings of patient and doctors. As a managed-care company, however, Health Net could counterattack. To strengthen its claim that the benefits of BMT were unproven, Health Net could challenge the oncologists' letters. The HMO could put forth its own assessment of Nelene Fox's condition, prospects, and options. It could even try to reorient her doctors to the HMO's way of thinking — in essence prying them away from their classic role as patient advocates. That is exactly what Health Net decided to do, even though its decision-making officials had never met Fox, let alone given her a medical examination. The HMO did have access to her medical records, and its administrators had their own views about the value of BMT. For Health Net that was enough knowledge to justify intervening in her treatment.

In mid-June Health Net's Dr. Ossorio jumped into action. He telephoned Dr. Camacho, the physician officially requesting a BMT for Nelene Fox, and questioned the community doctor's assessment of the case. Both men later reconstructed that crucial phone conversation while giving court testimony under oath. Their recollections differed slightly. But they agreed on the following particulars.

In that phone call Dr. Ossorio quickly established the agenda. He said he regarded Nelene Fox as a particularly bad candidate for BMT. He shared his own analysis of Fox's tests, including an assessment that cancer had spread farther into her bones than Dr. Camacho might have realized. And he urged Dr. Camacho once again to explain the risks of BMT to her. Dr. Camacho later recalled disagreeing somewhat with Dr. Ossorio's bleak assessment of Fox's condition. Still, at the end of the conversation, Dr. Camacho agreed to re-explain the risks of BMT to his patient.

In the next few days, people who spoke with Dr. Camacho encountered a changed man. Dr. Khan, the BMT specialist who was prepared to treat Fox, was one of the first to get a call from Dr. Camacho. "He was quite agitated and a little nervous," Dr. Khan recalled. "All enthusiasm was gone from him." Dr. Camacho relayed his conversation with Dr. Ossorio, including the assessment that Fox was an extremely poor candidate for BMT. Dr. Khan was left with the feeling that Dr. Camacho no longer favored BMT. Dr. Khan held his ground, saying that he didn't see any obstacle to continuing with the proposed treatment.

Shortly after Dr. Ossorio's phone call to him, Dr. Camacho met with Jim Fox, who also noticed a jarring transformation in the oncologist's outlook. As Jim Fox later recalled, Dr. Camacho said he now had some concerns about the transplant, adding that he doubted it was wise for Nelene to proceed directly to USC. Instead, Dr. Camacho said, he and Health Net would like to offer a different treatment plan. They proposed to have her reevaluated at a different nearby BMT center, City of Hope. If doctors there felt she was a good candidate, the transplant could then take place at a third center, UCLA.

Health Net may have regarded its counteroffer as a genuine attempt to meet the Foxes' wishes partway. But Nelene and Jim Fox saw the new proposal as bizarre, unhelpful — and perhaps even a sinister attempt to bog them down in delays and denials until Nelene's cancer worsened to the point that all therapy would be futile. As her medical records showed, her oncologists had already made phone inquiries in the spring about having her treated at City of Hope. But her doctors had quickly established that it was the wrong center for her; City of Hope's BMT specialists didn't handle patients whose breast cancer had spread to their bone marrow. For that reason oncologists had pointed the Foxes to USC/Norris, which did accept patients with Nelene's form of metastatic breast cancer. In Jim Fox's mind, the only reason to direct his wife to a second evaluation at City of Hope would be if someone wanted the referral to end in a rejection.

"Why would they send us back to someplace where we had already been denied?" Jim Fox pointedly asked Dr. Camacho during their meeting. Eighteen months later, under oath, Dr. Camacho said he remembered the question but not his reply. As Jim Fox remembered it, Dr. Camacho sat silently before him, with his palms up and his mouth open — before eventually saying, "I don't know."

Those exchanges destroyed the Foxes' trust in both Health Net and one of the physicians they had depended on, Dr. Camacho. On June 19 the Foxes sued Health Net, asking it to pay for BMT at USC/Norris. They staged a protest march outside Health Net's Woodland Hills, California, headquarters. And they pressed ahead with private fundraising to pay for treatment at USC/Norris, convinced that time was too precious to pursue the City of Hope offer. More than 1,000 friends and acquaintances contributed money to help pay for Nelene's treatment. The pastor at their local Lutheran church helped raise money. The Sizzler steakhouse and the yogurt shop in their hometown of Temecula pitched in as well, earmarking 20 percent of their proceeds each Monday night toward her treatment.

In late June 1992, Nelene Fox started preliminary treatment at USC, with the bone marrow transplant itself beginning August 17. The results were promising at first, and doctors pronounced her disease-free after the therapy. In February 1993, however, cancer was found again in her bone marrow. After that recurrence, doctors could do little to help her; she died in April 1993, just after her 40th birthday.

As Nelene Fox's personal tragedy played out, Health Net executives decided they needed a more systematic way to handle BMT cases. The HMO had achieved its main objective in the Fox case by denying payment, but it had done so in a messy, confrontational way. For several crucial weeks in the spring of 1992, control of the case had slipped out of the HMO's hands, leaving patient and doctors free to put together what Health Net regarded as a reckless treatment plan. That wasn't the way managed care was supposed to work. Health Net at that time was setting aside at least $8 million a year for various kinds of transplants; the HMO didn't mind paying for some very costly care, as long as it felt that the treatments were appropriate. If Health Net could find a way to control its breast cancer cases from the start, executives believed, they could avoid nasty clashes with doctors or patients, while ensuring that the "right" patients got the bone marrow transplants and the "wrong" ones did not.

Health Net's new initiatives sounded good — and, in fact, they were similar to the steps that helped many other health plans gradually resolve the breast cancer controversy. But the HMO's version of reform did not prevent additional disputes over the BMT issue.

Health Net began by turning to top BMT experts in its region for help. Doctors from UCLA, Scripps, and other research centers were appointed to a "transplant committee" that drafted formal guidelines on how Health Net would handle various types of transplant requests. These advisers produced a 19-page grid in January 1993, specifying the health plan's BMT policy for about a dozen forms of cancer in various stages of severity. In 38 of these situations, including all cases involving Hodgkin's disease and most leukemias, Health Net would routinely cover BMT treatment. Some other diseases would be evaluated case by case. And in 12 situations, Health Net would deny payment. The HMO then distributed this grid to all the primary-care doctors in its network, hoping to make them aware, right from the start, of how the HMO wanted cancer cases handled.

Health Net also tried to clarify its contract language so that members would have a more realistic sense of what the plan would cover. Instead of flatly listing bone marrow transplants as a covered benefit, Health Net in early 1993 asked California regulators for permission to describe BMT as covered "subject to exclusions for experimental or investigative procedures, as defined herein." Health Net also drafted a fuller definition of "experimental" and "investigative," terms that many doctors found maddeningly vague.

Both those steps had great potential to ease the breast cancer wars. By mid-1992 health plans had more research to digest — including a widely cited 1992 study by health-policy researcher David Eddy, suggesting that BMT generally didn't help breast cancer patients but might have "promising" potential to extend long-term survival in a few instances. By calling in the experts, health plans could reach more sophisticated judgments on each case, which greatly improved the HMO's relations with doctors and patients. The expert panels sometimes proved more lenient than HMO medical directors in approving transplants, but when the outside advisers said that BMT would be a mistake, patients and community doctors generally accepted their judgment.

As helpful as these changes sounded, Health Net's version of reform proved to be flawed. The HMO circumscribed its panel of experts so tightly that the treatment guidelines didn't really match California practice standards. Many top teaching hospitals by the early 1990s regularly treated some breast cancer patients with BMTs, both in formal research studies and in ordinary efforts to provide the best care. But when Health Net set up its definitions for treatment, it required such clear proof of efficacy or widespread acceptance that BMT for Stage IV cancer was tagged as an automatic denial, even though several doctors on its panel regularly provided patients with transplants. The HMO was creating conditions that could lead to two-tier medicine. Physicians could provide their other patients with BMTs, but for women covered by Health Net, the pioneering new treatment was to be off-limits.

Health Net's new system was a recipe for conflict — forcing doctors to choose between their classic obligations to their patients and a loyalty to the HMO that paid their bills. Before long a desperately sick young woman and her doctor found themselves caught in the middle.

The patient was Christine deMeurers, a southern California schoolteacher with Health Net coverage who was diagnosed with Stage IV breast cancer in 1993. Her local oncologists recommended that she consider a bone marrow transplant, and in early June of that year she was evaluated at the University of Colorado. But Health Net said it wouldn't pay for BMT at the out-of-state hospital, explaining in a letter that the treatment "is not uniformly accepted as proven and effective for the treatment of metastatic breast cancer." Within a matter of days deMeurers tried afresh, getting a consultation at the UCLA transplant center. This time she kept mum about her Health Net policy, saying instead that she wasn't sure about her insurance coverage and might try to raise money privately to pay for a transplant.

Her doctor was John Glaspy, a rising star at UCLA. He saw himself as a cautious proponent of BMT for breast cancer, hopeful that it would be an improvement over standard therapy but realistic about the new treatment's shortcomings. During deMeurers's initial visit, Dr. Glaspy spelled out BMT's risks, including a 5 percent mortality rate from the treatment itself and three months of low-quality life after the high-dose chemotherapy and transplant. But he opened the door for treatment, and Christine and her husband, Alan, thought they heard outright encouragement. "I remember him saying, 'This is the best course of treatment,'" Alan later recalled. The deMeurerses agreed to try to proceed as self-pay patients, hoping to raise the $92,000 needed to go ahead with the treatment.

A few weeks later it became clear that they couldn't raise the money fast enough on their own. They mentioned their Health Net coverage to Dr. Glaspy, putting him in a deep predicament. He told her he had an "obligation" to help her get a BMT if that was what she wanted. Even so, he told her, he was on Health Net's transplant panel, and the HMO's standards "do not call for coverage for people with metastatic breast cancer."

Struggling to find the right path, Dr. Glaspy called a Health Net administrator, explained his dilemma, and said: "There will be paper-work coming from me on the advocacy end." On September 13, he wrote Health Net, saying: "As a physician representing Christine, I have a responsibility to represent her interests and to help her achieve her goals in her health care."

Health Net had other ideas. It had spent months working with top doctors to set up transplant guidelines — and it wasn't about to see them disregarded. On the afternoon of Friday, September 17, Health Net's Dr. Ossorio called Dr. Glaspy's boss, Dennis Slamon, to discuss the case. Dr. Ossorio later said he didn't remember many details of that conversation, but Dr. Slamon provided a detailed account. He said the Health Net executive took him through a rapid-fire series of questions, about as follows: Are you aware of the Health Net panel's recommen-dations on transplants? Yes. Do you agree with them? Yes. Are you aware of the deMeurers case? No. Could you look into it and find out if it is in or out of the guidelines?

Within hours Dr. Glaspy began to feel new forces tugging on him. Dr. Slamon called him at home to discuss the case. As Dr. Glaspy later recalled, "He told me that Dr. Ossorio was upset and that he felt I had not stood strongly enough behind the guidelines that I helped him develop." A Health Net attorney called Dr. Glaspy, asking if he would file a legal declaration saying that he was on the Health Net transplant panel and citing the panel's guidelines. Dr. Glaspy agreed to do so.

On September 20, 1993, Dr. Glaspy filed a quite different, less enthusiastic statement regarding Christine deMeurers's case. He de-clared, "This procedure is of unproven efficacy in the treatment of metastatic breast cancer, and the results of clinical trials to date are not sufficient to establish beyond doubt that it is superior to standard dose chemotherapy." Dr. Glaspy later said that although he didn't view the second letter as being outright opposed to his patient's interests, he did assume it would be used to support Health Net's position. Most of all, Dr. Glaspy felt angry and frustrated by his predicament. No matter what he did, either Health Net or his patient would feel betrayed.

At UCLA, Dr. Slamon anguished over the medical mess that was unfolding. During the weekend after Dr. Glaspy filed his second let-ter, Dr. Slamon came up with what he believed was a just solution. Christine deMeurers could get a bone marrow transplant at UCLA, he decided, and she wouldn't have to pay. Neither would Health Net. Instead, UCLA would absorb the entire cost. It would be a stinging charge of more than $100,000 against one of his department's reserve funds. But it seemed to be the best way that the research center could uphold its competing obligations to the patient and the HMO, he later explained.

Christine and her husband quickly accepted, but they didn't quite feel that UCLA's generosity made everything right. The university's flipflops had made them question just how committed UCLA's doctors were to their case. Still, they had no other realistic medical options; starting afresh at another center would consume as much as two months, putting Christine deMeurers' health in further jeopardy. A few weeks later she began treatment at UCLA.

The entire controversy appeared to have only one winner: Health Net. It had tightened its rules on paying for bone marrow transplants in the year since the Fox case. And once again the HMO had prevailed, even when both a patient and her doctor at a renowned medical center initially wanted a costly procedure that wasn't on Health Net's approved list.

But the war of wills wasn't over by a long shot. Health Net was about to face massive legal challenges to its handling of the breast cancer cases. Leading the attack was Mark Hiepler, an Oxnard, California, attorney who was Nelene Fox's younger brother. He was a relatively recent law school graduate at the time, working as a junior associate in a midsize Los Angeles firm. What he lacked in experience, though, he made up for in intensity. Convinced that Health Net had wronged a series of women, including his sister, Hiepler spent more than a year developing a suit against the HMO. In December 1993, state court jurors in Riverside County, California, began to hear the case.

The suit, formally known as *Jim Fox and the estate of Nelene Fox v. Health Net,* accused the HMO of breach of contract, bad faith, and intentional infliction of emotional distress. Hiepler and his fellow attorneys argued that the HMO's contract did cover BMT for breast cancer and that it had been wrongly interpreted by the health plan. The attorneys also contended that Health Net had hurt Nelene Fox by coercing or improperly manipulating one of her physicians, Dr. Camacho.

In two weeks of testimony Hiepler brought out all the evidence about the HMO that he felt was most damning: its decision to pay for Janice Bosworth's BMT, the phone calls that Dr. Ossorio made to Nelene Fox's treating physicians, Health Net's formal denial letters, and the pathos of his sister trying to raise more than $200,000 from acquaintances while battling a terminal disease. In summing-up remarks to the jury, Hiepler portrayed Health Net as the villain. He asked for unspecified punitive damages so that "Health Net gets the message that this behavior cannot be tolerated. The doctor-patient relationship is something to be guarded. Insurance people who don't practice medicine should not be involving themselves." He added, "There are corporate boardrooms throughout the United States waiting to see what you decide."

Health Net's attorneys tried to focus the case away from its most emotional aspects, contending that for all the human tragedy of the case, the HMO hadn't done anything wrong. Health Net acknowledged that Dr. Camacho had changed his mind about the merits of BMT after talking to Health Net officials. But the HMO portrayed the oncologist's evolving skepticism as the right choice. On the witness stand, Dr. Camacho testified that he probably was too optimistic early on, when he encouraged Nelene Fox to think about a bone marrow transplant. "You might say I was lying to the Foxes," Dr. Camacho said.

In his concluding remarks, Health Net attorney Lyle Swallow said that the HMO's employees and executives simply did their jobs. "What you saw were intelligent, articulate, caring, honest people with nothing to hide," Swallow declared. "They made the best decisions they could under the circumstances. They didn't act in any malicious way or with any intention to harm Mr. or Mrs. Fox. . . . We contend it's investigative treatment, and that Health Net made the proper and reasonable decision in this case."

When the case went to the jury, Health Net's legal team thought it had a good chance of prevailing. To their astonishment, however, the jury hammered the HMO as hard as it could. It awarded Jim Fox and his wife's estate $12 million in actual damages and another $77 million in punitive damages. When television stations and newspapers rushed to interview jurors after the case, the media found a cauldron of populist, anti-managed-care sentiment. "You cannot substitute profits for good-quality health care," one juror told waiting cameramen. "The verdict was fair," another juror remarked. "It sends a message to all health carriers around the country."

Even though Health Net quickly negotiated a drastic reduction in the award — agreeing to pay about $5 million to settle the case — the

Fox case nonetheless was the landmark that the attorneys had predicted. Other HMOs began approving far more BMT requests, unwilling to risk an expensive, humiliating defeat in court. As the medical director of one East Coast HMO said, "This is a hot issue, and it just got hotter." Within a year of the Fox case, cancer specialists in various states reported that they could now get 80 percent of their BMT cases approved by insurers on the first try and could engage in a reasonable dialogue with health plans even when coverage initially was turned down.

In September 1994 the Federal Employees Health Benefits Program largely settled the issue by requiring all its health plans to cover BMT for advanced breast cancer. With 9.4 million employees and dependents, the federal program functioned as a trendsetter in the health-care market, setting standards for insurance coverage that smaller employers quickly followed. Some managed-care plans grumbled that they were being stampeded into paying for a treatment of dubious value. They brandished a study by a Plymouth Meeting, Pennsylvania, consulting firm, ECRI, arguing the HMOs' case that transplants often didn't help Stage IV breast cancer patients. But those objections were much feebler than before; when all the rhetoric was finished, managed-care plans generally paid for BMT for women with advanced breast cancer if patients and their doctors really wanted it.

At Health Net the legacy of the Fox case was clear to see. Transplant specialists at the HMO's main contracting hospitals continued to be guided by an advisory grid — but they no longer had power to designate whole categories of transplants as routine denials. Instead, the grid mainly identified types of cancer for which BMT would be routinely approved. All other cases were referred individually to a medical ombudsman who asked a new set of outside reviewers to look at the situation in detail. Those reviewers could then approve a transplant or tell the ombudsman that the case was hopeless. And even in the direst cases, a litigious patient might persuade Health Net to think twice. The new system was so clearly pro-patient that some doctors and HMO administrators wondered if it had overcorrected for its earlier faults. Even so, Health Net officials privately conceded, no one within the HMO wanted to fight the breast cancer battles again. In the wake of the Fox case, California's state legislature made BMT for breast cancer a mandatory benefit in all basic health plans, giving Health Net little maneuvering room.

Dr. Ossorio, meanwhile, left Health Net at the end of 1994. A year later he portrayed the departure as his decision but indicated that neither side was sorry about it. "I couldn't continue," he said. "They made me the fall guy [for the Fox case], and I never recovered from that." He set up shop as an independent consultant, doing some part-time work for PacifiCare Health Systems, another California HMO. Most of his work there involved new ways to evaluate the quality of doctors' work, a long-time interest of his. He stayed far away from breast cancer cases.

The three women who fought so hard to get Health Net approval for bone marrow transplants all eventually succumbed to breast cancer. Nelene Fox lived only eight months after her transplant, while Christine deMeurers survived for 16 months. In those two cases Health Net's doubts about the long-term efficacy of BMT may have been justified, even if doctors and family members were repulsed by the HMO's tactics to get its point across. But for Janice Bosworth, the former Health Net saleswoman, there is strong evidence that the hotly contested transplant meaningfully extended her life. She lived for more than two years after her BMT — longer than she could have expected with conventional chemotherapy. That gave her time to spend with her young son Christopher; he was four years old when she had her transplant, nearly seven years old when she died. Some people within Health Net scoffed at her chances all along; Dr. Ossorio in a July 1992 deposition said he believed she was doing "terribly." But for most of her post-transplant life, she was disease-free and able to eat normally, walk about, take her son to Disney World in Florida, and resume regular living. Even when her cancer finally recurred, it did not invade her liver, which Bosworth's oncologist, Lucille Leong, regarded as a sign that the costly therapy had stopped the ordinary progression of her disease.

Health Net, meanwhile, continued to face outside scrutiny over its conduct in the early 1990s, even though the HMO's tactics changed greatly after the Fox decision. In mid-1995 a California arbitration panel took up the deMeurers case at the request of Alan deMeurers, Christine's surviving husband. The panel looked into allegations that the HMO's contract interpretation was unduly restrictive and that the HMO had improperly lobbied UCLA about the handling of the case, thereby causing the deMeurers family emotional distress.

In October 1995 the arbitrators ruled in favor of the deMeurers claims, awarding $1 million and legal costs to Alan deMeurers and his wife's estate. The arbitrators faulted Health Net for its "ambiguous" definition of investigative procedures, which gave no clear indication of how that term would be applied. They also took issue with Health Net's call to Dr. Slamon, concluding that "the reason for the call was to influence or intimidate UCLA and Dr. Slamon, and through them Dr. Glaspy, to change Dr. Glaspy's conduct with respect to Ms. deMeurers' treatment."

Looking beyond the immediate facts of the deMeurers case, the arbitrators addressed the most fundamental question of all: how far can managed-care plans go in pressuring doctors to do their bidding?

The answer was illuminating. The arbitrators readily agreed that HMOs were permitted to have some influence over doctors' practices. But they said there is a line beyond which the plans ought not to step. The crucial distinction, they suggested, is between general, informational discussion of HMO policies — which are allowable — and something much more troubling: conversations with doctors about a particular patient after a treatment decision has been made and communicated between patient and doctor. Such patient-specific, late-in-the-game intercession "is clearly over the line," the arbitrators wrote. It can amount to an attempt "to influence or intimidate doctors into revising treatment decisions that had already been made."

For Nelene Fox, Christine deMeurers, and especially Janice Bosworth, such distinctions were much more than semantic niceties. They affected the way that life-and-death medical decisions were made. Recognizing the desperation of desperately sick patients trying to stay alive, the arbitrators wrote: "HMO actions designed and intended to interfere with an existing doctor/patient relationship constitute extreme and outrageous behavior exceeding all bounds usually tolerated in a civilized society."

8

Is This Really an Emergency?

THE SQUAT THREE-STORY office building at 300 Pearl Drive East in Boulder, Colorado, hardly seems like one of the great centers of emergency medicine in the United States. No ambulances ever screech to a halt in this suburban office park. No medical technicians rush stretcher-bound patients through the building's black metal doors. No doctors stitch up wounds, or analyze electrocardiograms, or wait anxiously for X-rays to come back from the radiology department. In fact, there are no physicians, medical supplies, or patients on the premises at all.

Yet for three million Americans with a sudden health problem, the Colorado office park is the first place they must go when they want medical attention. Cases arrive here by telephone at all hours of the day and night, directed into Boulder by managed-care plans across the United States. Callers hear a few brief clicks as their calls are bounced along by high-speed telephone switches — a system much like those used by United Airlines and L. L. Bean. And then a small squadron of nurses, sitting at computer consoles in a vast open room, begin to practice an eerie form of remote-control medicine. Each nurse briskly runs through a checklist of questions before performing the "telephone triage" of evaluating callers' complaints. The sickest patients receive instant approval to go to their local hospital's emergency room. People with less acute ailments are told to contact their doctor during normal business hours. Finally, patients who don't sound very sick at all are offered home-care remedies and told that they don't need immediate medical attention.

Even at 8:30 on a Sunday morning, the center is humming. Nurses in blue jeans and ski sweaters speak into telephone headsets and click away at computer keyboards, calling up software programs that help them sort out America's accidents, aches, and pains. Stray phrases waft across the sand-colored workspace partitions, creating a free-form concerto of medical diagnosis and advice. "Does he have any swelling? Is there any redness? OK. Here's what I want you to do. Take some warm tap water . . ." "Hello, my name is Robin and I'm a nurse. What seems to be the problem?" . . . "She sounds terrible. I'm going to give you an authorization number for the emergency department. Can you get her there safely?" . . . "Hello, my name is Kathy and I'm a nurse" . . . "On a scale of 1 to 10, if 10 is the worst pain you ever had, how much does this hurt?" . . . "Hello, this is Donna . . ."

Such large-scale phone centers are one of the boldest ways in which managed-care companies are trying to reshape emergency medicine by ensuring that fewer people in pain make a dash for the hospital. Each year Americans pay about 100 million visits to hospital emergency rooms, visits that generate about $14 billion in bills. Some of those visits involve life-and-death medical crises, but many do not. The managers of practically every major HMO, in fact, are convinced that half of all visits to the emergency room aren't really necessary. Academic studies have shown that almost any type of medical service, from a doctor's exam to a cardiac stress test, is about two and a half times as expensive in an emergency-room setting as in a primary-care doctor's office. Armed with such data, HMO executives argue that sprains, sore throats, and a host of other minor ailments ought to be dealt with out of the emergency room. Everyone would benefit, they say, if such conditions were treated more cheaply in a doctor's office or at home.

To make this point of view prevail, managed-care plans have systematically made it harder for members to reach the emergency room. Strict new definitions in members' coverage booklets warn subscribers that their HMO may not regard minor burns, vomiting, or other conditions as emergencies — and thus will refuse to cover unauthorized hospital visits for such symptoms. HMOs' sales representatives have been known to tell new members, "If you have to ask whether it's an emergency, it probably isn't."

When trouble does strike, HMO members often must check with their primary-care doctor or a nurse advice line before heading to the hospital. Those phone calls are meant to weed out noncrisis complaints and steer them toward slower, cheaper forms of medical care.

Companies such as Informed Access Systems, the operator of the Boulder telephone triage system, boast that they can redirect half of all callers away from the emergency room, saving millions of dollars annually for their HMO clients.

Even when health-plan members do get to the emergency room, many HMOs don't give up the fight. Health plans scrutinize bills after the fact, sometimes with the goal of denying coverage whenever possible. In 10 to 30 percent of all emergency-room visits, HMOs refuse to pay, leaving their members liable for the charges, on the grounds that there was no legitimate emergency in the first place. Taken all together, these tactics have helped managed-care plans cut their emergency-care bills by one third or more.

But the HMO crusade against emergency-room use has ominous implications for patient care even beyond sticking members, doctors, and hospitals with unpaid bills. This book began with the account of Lamona Adams and her feverish infant son, who suffered a medical disaster in part because their HMO didn't recognize just how sick little James Adams was. That crisis was hardly an isolated instance. In the past few years a growing number of HMO members with broken bones, severe lacerations, dangerous dehydration, and incipient heart attacks have run into managed-care obstacles in their efforts to get emergency care. In the worst of these cases, HMOs create a life-threatening climate of intimidation and delay. As Consumers Union discovered in a nationwide survey of 20,000 HMO members in 1992, emergency-care restrictions and payment denials are regarded as one of the biggest failings of managed care.

When emergency medicine began its big buildup in the late 1960s, no one was concerned about cost. The national priority at the time was to help people survive heart attacks, car accidents, and other calamities. Public pressure to upgrade emergency care came not just from doctors and hospitals but also from popular culture that glamorized medical rescues, including television shows such as *Emergency*. The heroic battlefield medicine practiced in the Vietnam war also spurred the campaign to improve emergency care. As author James Page put it, something was wrong when "a soldier wounded by enemy fire in Vietnam had a better chance of survival than the victim of a motor vehicle collision back home."

Congress responded with the Emergency Medical Services Systems

Act of 1973, which provided a framework for setting up 300 EMS systems around the country. Local telephone companies and ambulance services teamed up to create the "911" emergency phone system. People in a self-defined crisis could call a three-digit phone number at any hour of day or night and summon a rescue vehicle to their doorstep with lightning speed. Taxpayers or insurers would pay the bill. Hospitals, viewing emergency medicine as a prestigious and profitable specialty, scrambled to be designated as Level I trauma centers.

Governing this massive buildup was a belief that every distress call should be treated as a potential medical disaster until proven otherwise. The emergency room became a medical testing center, where doctors regularly used the best new diagnostic equipment to rule out stroke . . . to rule out heart attack . . . to rule out a brain tumor. Even if doctors thought a patient's symptoms were almost certainly unconnected to any serious illness, the ethos of emergency medicine was to keep running tests until a physician could say conclusively that the patient with chest pains was not having a heart attack or that the woman with a sore throat didn't have a rare, potentially fatal case of epiglottitis. Patients welcomed this approach, which treated even a routine illness as something special.

This buildup in emergency care became part of the overall explosion in medical costs, with an extra twist. Many emergency-room visitors were indigents with no insurance and no means of paying their bills themselves. For a while some hospitals tried to avoid treating such patients. (Doctors talked of performing "wallet biopsies," checking patients' insurance cards before deciding whether to provide care.) But Congress in 1986 required hospital emergency rooms to do medical assessments of all ER visitors and to stabilize the sickest ones, without regard to their financial status. That compelled hospitals to provide a lot of free emergency care, which led them to jack up charges for everyone. Patients with good insurance had to pick up the tab not just for their own treatment but also for a piece of the hospital's charity care. Charges skyrocketed to the point that some urban hospitals in the early 1990s demanded $250 or even $300 for a routine emergency-room visit. And that was only the base price; tests, medications, or sutures were extra.

When managed care entered the picture, HMO executives fumed at these spendthrift practices. They regarded hospital emergency rooms as financial black holes that would suck up premium dollars at a terrifying rate unless members could be kept away. As Gary Owens, a medical director at Philadelphia-based Keystone Health Plan East, put it, "We inherited a system in which the ER was the 7-Eleven of medicine. It was open all the time. It was convenient; you didn't have to make an appointment. But there was a premium to be paid for staffing it 24 hours a day, seven days a week."

HMOs started to address this cost issue by insisting on emergency-room discounts in their negotiations with hospitals. But many managed-care plans wanted to go further. The whole philosophy of managed care was that the primary-care doctor, working as a gatekeeper, would oversee and control almost all medical needs. Heavy use of the emergency room made a mockery of the entire managed-care system. Inside many HMOs, executives began talking about making members use the emergency room more responsibly. Before long a series of initiatives took shape.

One way for HMOs to tighten up was by changing their definition of a covered emergency. Under the 1973 HMO Act, federally chartered HMOs were required to pay for members' emergency care. But drafters of that statute neglected to spell out a precise definition of the term "emergency." So managed-care plans began paring back definitions to help restrain costs.

In Philadelphia, Keystone Health Plan mailed a patient-care manual to its network doctors in 1994, explaining that while it regarded heart attacks, strokes, and poisonings as emergencies, it considered twisted ankles with no open wound, minor burns, or abdominal pain lasting one day or more to be "non-emergent conditions." A true emergency involves severe symptoms requiring immediate care that "must occur suddenly and unexpectedly," Keystone added. To make sure that its participating physicians didn't miss the point, the HMO told them to "use the ER judiciously."

In Worcester, Massachusetts, an 80,000-member HMO, Central Massachusetts Health Care, opted for an even more stringent definition. In mailings to its members, the HMO explained that "a medical emergency is an immediate threat to life, limb or vital body function such that the need for medical intervention is so immediate that time may not be taken to contact your primary care physician." Lesser medical problems amounted to "urgent care," the HMO told its members. People needing urgent care were directed not to go to a hospital emergency room without permission, but to call their primary-care doctor and await instructions on appropriate care.

Occasionally HMOs attacked the widespread use of emergency rooms so belligerently that subscribers mutinied. When Mid-Atlantic Medical Services in 1994 decided that emergency costs were too high, the Rockville, Maryland, health plan sent its members a leaflet entitled *Why I Can't Go to the Emergency Room Anytime I Think It's Warranted.* That flyer declared that vomiting, diarrhea, earache, sore throat, flu, small cuts, poison ivy, and rashes all would be regarded as nonemergency conditions because they could be taken care of by primary-care doctors. Even if those conditions arose on weekends or late at night, the HMO said, members should consult their regular doctor, who could handle after-hours calls. In its mailings the HMO contended that this new arrangement would actually mean improved care. "When you go to an ER," the health plan wrote its members, "you are interacting with a provider who knows nothing about you, in a hectic setting. In order to compensate for the lack of clinical information in this busy setting, the physician will often order time-consuming and costly tests. In your physician's office, he or she knows you . . . and can appropriately diagnose your problems."

Within a few months Mid-Atlantic Medical was forced to abandon its tough new rules. "We got such feedback and complaints that we rolled it back," explained Paul Dillon, an executive vice president at the company. A year later Mid-Atlantic Medical put forth a much more lenient definition of an emergency: it would cover treatment whenever a prudent layperson believed that the absence of immediate medical attention could "place the patient's health in serious jeopardy."

More often, though, HMOs called the shots. In California, Kaiser Permanente came up with an especially artful definition of a covered emergency: "medically necessary health services for unforeseen illnesses or injuries that require immediate medical attention as determined by Health Plan." Under that definition Kaiser could be as liberal or as stingy as it wanted. It both administered and defined the benefit, case by case.

HMOs also decided to push much more of the cost of emergency-room visits onto their members. For regular doctors' visits, managed-care plans required only a trifling $2 or $5 copayment. That was one of the HMOs' big marketing advantages against fee-for-service health plans. For emergency services, however, different rules applied. HMOs warned members that the first $25, $50, or even $100 of most emergency-room visits would come out of the patient's own pocket. When asked, HMO executives defended this practice as smart management. "We call it a hesitation fee," explained Peter Kilissanly, president of Physicians Corporation of America, a Miami-based HMO. "If it's going to cost you to visit the ER, maybe you'll wait."

How have those strict new policies changed things? In some HMOs they have shrunk emergency-room use as much as 40 percent from earlier levels. But the cases that stay out of the emergency room aren't limited to earaches, poison ivy, and other minor ailments. The HMOs' new barriers can be so rigid that they overwhelm people at their most vulnerable moments.

Consider the case of John McGirr, a retired New York City sanitation worker living in the Long Island town of Cutchogue. He and his wife, Mae, got their medical coverage through Health Insurance Plan of Greater New York, an HMO that they both regarded as "pretty good." The one notable time that HIP denied coverage for the couple was in 1984, when Mae McGirr fell off a chair at home while hanging curtains. She broke her right arm in two places and was in such excruciating pain that she asked her husband to call 911 and summon an ambulance at once. HIP promptly paid to have her bones reset. But the $200 ambulance bill was bounced back into the McGirrs' hands on the grounds that they should have checked with the HMO at the time to see whether such a costly dash to the hospital really was warranted. From that experience Mae McGirr took away a fateful lesson: if sudden medical problems arise, call 1-800-HIP-HELP instead of 911.

On September 20, 1995, Mae McGirr woke up just before dawn and found her 78-year-old husband in bad shape. He was making gurgling sounds, staring ahead with glassy eyes, and holding his mouth wide open. Mae was frightened and unsure what the problem might be. "I thought it might be his ulcers, or perhaps another attack of pneumonia," she recalled. But she was determined to do the right thing. She called her HMO's help line and relayed her husband's symptoms. A physician told her he would decide what to do. And then Mae McGirr waited for help to arrive.

Minutes ticked by. An out-of-town ambulance company called, saying it had been sent by HIP to find her house but had got lost in the wrong town. After perhaps twenty to thirty minutes, a local policeman arrived; then, seconds later, an emergency medical crew from the fire department. Medical technicians rushed into John McGirr's bedroom, squeezing past his wife, who retreated to the hallway. As she watched the rescue squad frantically trying cardiopulmonary resuscitation, the unthinkable began to sink in. She heard a voice call out, "No vital signs." A few minutes later the fire chief walked over to her and said, "I'm sorry, but John passed away. It was cardiac arrest."

Five months later Mae McGirr saw herself as having been trapped by an invisible wall of HMO rules. "Calling their number first in a case like John's has to be the stupidest damn thing," she said. "I should have had access to 911." In theory, of course, she could have called 911 and gotten the fastest help possible. Her hometown fire department would have been dispatched instantly, avoiding the lost minutes caused by HIP's effort to bring an out-of-town rescue service to the scene. And with John McGirr's life at stake, HIP doubtless would have paid for the ambulance. But such issues seem clear only in hindsight. At 5:55 A.M., when an elderly man is once again sick and the sun hasn't yet come up, his wife's first response will be determined by habit. In the McGirrs' case, their habit — taught by earlier dealings with their HMO — was to follow the rules, even if medical care wouldn't arrive as fast.

In Silverton, Oregon, family practitioner Curtis Climer watched helplessly in June 1995 as a similar drama unfolded with a female patient who belonged to one of the state's managed-care plans for low-income people. In a letter shortly afterward to *American Medical News,* Dr. Climer recounted the case as follows:

A patient of mine who had only mild asthma became depressed in the past three months. I was unaware of her condition. In an effort to lift her spirits, her husband took her to Los Angeles for her 30th high school reunion. While there, her depression worsened. She had lost 15–20 pounds and was unable to walk across the room. Her husband realized she was getting into serious trouble.

His first thought was to telephone her managed care plan and try to get her some help in the Los Angeles area. After several hours and numerous conversations with people, he called me. He described her as being in a condition I would characterize by phone as one of severe dehydration and impending circulatory collapse. I advised him to call an ambulance and have her transported to the closest hospital. He felt this might be a problem because he had been advised the Oregon Health Plan had contracts with certain hospitals in the Los Angeles area, but neither of us knew where or who they might be. He wondered if he shouldn't put her in the car and drive back to see me since I was her primary care physician. I advised strongly against this and told him to call an ambulance and we could sort this out later.

In about 45 minutes I received a call from an emergency room physician advising me that my patient had just come in in full arrest and died. The next call I received was from the L.A. County coroner wanting to know if I had any idea why my patient had died. Would it be fair to say she died because the managed care plan had done such a good job scaring this family about the proper way to use the system that they were unable to actually access the care needed when it was needed?

Many HMO executives bristle at the idea that they are to blame in any way for such disasters. The standard HMO response is to portray these deaths as freakish bursts of bad luck that would occur with or without managed care. No broad lessons should be drawn from such calamities, the executives maintain — sometimes adding that their rarity means that HMOs' cost-control measures generally work fine. "If we were really screwing up, there should be hundreds of these cases," states Richard Cornell, senior medical director at Blue Cross–Blue Shield of Massachusetts.

One by one, though, allegations keep mounting that HMO emergency rules lead to unnecessary deaths. Consider the final hour of life for Stephen Cummins, a 35-year-old engineer who lived in Atlanta with his wife and two small sons. On the afternoon of July 28, 1994, he was mowing the lawn when he experienced sharp chest pain and numbness in his left arm. His wife, Janis, called their HMO, Kaiser Permanente, at 5:02 P.M. and described his symptoms. In a lawsuit she later filed in Georgia state court, Janice Cummins accused Kaiser of "negligence" in handling her husband's case. An HMO representative, she alleged, first recommended that her husband take an antacid, then called back and advised her to take him to Northside Hospital, 16 miles away.

Statistically, the odds of a heart attack in a man so young are minuscule. The vast majority of heart attacks occur in middle-aged or elderly people. But while cases in people under forty are highly unusual, that isn't the same as impossible. And in the next few minutes that afternoon in Georgia, disaster struck. Before the couple could leave for the hospital, Stephen Cummins vomited, collapsed to the ground, and stopped breathing. Bypassing Kaiser, his wife phoned 911 at 5:28 P.M. A fire department rescue unit arrived within 10 minutes. Paramedics found Cummins in cardiac arrest; they attempted to revive him but failed. At 6:25 P.M., doctors at a nearby hospital pronounced him dead. In her suit Janis Cummins accused Kaiser of negligence that resulted in her husband's untimely death.

All these cases reveal some dangerous blind spots in the managed-care model. HMOs want to believe that they can skillfully and instantly sort patients' situations into emergencies and nonemergencies and erect barriers to stop the needless dashes to the hospital without obstructing or delaying any of the vital ones. Such models work so nicely on paper that managed-care executives sometimes forget the chaotic, fast-moving conditions in which real-world emergencies occur. Some patients are confused or panicky; others are unnervingly stoic; some don't explain their symptoms clearly; some simply don't fit neatly into a particular emergency category. Without extra leeway, all those people are in peril. They may be brushed aside when they most need care, ending up as another supposedly rare casualty of managed-care guidelines.

Dr. Climer, the Oregon physician, has thought hard about the lessons from such tragedies. He isn't particularly pleased with his conclusion, but he regards it as inevitable. "If you're conscientious and follow the rules," he says, "you may get yourself in trouble. Sometimes you're better off getting the best care you can and letting the chips fall where they may."

A handful of paramedics, doctors, and other medical professionals are so scornful of managed-care protocol on emergency care that they go out of their way to defy the rules. Typical of the people in that camp is Darryl Hinthorne, a Boston ambulance paramedic who has fielded distress calls from HMO patients since 1981. Some of his favorite moments, in fact, involve clashes with HMO bureaucracy about ambulance calls — in which his own view has prevailed.

Twice in downtown Boston, Hinthorne says, he has been called to a Harvard Community Health Plan clinic to pick up a patient in distress. One case involved a middle-aged man with chest pain; the other, a young child having a severe asthma attack. Each time Hinthorne says he was told to take the patients to Brigham and Women's Hospital, the HMO's preferred hospital, which is about a five-mile drive through tortuous traffic. Each time, however, the patient appeared to him to be too sick to make such a long drive prudent. So in both cases Hinthorne headed straight for Massachusetts General Hospital, about a mile away — daring health-plan officials to stop him. As he roared away from the HMO clinic, he shouted, "We're going to the closest hospital! If you want UPS, call them. This is the guy's life you're messing with!"

Such defiance is exciting but hardly typical. Many cases are hard enough to diagnose that there is no dramatic showdown between medical professionals on one side and HMO bureaucrats on the other. Instead there are a number of drawn-out conversations as a case unfolds, concerning what sort of treatment makes sense, given the HMO's budget constraints. Providers dare not push the health plans too far for fear of being stuck with a big unpaid bill — and perhaps being frozen out of the HMO's network for years to come. What is more, most doctors and health-care workers aren't looking for a fight. They grudgingly accept the idea that insurers can have a say in how patients are treated, though front-line medical professionals may grumble about a dubious call for months to come.

Cardiologist Leslie Saxon encountered one of those exasperating moments in late 1994, when she was treating an emergency case at UCLA Medical Center in Los Angeles. The patient, a middle-aged man, had arrived at the hospital by ambulance suffering from ventricular tachycardia, a racing heartbeat suggestive of serious cardiac disease. The doctors stabilized the patient and were ready to do a full electrophysiological study, which might have cost $8,000 or more. But Cigna, the patient's managed-care plan, refused to pay for the treatment at UCLA; it insisted that the patient be transferred to Hospital of the Good Samaritan, about 20 miles away, where Cigna had negotiated better rates. Dr. Saxon lashed out at Cigna, arguing that the transfer would be enormously upsetting to the patient and that the ambulance ride to another hospital carried its own risks. But in the end she had to concede that the transfer wasn't likely to endanger his life. Once she made that concession, she couldn't budge the HMO. And in that case, she acknowledges, the gamble paid off; the patient survived the transfer and was treated at lower cost.

In Toledo, Ohio, emergency-room physician Bruce Janiak faced a tougher version of the same quandary in November 1995. He had begun to treat Beatrice Luna, a 45-year-old Chrysler auto worker, who had arrived at Toledo Hospital a few minutes earlier complaining of chest pain. Dr. Janiak quickly got an electrocardiogram and asked the cardiologist on duty, James Bingle, to help him analyze it. The two men agreed that her EKG looked normal, but both doctors remained concerned about her heart. Dr. Bingle proposed that he perform a cardiac catheterization and angiogram so that he could analyze her condition much more thoroughly — and be ready to perform an angioplasty or deliver clot-dissolving drugs at once if there was any sign of a heart attack in progress.

Beatrice Luna hesitated. She wasn't afraid of the procedure itself, but she was worried about its cost. She belonged to a local HMO, Medical Value Plan, that required her to get care from doctors in its network. Dr. Bingle wasn't in the network; it might cost her $6,000 or more of her own money for him to treat her. Rather than get immediate care, she decided, she would work through her HMO, waiting for it to authorize Dr. Bingle or another cardiologist to take over her case. Then all of her treatment would be covered. No one was immediately available, but indications were that an HMO cardiologist would stop by the hospital before long. Then all her treatment would be covered.

Later that day, Beatrice Luna's health plan authorized an out-of-plan cardiologist, Roger Miller, to perform angioplasty on her. By the HMO's account, the decision to pay for Dr. Miller's services was made quickly and automatically. But Luna and Dr. Janiak tell a different story. Both of them recall an hour-long wait to get coverage approved. During that period, the electronic tracings of Luna's heart waves showed the unmistakable signs of a heart attack in progress. Ultimately, she was very lucky. Doctors rushed her into the catheterization lab and began treatment right away. The damage to her heart was quite small, and a few days later she was able to leave the hospital.

Several months later, Dr. Janiak turned sharply critical when he thought about managed care's impact on the case. "I used to work for a managed-care company," he confided. "I've denied care. But this is the dark side of the business. I don't think anyone with her symptoms should have to wait an hour to get treated. We're very lucky that she ended up with minimal damage. But if she had been treated right away, there could have been no damage at all."

In other situations, patients and their families sometimes fight very hard for quick access to the emergency room. The ones who succeed — and avoid the types of tragedies that befell Stephen Cummins, James McGirr, and others — seldom get much in the way of thanks from their HMO.

Todd Buehler, for example, was certain he had done the right thing at 1:30 A.M. on a December night in 1995, when he brought his wife, Donna, to the emergency room of their hometown hospital in Milford, Massachusetts. For more than a day Donna had been wracked with vomiting and diarrhea. When she got up in the middle of the night, she briefly passed out, fell, and cut her chin. She regained consciousness for a bit, then fainted again. "I knew the cut was going to require stitches," Todd recalled, "but the passing out was more alarming than anything." When the couple reached Milford-Whitinsville Regional Hospital, they learned that Donna was so dehydrated that she needed two intravenous lines to restore her normal fluids.

When Todd Buehler called the HMO from the hospital to brief the health plan on his wife's situation, his call was routed to a Providence, Rhode Island, hospital that provided nighttime coverage for plan members. That facility was at least a 40-minute drive from the Buehlers, but the couple was told that they should have gone to Rhode Island. Todd Buehler came away from the call upset, and his wife's treating doctor in Milford, Mary Burke, was outraged. As Dr. Burke later said, "I told the people in Providence: would you mind repeating your position while I tape-record it? I think the *Boston Globe* would be very interested in what you want us to do."

Eventually the HMO and its cut-price hospital in Rhode Island backed down, letting Donna Buehler get full coverage for treatment in her hometown. "But they were quite rude about it," Todd Buehler recalled. "And there was a real suggestion that we had done the wrong thing."

In McKees Rock, Pennsylvania, Edmund Popiden waged a much more protracted coverage battle with his HMO, Aetna Health Plans of Western Pennsylvania. "They treated me like a slab of meat," Popiden later remarked. It took him seven months — and the intervention of the Pennsylvania Department of Health — before he got what he regarded as reasonable insurance benefits.

The case started on a Sunday afternoon in August 1992, when Popiden, at home, began feeling chest pains. At first the 64-year-old government worker tried to disregard them. He didn't want to be sick that day; he was enjoying a visit by his daughter and son-in-law. But the pains kept getting worse. "It was an unbelievable burning sensation," Popiden later said. "Like someone was holding an acetylene torch to my chest." Finally his son-in-law announced he would drive Popiden to St. Francis Medical Center in Pittsburgh, a hospital about 20 minutes away that was known for its cardiac-care unit. When Popiden got there, doctors grimly told him, "You've come to the right place." He was in the midst of a heart attack, and every minute was precious in saving as much of his heart muscle as possible. St. Francis physicians quickly performed an emergency angioplasty to unclog three arteries and kept Popiden in the hospital for five days. When he was discharged, he asked Aetna to pay the bill.

Aetna refused. Popiden hadn't called ahead for approval to use St. Francis, the HMO explained. He thus had failed to find out that the HMO wanted him to use a smaller hospital that was near his home and was in Aetna's cut-price network. Popiden — better known to Aetna as Plan Member 3001-895-78 — had violated two managed-care rules. In a terse letter to St. Francis, Aetna medical director Frank Keller explained that because of those infractions, "the above-captioned member is responsible for the billed charges of $20,254.90."

Ed Popiden was furious. "Do you have any idea what the wife and I have been going through in the last few months?" he pleaded with Aetna during a grievance hearing in December 1992. As he saw the case, the main issues were clear. He was in the midst of a medical emergency and needed care. He got it. His HMO had previously let him go to St. Francis for minor surgery, and he didn't know that the Pittsburgh hospital had since been dropped from Aetna's network. During a crisis, could he really be faulted for putting his own life ahead of managed-care procedures?

In its internal grievance hearing, Aetna upheld its refusal to pay for Popiden's heart care. But Joe Lucia, Pennsylvania's public health program administrator, saw the case differently. In a stinging April 1993 letter, Lucia ordered Aetna to pay all of Popiden's bills. He explained, "The public interest in saving Mr. Popiden's life . . . and encouraging prompt diagnosis and treatment of heart attacks far outweighs Aetna's limited interest in teaching Mr. Popiden a lesson to use a participating hospital even in an emergency." Lucia added, "Aetna's position reflects the very worst alleged negative impression of managed care and HMOs: that rules are more important than providing members needed and timely quality health care."

Across the United States, emergency-room doctors say they are running into similar conflicts between patients' desire to get care and HMOs' unwillingness to pay for it. Legislatures in California, Maryland, and several other states in 1994 and 1995 passed laws requiring managed-care plans to pay for care in situations where a "prudent layperson" would regard a patient's symptoms as justifying an emergency-room visit. In most states, however, HMOs can deny emergency claims with impunity after the fact. That leaves the Ed Popidens or their doctors and hospitals stuck with the bills.

In New York City, Lewis Goldfrank, head of the emergency department at city-run Bellevue Hospital, often treats people in such dire shape that their identity is unknown when they arrive. They include stroke victims, people with seizures or psychotic episodes, and victims of brutal robberies. As these patients recover, the Bellevue doctors learn their names and then can make inquiries about their insurance coverage. In nearly 100 cases during a six-month span in 1995, however, managed-care plans refused to pay for such patients' treatment. The reason: Bellevue didn't notify the HMOs of the patients' status within 48 hours of admission. By filing appeals, Dr. Goldfrank and his colleagues were able to have insurance coverage reinstated in about half the cases. Yet in many cases the managed-care plans took a rule written for one set of circumstances — the stable patient who can be transferred after a day or so in the emergency room — and used it to deny coverage for people on the verge of death. "You end up getting mugged by the bad guys and the insurance companies too," Dr. Goldfrank concluded.

In Gainesville, Florida, emergency physician John Stamler has kept track of all the cases that managed-care plans have refused to cover, either because they were deemed nonemergencies or because the HMOs weren't notified promptly. His collection includes a 51-year-old man with a fractured ankle; a 48-year-old man who arrived at midnight with a six-centimeter scalp wound that had to be sutured shut; a 74-year-old woman who had fainted for 15 minutes and had numbness on her left side; and a six-year-old boy with appendicitis who needed to be hospitalized and undergo surgery. "The insurance companies are denying payment and getting a free ride from us," Dr. Stamler remarked. "They have designed definitions that are so very narrow that when people go in for things that you would normally expect emergency care, the companies can write back and say: That doesn't fit our definition."

In Neptune, New Jersey, emergency physician Robert Sweeney in early 1995 made what he thought was such a clear-cut medical decision that he didn't bother to clear it with the patients' managed-care company at the time. Dr. Sweeney was treating a family poisoned by carbon monoxide from a faulty heater in their home. While he could help them slightly by administering oxygen through a face mask, he knew that a full cure required placing the victims in a special high-pressure cell known as a hyperbaric oxygen chamber, which would do a much better job of flushing the carbon monoxide from their bloodstreams. His hospital didn't have such a chamber; the nearest accessible one was in Philadelphia. So Dr. Sweeney called an air ambulance, which flew the family to safety. Several weeks later his billing service told him that the $5,000 helicopter charge was being denied, on the belief that a cheaper road ambulance would have gotten the patients to Philadelphia on time. Doctors who worked on the case were shocked; they regarded every minute saved as essential when trying to prevent lasting neurologic problems from the carbon monoxide poisoning. But under the letter of the HMO's coverage, payment could be denied with impunity.

One of the few people who can analyze the emergency-medicine controversy from the patient/doctor perspective and also from the HMO perspective is Keith Ghezzi, an emergency-room doctor in Washington, D.C., who also sits on the board of George Washington University Health Plan. "Managed-care plans are putting up more and more impediments in the way of patients' getting care," Dr. Ghezzi observes. Yet he believes that HMOs could do a far better job of handling medical emergencies if they made three major changes.

First, he says, the plans need good enough primary-care networks that members can get most of the care they need at their regular doctors' office. In their advertisements and brochures, HMOs like to play up the importance of primary care. But in many cases, Dr. Ghezzi finds, "HMOs are growing faster than they can add primary-care doctors." As a result, health-plan members end up at the emergency room because their designated primary-care doctor is so overloaded that he or she can't schedule an office visit promptly and can't return patients' calls seeking medical advice. Patients in such a predicament would gladly see their regular doctor if good service existed. They use the emergency room as a last resort.

Second, Dr. Ghezzi says, managed-care plans often are too optimistic about sick patients' ability to navigate the system. Many people facing a medical emergency are scared, or far from home, or otherwise not at their best. Rules that may make sense on paper become bewildering in a crisis. That predicament led to the creation of the "911" emergency-response system. With one simple call, patients or their families knew that help was on the way fast. Many managed-care plans, to save money, act as if 911 doesn't exist. They don't mention the service in their brochures or educational flyers for new members. A survey of Chicago HMOs, in fact, found that only three out of twenty-five plans explicitly told their members that it was all right to phone 911 in a crisis.

Finally, Dr. Ghezzi observes, many managed-care plans don't take the trouble to explain emergency-care rules to new members in a way that puts the patient's interests first. "There needs to be a massive educational campaign in this area," he says. Face-to-face briefings, instructional videos, and other teaching methods could do a lot to get members comfortable with the idea of seeking nonhospital alternatives for minor ailments while still depending on ambulances and 911 for true crises. Currently, however, HMOs don't do much beyond mailing out rule books, which often don't get read. As a result, HMOs find themselves locked into a system in which some members overuse the emergency room (and grow angry when claims are denied) while other members become so wary of breaking the rules that their own lives may be jeopardized.

At the phone triage center in Colorado, all those tensions and conflicts arise daily. "If this were easy, we wouldn't need nurses at all," observes Barry Wolcott, a physician who helped design the medical-diagnosis software packages used at the center. "We could simply switch everyone into voice mail and have them punch a few buttons. You need people — experienced, caring, medically smart people — to handle all the hard cases."

To the degree that remote-control medicine can work, the Boulder center gets high marks from consultants and physicians, including Dr. Ghezzi's HMO. Executives at Informed Access Systems, the company that runs the Boulder center, say their diagnostic software is meant to mimic the way a good emergency physician would think. That is, it initially focuses on the worst possible causes for a patient's main symptom, even if such diseases are quite rare. Nurses then ask probing questions that point to appropriate emergency treatment if the condition might be life-threatening. Only after nurses rule out rare, dangerous problems do they start focusing on the most likely prospects — the ordinary, manageable illnesses that cause most symptoms. In a reenactment of the James Adams tragedy, the issue of the baby's breathing problems surfaced within 15 seconds; a nurse promptly recommended calling 911.

In real life, though, managed-care checklists don't always work as smoothly as the simulations might suggest. Nurse Deb Rogalski in Boulder learned that lesson during a series of calls from a Washington, D.C., mother whose four-month-old son had been sick with diarrhea for a week. The boy had already visited the doctor once, and his mother worried that he was recovering more slowly than she had expected. Unsure what to do on a Sunday afternoon, the mother called for help.

Rogalski asked some questions about the boy's fluid intake and his ability to form tears. Then she reassured the mother that the boy didn't sound dangerously dehydrated. "You're doing a real good job of getting fluids into him," Rogalski said. "But with him still being sick, I'm going to recommend you get in touch with a doctor." A more detailed assessment from a physician was needed, she explained to a visitor. The boy quite likely was making a regular, somewhat protracted recovery. But it wouldn't hurt to have a local doctor give that judgment officially. Rogalski gave the mother a special phone number for the HMO's weekend on-call doctor and hung up, assuming that the case had been resolved.

A while later the mother phoned back. She had tried the doctor's line repeatedly and could not get an answer. When she called the HMO's regular business line, a clerk told her that no doctors were available on the weekend. Meanwhile, her son's diarrhea continued and he was unable to eat regular food.

"I don't know what to do," the mother told the telephone-service nurse, 1,500 miles away. "I'm worried. Do you think I should take him to the emergency room?"

9

HMOs and Mental Health

EVERYTHING IS FINE. There are no problems here.

Throughout late 1994 and early 1995, Rhode Island state investigators Linda Johnson and Alison Woodbine kept hearing that message from executives as they scrutinized United Behavioral Systems of Rhode Island. Executives at the managed-care company wrote testy letters and made chilly remarks whenever Johnson and Woodbine pressed them about growing complaints that UBS was shortchanging its members. Their righteous defense sounded plausible at first. UBS was a newcomer in New England, having arrived only in 1993. But it was part of a well-regarded multistate HMO, Minneapolis-based United HealthCare. Within the United empire, UBS played a limited yet crucial role in more than a dozen states. It was a "carve-out" company, one that takes a specialized piece of the health-care market — in this case mental health — and applies managed-care principles to it.

Like any managed-care company, UBS was a powerful rulemaker, deciding exactly how much treatment it would underwrite for each patient. Some people wanted weekly or monthly therapy sessions to deal with depression, anxiety attacks, or other problems. Some were candidates for psychiatric hospitalization or multiday stays at alcohol-treatment centers. All these cases were funneled to UBS, which decided who deserved coverage, who didn't, and how many therapy sessions or hospital days it would pay for.

In its marketing materials UBS implied that good care and saving money went hand in hand. "Our goal," the company declared in one brochure, "is simply stated: To help people receive appropriate and coordinated care sooner, improve faster and stay well longer at a lower cost than they would in any other system." And on paper UBS's system looked impeccable. Soon after entering Rhode Island, the company hired a well-known local psychiatrist, Daniel S. Harrop III, as its state-wide medical director. Local employers rushed to sign up with United HealthCare and UBS, attracted by low rates and seemingly generous benefits. UBS grew rapidly, providing mental-health coverage for nearly 200,000 people in mid-1994. Clients included Fleet Financial, the Hasbro toy company, and the state of Rhode Island itself.

Nonetheless, disturbing reports about UBS's methods surfaced in 1994, during the program's second full year in Rhode Island. The managed-care company was saying no to mental-health treatment far more often than Rhode Islanders had expected. In some cases UBS's denials were so blunt and unexpected that angry patients and psychiatrists took their grievances to the state Department of Health. As complaints mounted, two state officials began to investigate. Linda Johnson, a one-time HMO manager herself, had worked for the state of Rhode Island since 1987, looking into all aspects of wrongdoing in health care. She became the "tough cop." Everything about her — her aggressive questioning, no-nonsense suits, jet-black hair, and slightly raspy voice — suggested that she wasn't someone to tangle with. Her younger associate, Alison Woodbine, came across as the earnest rookie investigator, calmly but persistently pressing her inquiries.

In February 1995 Woodbine made full use of Rhode Island's authority: she asked to inspect complete medical records for more than 40 randomly chosen cases in which UBS had denied care. Officials at the managed-care company stalled at first. The records weren't available. They hadn't been filed. It would be hard to locate them. In early March, however, when UBS's Rhode Island executives were in Minneapolis for a management strategy session, a lower-level UBS employee relented. With a wave of his hand, he allowed the state investigators to step inside the company's medical-records room — and hunt down cases themselves.

A few minutes later Johnson and Woodbine were kneeling on the green carpeting of UBS's medical-records room, pulling out confidential patient folders from filing cabinets. As they thumbed through the manila folders, the two investigators began shaking their heads in horror. In case after case, Johnson recalled, doctors' hand-written notes spelled out the intimate details of human crises: a man plagued with thoughts of suicide, a mother hearing voices telling her to kill her own children, adults wrestling with ferocious addiction problems. UBS had repeatedly rejected doctors' pleas for insurance coverage to pay for more therapy, hospitalization, or medication in these cases. The standard explanation: "Does not meet medical criteria."

Two denials were near brushes with catastrophe, Johnson and Woodbine discovered. One involved a manic-depressive woman who had struggled for years to control her illness with lithium. Now her mental equilibrium was coming unstuck because she was pregnant and couldn't adjust the dosages of her medicines without fear of damaging the fetus. Her psychiatrist admitted her to a local hospital so she could be watched around the clock while doctors tried to determine a safe, effective dose of medicine. Partway through the hospital stay, Johnson recalled, UBS stopped its coverage, even though medical records showed that the woman was in a "chaotic" state at the time. To save the woman and her unborn child, Johnson recalled, her husband ended up paying the hefty hospital bills himself — and scrambling to find a different insurer that could provide better coverage.

In another case a despondent handgun owner worried that his thoughts of suicide might lead him to use the weapon on himself. "He gave the gun to a friend," Woodbine recalled, "and told him, 'I'm going through a tough time. I think you'd better keep this for a while.'" That turned out to be a tragic mistake. "The friend shot his own wife and killed himself," Woodbine recalled. "Now the man was overwrought with guilt. He wanted treatment." UBS turned down an extended treatment plan, according to a psychiatrist who later reviewed the case; the company limited its coverage to an initial assessment and several outpatient visits. The care he received appeared to have prevented another suicide, but Woodbine never felt reassured. When she asked, out of compassion, about the man's eventual fate, she got what she regarded as inadequate answers. "The best that UBS could tell me was that he was no longer a plan member," she later remarked, "and that they thought he had moved out of state."

Armed with such examples of managed care gone wrong, the Rhode Island Department of Health took aim against UBS and its parent company's other HMO operations in Rhode Island. Behind closed doors, state officials talked about freezing the offending health plans' enrollment or perhaps holding hearings on their fitness to be licensed as health insurers. United and UBS officials insisted at first that they hadn't done anything wrong. As the depth of UBS's problems became clear, however, the company negotiated a settlement with state authorities. In mid-1995 UBS agreed to oust its top two Rhode Island executives, including Dr. Harrop, the medical director; to embark on a wide-ranging corrective program; and to pay $66,000 in fines and legal fees to the state.

For Johnson and Woodbine the outcome of their investigation was bittersweet. The fines and the management shakeup were hailed by patients and doctors as a triumph of regulation and a warning to managed care. But their peek inside the dingy UBS medical-records room left the two investigators worrying about problems far beyond the one-company settlement. What kinds of people were applying managed care to the nation's treatment of depression, schizophrenia, and other mental illnesses? How much did these executives care about their members' well-being? Was UBS of Rhode Island an isolated case — or were untold human tragedies locked inside medical-records rooms across the country? Most fundamentally, could managed care work well at all in a specialty as murky as mental health?

Of all the free-spending areas of medicine that invited managed care's discipline in the late 1980s and early 1990s, mental health may have been the ripest target. The cost of care was escalating 12 percent a year, double the rate of general economic growth plus inflation. Within that total some of the fastest-growing subspecialties engaged in practices bordering on fraud. Overweight women from the Midwest were lured to Florida for "free weight-loss spas" — which promptly diagnosed the women as bulimic, suicidally depressed, and in need of 30 days of inpatient psychiatric care (in a pseudo-spa setting). Treatment stopped when participants' health-insurance coverage ran out. In an even more notorious abuse, as many as 300,000 teenagers a year were sent to psychiatric hospitals for multiweek stays for treatment of routine adolescent problems. Guidance counselors in some states were offered bonuses if they steered troubled teens toward certain for-profit hospitals. By one estimate as many as 75 percent of teenage psychiatric patients in the early 1990s really didn't need to be hospitalized at all.

Employers, not surprisingly, became disgusted with psychiatrists and counselors, convinced that those professions put their own greed ahead of the public interest. Companies such as Xerox, IBM, and Time discovered to their chagrin that 10 percent or more of health-care premiums were being spent on mental illness, without any clear sign that employees and dependents needed such extensive care or were benefiting greatly from it. "We had some employees going [to therapists] twice a week at $150 a visit," recalled Xerox's health-benefits chief, Helen Darling, "with no end in sight." The culprit, she came to realize, was Xerox's liberal and unsupervised benefits package, which provided open-ended reimbursement of almost any bill submitted. As Darling acidly put it, "There was a powerful incentive for therapists to find problems."

A few employers tried to clamp down by directly overseeing their workers' treatment for mental illness. But that brought messy problems involving redesign of benefits, employee confidentiality, and the need for in-house expertise to review cases. A much easier strategy, adopted by thousands of employers in the late 1980s and early 1990s, was to hire outside experts to do the hard work.

That created boom conditions for a handful of doctors, psychologists, and insurance executives who set up mental-health carve-out companies. These managers promised to take charge of companies' mental-health and drug-abuse programs. Costs would be controlled through a new system in which spending power was taken away from doctors and therapists. Instead, managed-care staffers would decide, right from the start, how much covered treatment each patient could receive. From a tiny beginning in the early 1980s, mental-health management companies grew to cover 80 million people in 1993 and more than 100 million in mid-1995. Venture capitalists poured money into these businesses, convinced they had found a major growth industry. They were right.

Companies such as Value Behavioral Health, MCC Behavioral Care, Human Affairs International, Merit Behavioral Care, and Green Spring Health Services took command of 10 million or more subscribers apiece. Each company generated yearly revenue of $200 million or more. Insurers such as Aetna and Cigna acquired mental-health carve-out companies for premium prices. Even Kohlberg Kravis Roberts, the leveraged buyout firm known for its 1989 takeover of RJR Nabisco, jumped into the mental-health business, buying Merit in mid-1995 for $340 million.

From a pure business perspective, the carve-out companies delivered everything they promised. They cut mental-health benefits costs at many companies to as little as 3 percent of overall health insurance premiums, saving $1 billion or more a year for their clients. Xerox —

which used an assortment of carve-out companies — reported a 38 percent drop in psychiatric hospitalizations of its employees between 1987 and 1994. The average hospital stay shrank even more drastically, from 33.7 days to 9.9 days. Benefits chief Darling pronounced herself "well satisfied" with the results.

As managed-care companies hacked away, however, concerns grew that the efficiency patrol was indiscriminately attacking any kind of mental-health spending, whether wasteful or essential to patients' well-being. Kenneth Wells, a Rand Corporation analyst, found evidence that depressive patients got fewer therapy sessions under managed care and sometimes didn't fare as well as those covered by fee-for-service insurance. In a widely read article in the *New England Journal of Medicine* in January 1996, John Iglehart, editor of *Health Affairs,* expressed concern that managed care's tight control of mental-health spending had a "very real potential for stifling the development of new drugs and other clinical improvements that could benefit the mentally ill."

The fiercest outcries against carve-out companies came from psychiatrists. Their protests inevitably have been tinged with self-interest; managed care's retrenchment often has meant less autonomy, more outside supervision, and lower incomes for these doctors. Even so, psychiatrists have filled professional journals with accounts of patient treatment threatened by managed care. In the spring of 1995 Stephen Sharfstein, the sitting president of the American Psychiatric Association, who favored some sort of accommodation with managed care, lost his reelection bid to one of the most vocal critics of the carve-out industry. The new president, Maryland psychiatrist Harold Eist, denounced managed-care companies as "greed-driven sharks in a feeding frenzy" and vowed to fight for legislation to restrain them.

While carve-out companies say they are improving America's mental-health system, large-scale examples of hurtful stinginess have surfaced throughout the United States. In July 1995 *Wall Street Journal* reporters Ellen Pollock and Carol Hymowitz chronicled Ohio's problems with American Biodyne, a predecessor company to Merit Behavioral Care. In 1990 American Biodyne won a $7 million-a-year contract to cover 21,900 of Ohio's state employees, promising to improve service while trimming costs 30 percent from the previous $10 million-a-year level. But when the program was audited in mid-1992, inspectors found alarming signs of undercare. New patients had to wait an average of 14 days before beginning therapy sessions instead of the promised five days. One third of Ohio's 88 counties had no substance-abuse counselors, even though American Biodyne had promised to find one for each county. Overall, American Biodyne was spending less than $3 million a year on direct patient care, even though it had told the state it would spend $4.5 million. American Biodyne disputed many of the audit's findings but agreed to cut its yearly price $1 million and return $320,000 to the state when it negotiated its 1993 contract.

In government-run Medicaid programs for poor people, too, the carve-out companies' practices have come under fire. Iowa in 1994 awarded a two-year, $100 million contract to Merit Behavioral Care to handle mental-health services for 175,000 Medicaid recipients. But after a few months the state became concerned about the program's performance. Hospital administrators and psychiatrists accused Merit of denying essential care, signing up too few providers, and burdening doctors with excessive paperwork. "There have been some bumps in the road," a Merit executive acknowledged, though he said the company was doing its best to respond to major criticisms. Similarly, Massachusetts officials in mid-1995 told Medicaid managed-care companies that they weren't spending enough on mental health; studies showed that children and adolescents, in particular, appeared to be getting shortchanged.

"Mental health services have long been the neglected stepchild of health services," ethicists Philip Boyle and Daniel Callahan argued in a 1995 essay in *Health Affairs*. As managed-care companies enter the picture, there is a temptation to declare persistently ill people untreatable, while labeling the worried well as not requiring coverage. Taken to its extreme, such an approach can slash costs to zero by creating an unusable benefits plan in which everyone is either too sick or too healthy to warrant attention. Even if managed-care companies do try hard to treat the full spectrum of mentally troubled patients, all the usual tradeoffs between efficiency and medical quality arise, along with several unique challenges.

Something as simple as a person's first request for treatment can be problematic. Most carve-out companies require members to call an "800" number and speak with a case manager, usually a nurse or social worker. The case manager then decides whether the member should see a psychiatrist (who has a medical degree and can prescribe drugs or provide psychotherapy), a psychologist (who has advanced therapy training but no medical certification), or a counselor/social worker with less formal training. During the initial call or after a first "assessment" visit to a therapist, the case manager also decides how many outpatient visits the company will cover. In the best-run health plans, well-trained case managers can guide members to the right specialist in a compassionate way. But in other cases phone clerks mechanically zip through checklists of questions — expecting that patients will volunteer details of secret addictions or suicidal thoughts with no more embarrassment or hesitation than if the clerks were asking for details about diabetic symptoms or a twisted knee. Such impersonal screening systems have become widely lampooned in cartoons and on electronic bulletin boards; they reinforce patients' and therapists' worst images of managed care. In a particularly egregious case, says California psychiatrist Mark Levy, a college student's confidentiality was betrayed when she sought therapy regarding problems with an abusive father. The health plan let the father know about the visits; he angrily put a stop to further care.

Managed-care companies also face tough choices as they try to assemble cost-effective networks of psychiatrists, psychologists, and hospitals. After the abuses of the 1980s, carve-out companies see tremendous potential for saving costs and improving care by weeding out incompetent or fee-hungry doctors. "The goal is to get as many patients better as you can, as fast as you can," contends Ian Shaffer, chief medical officer of Value Behavioral Health. "Will someone please show me the literature where hurting longer is a good thing?" Yet if cheap, short-term care becomes the overriding concern, patients' well-being may suffer. Outpatient therapy can be truncated to the point that short-term suicide prevention becomes the only goal, with little effort to help a person regain the stability needed to succeed in the workplace or function well in everyday life. Barriers meant to prevent excessive use of psychiatric hospitals can rise so high that even the truly sick aren't admitted for overnight stays or are discharged too soon.

UBS's experience in Rhode Island shows all those tensions at work. By financial yardsticks the mental-health plan was a great success in its first two years. But it never won patients' trust or the respect of Rhode Island's many therapists. Coverage standards for mental illness — ranging from outpatient antidepression therapy to hospitalization for alcohol or drug dependency — were far more stringent than patients and their doctors had expected. The health plan banged out benefit-denial letters and, when disputes broke out, held its ground, making little effort to compromise. That policy saved money in the short term. In the long run, however, UBS's frugal ways were anguishing for patients, disruptive of relations between the company and local doctors, and ultimately embarrassing for the health plan itself.

The Rhode Island saga started in 1991, when United HealthCare moved into New England. The Minnesota company acquired a small Rhode Island HMO, Ocean State Health Plan, and installed new management to spark growth and profitability. That strategy proved astute; the Rhode Island plan, renamed United Health Plans of New England, tripled its membership and slimmed down its medical-loss ratio by several percentage points in its first three years under new ownership.

In overhauling the Rhode Island plan, United executives took a hard look at its mental-health provisions. The plan had contracted with two local psychiatrists, Paul Alexander and Louis Hafken, who provided much of the care themselves and farmed out other cases to colleagues. That ad hoc arrangement needed to be changed; with 160,000 members in 1993, the HMO wanted to have a bigger network of mental health specialists and greater oversight of their work. United also hoped to save money. Although mental-health care consistently amounted to less than 3.5 percent of total premiums, the cost was creeping upward. It reached $7.3 million in 1993, up from $5.5 million the year earlier. By that time, United HealthCare already operated its own mental-health benefits company, known as United Behavioral Services (UBS), in nearly a dozen states. Rhode Island seemed like a logical new market for UBS to enter. So United executives leased some office space just south of Providence and set up shop as United Behavioral Services of Rhode Island. The company hired John Chianese, a local managed-care administrator, to be executive director; key patient decisions would be made by a different employee, a psychiatrist serving as medical director.

An eager candidate for the medical director's job emerged in late 1993: Daniel S. Harrop III, a 39-year-old former colleague of Dr. Alexander's. Dr. Harrop had a part-time teaching position at Brown University and a fearsome reputation among psychiatric patients. "I used to tease him that his adolescent patients would go in and out of the hospital faster than anyone else's, simply because they hated dealing with him," recalls Rhode Island social worker Cathy Clark. "And I meant it as a compliment." Dr. Harrop's icy, edgy style apparently was what United wanted. UBS signed him up in December 1993 as the Rhode Island plan's first full-time psychiatrist, handling its hospitalized patients in the mornings and serving as medical director in the afternoons. His starting pay was nearly $150,000, about 40 percent more than the average psychiatrist in private practice earns. If things worked out, Dr. Harrop was told, he could look forward to stock options and a 20 percent bonus.

From the beginning Dr. Harrop braced for clashes with the practicing therapists who had been his colleagues. "I didn't go in thinking that the mental-health community would get comfortable with managed care," Dr. Harrop later said. "It's difficult to get people to change. It isn't so much that they minded short-term care. They did not like someone looking over their shoulder." But Dr. Harrop wasn't about to shy from confrontations. Proud of his own clinical record and his professional credentials, he believed he could make wise treatment choices, even if other people disagreed with him. "You always have to do what's best for the patient, even if that isn't always what the patient wants," he would tell skeptics.

Dr. Harrop settled quickly into his new job. He collected computer printouts showing how long each psychiatrist kept patients in the hospital, so he could identify doctors who allowed unusually long average stays. Then he urged them to look for ways to bring the length of treatment down to local averages. He also checked out the backgrounds of therapists in the plan and kicked out several whom he believed were romantically entangled with their patients or were doing a poor job of monitoring suicidal patients. Such problems traditionally have been handled by state medical boards, whose disciplinary proceedings can take years. Dr. Harrop, to his satisfaction, found that as a managed-care medical director, he could move more quickly than the state licensing authorities to stop using therapists that he didn't trust.

These initiatives were accompanied by cost cutting. Before UBS arrived, alcoholic members needing inpatient care had been sent to Rhode Island's most renowned psychiatric facility, Butler Hospital, where they were treated for $600 a day. Dr. Harrop knew Butler well; he had done part of his residency training there. When he looked at UBS's contracts, however, he found he could get per-day rates as low as $110 by sending alcohol-dependent members to two less distinguished facilities just across the Massachusetts state line. The savings looked so compelling that Dr. Harrop switched all of UBS's alcohol-rehabilitation contracts to the Massachusetts facilities — which alarmed his old colleagues at Butler. Among the people who felt taunted was Dr. Hafken, the previous overseer of the health plan, who had since returned to private practice at Butler.

"I remember Dan Harrop coming to talk to us and telling us: 'We're going to close down one or two of your units,'" Dr. Hafken recalled. It wasn't a message that Butler's staff physicians wanted to hear. Dr. Harrop was "very much like a smoker who quits," Dr. Hafken observed. "He came on pretty strong to people and antagonized a lot of them."

UBS also attracted controversy with an aggressive program to save money by shortening outpatient therapy. Officially the carve-out company offered most members 20 covered sessions a year. But former case managers say they repeatedly were told that most patients didn't need more than six or eight sessions and that longer-term therapy seldom accomplished much. An outside audit later found one UBS case manager who believed therapy should be halted after three sessions if the patient didn't improve. A therapist who asked for 12 sessions to help an out-of-work, depressed patient rebuild her self-esteem was turned down. A UBS case manager sent the therapist a form letter with a hand-written note saying that the mental-health plan had recently "clarified" its benefits and now covered only "short-term crisis intervention."

Some therapists and patients appealed those denials, but they seldom succeeded. Contested cases were reviewed by Dr. Harrop or outside psychiatrists whom he had chosen; those reviewers upheld UBS's original ruling more than 80 percent of the time. Other therapists dodged confrontation by telling patients that if they wanted to continue treatment, it would be at their own expense — because the odds of winning a coverage battle with UBS were too low to justify the upheaval. Therapists who did battle UBS for more coverage worried, with some justification, that they might be blackballed by the managed-care company.

Within UBS's headquarters case workers were directed to look each day at a large blackboard listing the dozen or so therapists currently favored by the plan. Therapists who periodically made the list could expect lots of cases; those whose names never appeared would be starved for business. "Some of the list was based on quality, but some of it was based on efficiency," recalled Peter Cannata, a former UBS case manager. "They kept listing one person who treated everyone in three sessions. They thought that was wonderful."

As it happened, Dr. Harrop had a direct financial interest in the quick handling of outpatient cases. Part of his annual bonus was based on how well the Rhode Island office met various corporate budget goals, one of which was limiting 80 percent of outpatient cases to 10 or fewer therapy sessions. State regulators frown on explicit quotas and regard such bonus clauses as open inducements to undertreat patients. When Rhode Island regulators learned about that clause in the spring of 1995, they regarded it as further evidence of problems at UBS. By that time, however, Dr. Harrop had been in office nearly 18 months.

From United's perspective, Dr. Harrop in 1994 appeared to be off to a fine start. Costs of mental-health care, which had climbed 30 percent in 1993, inched up only 4 percent in 1994. United asked an outside psychiatrist, Harold Davidson of Massachusetts, to review some of Dr. Harrop's decisions once a month, just to make sure there weren't any quality problems. Dr. Davidson consulted frequently to HMOs but believed he could deliver an objective view of the Rhode Island plan. "Opposition and resistance can be expected from a large and vociferous group of private practitioners in the face of great change," Dr. Davidson wrote in one evaluation. "I have been very impressed with the work done at UBS. The case managers are very thorough, clinically astute and consult easily with the Medical Director."

UBS's style seemed much more menacing to patients and their advocates. Starting in mid-1994, protests about the managed-care plan poured into the offices of Ruth Glassman, the state's mental-health advocate, and Bill Emmet, head of the Rhode Island Alliance for the Mentally Ill. "People thought they had coverage, and then they kept getting denied," Emmet recalled. "These were suicidal or depressed people or their families. They didn't know where to turn. We kept a record of their complaints, and pretty soon we decided there was enough going on to turn it over to the state."

In November 1994 Glassman, Emmet, and Jim McNulty, president of the Rhode Island Manic-Depressive and Depressive Association, sent nearly 20 documented patient complaints to state authorities. There weren't any headline cases involving murders or suicides, yet the advocacy groups felt that these stories of despair and frustration deserved regulatory attention. "There was a nasty, insulting quality to some of the denials," Glassman recalled. "It was more than an inconvenience to patients. These things touch at the essence of the relationship in psychotherapy." Bolstering their complaint files were three cases documented by Michael Ingall, a Providence psychiatrist who had helped train Dr. Harrop in medical school. Dr. Ingall contended that his one-time pupil had been unreasonably stingy with coverage for some depressed patients, a charge that Dr. Harrop steadily denied.

Over the next six months, state regulators and an outside auditing team from the health-care consulting firm of William M. Mercer picked over UBS's way of doing business in Rhode Island. What they found wasn't a pretty sight.

The Rhode Island plan had some of the most extreme "underutilization of care" encountered in more than 100 audits, Mercer's reviewers wrote. UBS on average approved just 7.2 outpatient therapy sessions for members — barely one third of the full benefit offered in its brochures. If members needed hospitalization, Mercer found, UBS paid for an average stay of only 4.5 days. That compared with an average of 15.5 days for psychiatric hospitals across the United States and 7.8 days for other managed-care plans studied by Mercer. As Rhode Island regulator Don Williams later said, "Their regular practice was to deny medically necessary care, day in, day out."

UBS's hiring standards for case managers also provoked an outcry. Some of its recruits were recent graduates of nursing or social-work programs with limited clinical experience. Others were still completing degree programs. As the Mercer audit dryly put it: "There were some inconsistencies noted in the sophistication and training of staff." One psychiatrist discovered, to her dismay, that two of UBS's case reviewers were former patients of hers with borderline personality disorders. "I wouldn't want a reviewer's personality disorder affecting my treatment plan," she remarked. UBS executives later said they weren't aware that any Rhode Island case managers had histories of mental illness, but added that they would check employees' credentials more carefully in the future.

Among the patients complaining about UBS was Larry O'Brien, a middle-aged executive recruiter in Providence who at several stages in his life had suffered from manic-depressive illness. He got health insurance through his wife's job; when her company switched to United and

UBS in early 1995, he called the health plan to see what it could do for him. O'Brien asked for coverage approval to see a psychologist regularly and a psychiatrist twice a year. He was turned down at first, he later said, because his condition wasn't severe enough to require regular medication. "They were only interested in treating acute episodes. I was trying to avoid an acute episode, but I didn't fit any of their categories." After a series of arguments over the phone with a UBS case manager and then with Dr. Harrop, O'Brien finally got the permissions he wanted. But the dickering galled him. "These people want to collect our premiums and then not pay claims," O'Brien later remarked. "I say the hell with them."

Eileen McNamara, a psychiatrist who dealt with UBS during Dr. Harrop's tenure, was unnerved by the plan's handling of several cases involving people with alcohol or drug-abuse problems. At a state hearing in September 1995, she testified about a case in which a depressed alcoholic man called UBS on a Friday and was told over the phone that he didn't meet the criteria for treatment. "He was told to consult the Yellow Pages for two names of people who could see him on Monday," she declared. That cavalier response was grossly inappropriate, she said, explaining that a quick phone conversation can't accurately gauge how badly off such patients may be. "If I practiced medicine the way managed care practices it," Dr. McNamara asserted, "I would lose my license."

The Mercer auditors, in more muted language, also questioned UBS's handling of alcohol-related disorders. "What appeared to be clear evidence of possible substance abuse was overlooked," the auditors wrote in their report. They cited an instance where a UBS case manager briefly noted, without probing further, that a member denied substance abuse. When the man was admitted to a detoxification program a few months later it emerged that he had been drinking two liters or more of gin each week.

As resentment intensified about UBS's clamping down on benefits, some of Rhode Island's psychiatrists and psychologists began fighting the managed-care company with a civil disobedience campaign of sorts. Their main tactic was to describe patients' symptoms in the grimmest or "juiciest" possible terms, so that treatment could be approved even under UBS's strict rules. A bit of such gamesmanship has existed in American medicine for decades. But people on both sides of the UBS/therapist divide in 1994–95 portray the Rhode Island uprising as a particularly fiery clash, marked by each side's utter contempt for the other's position.

To therapists, Dr. Harrop was the villain — the man they nick-named "Dr. Deny" — and almost any ruse was permissible if it helped patients get the care they needed. "There was an overstatement of suicidal risk to get people hospitalized," conceded psychiatrist Michael Ingall, one of the feistiest critics of UBS. Yet Dr. Ingall contended that in the big picture such ploys were justified. Good psychiatric care means more than heading off a suicide with a quick hospital stay, he argued; doctors need to remain on the case until they have tried to tackle the underlying issues causing a patient's despair. Companies such as UBS refused to see that, he maintained, adding, "If you tell them that a person is no longer suicidal, they say, 'Fine. Treatment's over.'" Rather than play by managed care's rules, he and other Rhode Island therapists followed what they regarded as a higher law.

For Dr. Harrop and some of his colleagues, the therapists' uprising was shocking, inexcusable — and proof that mental-health providers couldn't be left unsupervised. "I remember one provider pushing me to authorize extensive outpatient treatment," Dr. Harrop later said. "I told him, 'You're right. This patient needs care. I will authorize admission to the hospital.' Well, suddenly the patient wasn't so sick after all." Examples like that reinforced Dr. Harrop's belief that some thera-pists were trying to take advantage of the system and that he needed to stop them. "When you know the cast of characters, that becomes part of how you do your job," he remarked.

Those battles turned especially heated when psychiatric patients were admitted to the hospital. Outpatient therapy typically costs a managed-care plan $60 to $90 per session, assuming a discount of about 30 percent from therapists' standard rates. A one-day psychiat-ric hospitalization, in contrast, may carry a base charge of $500 or more. If the doctors prescribe medicines, run blood tests, or order brain-imaging studies, bills can soar to as much as $2,000 a day. Such expenses can chew up a managed-care budget at an astonishing rate; as a result, most carve-out companies keep a tight watch on hospital stays. UBS's monitoring was especially strict; the Mercer auditors later faulted the plan for "evidence of premature decertification of care" — in essence, cutting off payment for hospital stays before patients were stable enough to be safely discharged.

Terry Lusignan, a Providence resident, discovered how strict UBS could be when she tried repeatedly in July 1994 to have her manic-depressive sister admitted to a psychiatric hospital. At that time, Lusignan later said, the sister was having hallucinations that she was being stalked by a murderer; she also was crying uncontrollably, was unable to eat or sleep, and was reacting badly to her medications. "She needed immediate help," Lusignan recalled. But, Lusignan said, UBS refused three times to authorize any overnight hospitalization. By the end of the process Lusignan herself was in tears, telling the UBS case managers that she didn't feel capable of shepherding her sister through another night. Unable to budge the managed-care company, Lusignan and other family members got the woman admitted to Rhode Island Hospital at her own expense — $7,648 for an eight-day stay.

For months afterward Lusignan tried to get UBS to reconsider its initial denial and pay the hospital bill. In a September 1994 letter to state insurance regulators, UBS acknowledged that the patient had been "agitated" and hard to care for during the July crisis, but said that she nonetheless failed to meet the company's standards for hospitalization. Lusignan filed a formal appeal, which was turned down in a January 1995 letter from Dr. Harrop. He wrote that an outside reviewer had looked at the case and "determined that there is nothing in the record to indicate the patient needed 24-hour level of care. She did not appear in imminent danger to herself or others." Only after Dr. Harrop was ousted from his job did UBS finally reimburse Lusignan's family for the hospital bill, as well as $2,500 in legal fees associated with the case. The delayed payment did little to soothe Lusignan's worries. "I don't feel that my sister's future is secure," Lusignan told a Rhode Island state hearing on mental-health issues in September 1995. "Nothing has changed to guarantee that she will get her benefits today — without a fight."

During Dr. Harrop's tenure as medical director, UBS concentrated an extraordinary amount of power in his hands. Not only did he set policies on hospitalization, review them, and handle first-level appeals from members and doctors, but he also was the treating doctor for some patients as well. Nurses at Rhode Island Hospital, where Dr. Harrop worked part-time in late 1994 and early 1995, were told that some UBS-enrolled patients were to be assigned to Dr. Harrop, who regularly made morning rounds. He would decide how long those patients should be hospitalized, a privilege that troubled patients' rights groups. "Patients would come in at night and he would attempt to discharge them in the morning," recalled Ruth Glassman, the state mental-health advocate. "We got several of these complaints; we called them his 12-hour specials. A lot of people would fight this. He felt people had no medical necessity to be in the hospital."

Dr. Harrop later acknowledged that some patients and psychiatrists disliked his coverage decisions. But he said he didn't believe that his denials hurt patient care. "I'm not aware of any suits against the plan or its providers while I was medical director," he said in an interview after leaving UBS. "There was no case of someone throwing themselves off a bridge or off the roof of the Westin Hotel." Three patient complaints were aired at one point on a *CBS News* report, but Dr. Harrop maintained, "If those cases are the worst that they could come up with during my 18 months, then I'm happy with what I did."

By the spring of 1995, however, Rhode Island regulators believed they had a mighty case against UBS. They gathered 25 examples of benefits denials and asked two renowned psychiatrists affiliated with Harvard Medical School to review them. The reports that came back were blistering.

William Falk, who examined nine inpatient records, reported that in each case, treatment was medically necessary under UBS's own criteria, even though the company had denied benefits on the grounds that it wasn't necessary.

Ronald Schouten, the psychiatrist who examined 16 outpatient denials, declared that in UBS's system "individuals with disabling mental illness are excluded from coverage." In five cases, he wrote, care was medically necessary even though UBS said it wasn't. In a further eight cases, Dr. Schouten added, UBS was applying criteria that hadn't been disclosed to regulators beforehand. Patient care appeared hamstrung by a series of unwritten rules, such as: "Only crisis intervention is covered," "No psychotherapy can last longer than 10 sessions," and "The condition of the patient is much less important than the treatment plan." If those standards were applied to general medicine, Dr. Schouten suggested, they would be so repulsive as to be unthinkable. Stroke patients could be denied coverage for recuperative physical therapy because they were no longer in crisis. Patients with emphysema could be barred from seeing doctors because treatments can't cure the diesease, only slow its damage. By applying such strict standards to psychiatric cases, Dr. Schouten concluded, UBS was acting as if "mental illness is not real, and is certainly not to be given parity with other problems."

As expert opinions rolled in, so, too, did fresh tales of agony from UBS members. A distraught father called the Rhode Island Department of Health one afternoon, complaining that his three-year-old daughter had been raped a week earlier and that UBS was refusing to pay for special counseling with a child psychologist. State investigator Linda Johnson, who took the call, immediately phoned UBS, asking for details about the case. But because the man hadn't given his name during his call to the state, Johnson later recalled, she was told by UBS officials that they couldn't locate the case and thus couldn't check to see how it was handled. "I kept saying, 'How many three-year-old rape cases do you get?'" Johnson later said. "'You've got to know which case this is!' But they were adamant. It's times like those that make you want to reach through the phone and grab someone."

On June 1, 1995, state officials had enough evidence to file a 15-page Statement of Deficiencies regarding UBS, listing more than two dozen alleged violations of state Health Department rules. Unknown to UBS, some of the most damaging evidence came from two of its own employees, who had quietly contacted the Department of Health and said they wanted to help regulators with the probe. For more than a month one of those informants had been meeting after hours with Johnson and Woodbine, signing affidavits and sharing an insider's view of UBS's operations.

Once the deficiency report was filed, the next move was up to UBS and its corporate parent, United HealthCare in Minnesota. Under Rhode Island law the Department of Health could hold hearings on the charges spelled out in the Statement of Deficiencies — and could impose sanctions, including a membership freeze for United's Rhode Island plans or even a license revocation. Some Minnesota-based UBS officials wanted to contest the case, thinking they could beat back the little New England state's challenge. "We are absolutely confident that when we speak with them, we will be able to adequately refute the allegations with the facts," UBS's chief operating officer, Deborah Trout, told a reporter in early June 1995. Some senior officials at the parent company took a different view, observing that a drawn-out public fight would be hurtful to the company's image. And, bravado aside, there was no assurance that United and UBS would win. Rather than contest the state's charges, they argued, it might be wiser to settle.

Partway through June, United's top corporate negotiator, executive vice president Travers Wills, went to Providence with an interesting proposition. If UBS purged its management in Rhode Island — Dr. Harrop and executive director John Chianese — and if it agreed to pay some modest fines and embark on a program of corrective action, would the state be satisfied?

The answer, ultimately, was yes. "We didn't ask them to get rid of Harrop and Chianese," recalled Don Williams, the associate director of Rhode Island's Department of Health. "They offered them up all by themselves." Some minor haggling remained about the size of the fines and the terms of the remedial program, but the outline of the deal had been struck.

On June 15 — Dr. Harrop's birthday — the Minneapolis-based chief executive officer of UBS, John Tadich, phoned the company's Rhode Island office and asked to talk to both Chianese and Dr. Harrop on a speakerphone call. "This can't be good," Dr. Harrop told himself as he walked into Chianese's office. For the medical director the news was bad indeed. Tadich explained the provisional settlement, the key feature of which was dismissal of the plan's top two Rhode Island executives. "I'm sorry," Tadich said. "I don't think you've done anything wrong. But we need to do this to move on." The phone call wrapped up in about 10 minutes, but Dr. Harrop sat, stunned, in Chianese's office for another hour and a half, slowly coming to terms with the fact that his short, powerful career at UBS was over.

During the rest of 1995 UBS reshaped its Rhode Island operations in an effort to keep regulators, therapists, and patients at peace. The company hired a new executive director, Maria Sekac, a social worker with a strong pro-patient record in mental health. UBS installed new appeals procedures that were meant to be much easier for patients and doctors; it also stepped up its training of case managers. The company delayed finding a permanent replacement for Dr. Harrop, but it advised its acting medical directors to be lenient in their coverage decisions. Spending on mental-health services climbed to about $1 million a month, up more than 30 percent from 1994's stringent levels, though still less than 4 percent of United's total health insurance premiums in Rhode Island. As a United official told the *Providence Journal-Bulletin* in August 1995, "We basically have backed off from trying to manage much at all." Eventually, though, UBS planned to bring in a new medical director. Then the company would try afresh to explain its theories of managed care to Rhode Island's therapists — and see if it could find a better way to hold down costs without ending up in regulatory trouble.

Dr. Harrop remained in Providence, teaching a group psychotherapy course part-time at Brown and hoping to find a new job in managed care. "If I had it over, I'd still have worked for UBS," he said in early 1996. "I just would have preferred a different ending." He turned down an offer to relocate to Illinois and instead concentrated on negotiating a sizable severance award from UBS. State investigators Linda Johnson and Alison Woodbine, meanwhile, focused on Rhode Island's other big managed mental-health company, Green Spring Health Services. Once again they found evidence of administrative deficiencies and some questionable denials of coverage, leading to a fresh disciplinary case.

Publicly UBS officials veered between apologizing for their problems in Rhode Island and portraying the Rhode Island company as a well-run business whose only fault was to lose a power struggle with old-guard, anti-managed-care therapists. In a 1995 newspaper interview, Travers Wills, the United executive vice president who negotiated the Rhode Island settlement, declared, "We are witnessing providers who have got the ear of the Health Department." UBS didn't admit wrongdoing in the settlement, he observed; it simply decided that things would "go forward faster" if it resolved the dispute than if it went through the negative publicity of open hearings.

Top-level UBS and United officials even took some cheer from the Mercer audit, conducted in May 1995 while the state investigation was under way. The study faulted UBS for a wide range of practices, yet Mercer's auditors said the carve-out company was "within the mainstream of managed care." On a typical audit of a mental-health company, Mercer explained, quality-of-care problems surface in 15 percent to 40 percent of cases under review. UBS matched its peers, Mercer said. One quarter of its audited cases "contained indications of problems in the quality of treatment services being provided to the patient."

For the Department of Health's Linda Johnson, the idea that managed-care companies could regard a 25 percent defect rate as tolerable was one of the most chilling parts of the whole investigation. "The thing that bothers me most about the UBS case," Johnson said, "is that they still don't think they did anything wrong. I'd like to get Travers Wills on the phone with the father of the three-year-old, or talking with the man with the gun. I'd like to have him do some front-line work and see what shape these people are in."

10

When the Elderly
Fall Sick

"TAKE THAT THING AWAY!" Belva Johnson snapped as she stared at a four-pronged cane designed to help elderly people keep their balance. "I don't need it!"

"I'm sorry, Mother, but you do need it," her son Richard replied. All around them, nurses and therapists at the Hillhaven-Brookvue skilled-nursing facility in San Pablo, California, broke into knowing smiles. The 88-year-old widow was hardly the facility's easiest patient. She chided her nurses for taking too many breaks. She scolded her speech therapist for asking repetitive, nosy questions about the Johnson family tree. And when a well-meaning therapist took Belva into a model kitchen and asked her to reach for food on the top shelf as a stretching exercise, the small patient in the light-brown housecoat quickly dismissed such foolishness. "I don't keep any food on the top shelf in *my* kitchen," Johnson declared. "I haven't had anything there in 10 or 15 years. I took it all down. I didn't like reaching for it. I don't stretch for it in my home, and I'm not going to stretch here."

For all her fussy, headstrong ways, Belva Johnson was one of Hillhaven's major successes. When she arrived at the skilled-nursing facility in early October, she had just been discharged from an acute-care hospital after suffering a major stroke. Her right foot was bent and hard to move. Her right arm wasn't responsive; it would flap aimlessly when she tried to move it. Her slurred speech would tail off in midsentence; her usually strong memory was disorganized. Beyond those stroke-related problems, she also suffered from a bladder infection, a heart condition, and severe deterioration of her right hip. In those first days at Hillhaven, her children feared she would never leave the nursing facility alive.

Gradually Hillhaven's therapists helped Johnson mend. By December her strength and balance had improved enough that she could take short walks along the corridors accompanied by a relative or an aide. Her bladder infection cleared up; her heart and hip problems stabilized. She regained enough control of her right arm and hand to sign her name with difficulty. Her memory lapses became less severe — she knew she had two grandsons named Larry, though she couldn't always tell them apart. After three months at Hillhaven she was ready to go home and enjoy her garden, her own bed, and her sensibly designed kitchen. The medical crisis had left her much frailer, but Johnson stubbornly believed she could overcome more of the stroke's damage. When she reluctantly sold her 1968 Mercury sedan to one of her grandsons for $200, she made him promise that if she improved enough to drive again, she could reclaim the car.

Belva Johnson's recovery could have been a showcase example of her HMO's willingness to stand by its older members during a costly illness. It wasn't. At a crucial stage in her recovery, her HMO denied coverage for further treatment, even though conventional Medicare would have continued to pay. Only by hurriedly plucking their mother out of managed care could her children avoid what they viewed as a looming medical or financial catastrophe.

Like millions of Americans age 65 and over, Johnson belonged to a Medicare HMO, a managed-care health plan for older people. She had signed up with Health Net, the big California HMO that was part of Health Systems International. "Members receive high quality, appropriate and cost-effective managed care," Health Net's brochures promised. That slogan seemed apt during Johnson's first few years with the HMO, when she needed little care and generally liked what the plan provided. Even after she had her stroke in late September 1994, Health Net paid for her brief hospitalization and approved the transfer to Hillhaven for her recovery. Then came an unexpected jolt. After Johnson had been at Hillhaven for less than 20 days, the HMO sent a messenger to her bedside with a stiff, two-page letter that amounted to a nursing-home eviction notice. "Health Net has determined that the care you are receiving at Hillhaven-Brookvue no longer meets Medicare guidelines or Health Net Senior Security guidelines," the letter stated. "If you remain in the skilled nursing facility, you will be responsible for all services provided to you by that facility after October 25, 1994."

When Johnson's children found out about Health Net's letter, they seethed. "Mother was helpless at the time," recalled Marilyn Blackwood, Johnson's oldest daughter. "She needed round-the-clock care. She couldn't get up to go to the bathroom by herself. She could hardly talk. She couldn't eat by herself. She wasn't sleeping well. All of her children were willing to do certain things to help her. But we couldn't figure out anyone who could stay with her day and night. If we'd taken her home, it would have been unthinkable." Health Net did tell the family that they could appeal its denial of coverage, but the process could take weeks, even months. Although the Johnsons eventually filed appeals, they believed they needed a different strategy to deal with their mother's immediate needs.

Two of Belva Johnson's five children visited Hillhaven to plead the family's case, in hopes that the nursing home could then sway the HMO. Fifty-seven-year-old Richard Johnson, the angriest member of the family, confronted his mother's care team in the nursing-home lobby. "She needs medical care!" he declared. "Is there anyone here who can tell me that she's ready to go home?" A long silence greeted him. "Well," he muttered, "I guess this is all about money, and not about health care." No one argued the point, he later recalled; Hillhaven officials simply asked him what he proposed to do.

Richard declared that if Health Net wouldn't pay for his mother's further care, her family would. Hillhaven officials told him to check their daily rates before making such a promise. The skilled-nursing facility charged $700 a day for private patients getting full therapy (though it offered discounted prices of about $420 a day to patients with Medicare or HMO insurance coverage). At those rates, the Johnson children realized, they could pay for a week or two of further care. An extended stay would devastate them.

While the family debated their next move, a Hillhaven nurse gently interrupted them. "You can get your mother out of the HMO and back on regular Medicare," the nurse whispered. "If you do that, 80 percent of the bill will be covered." That murmured advice turned out to be a godsend. The Johnsons kept their mother in Hillhaven but quickly disenrolled her from Health Net. Then they reinstated her in conventional Medicare, the federal health insurance program for older Americans. The switchover had its costs; Hillhaven later billed Belva Johnson for $6,202 of copayments on Medicare bills incurred after she left Health Net. Even so, the change allowed Johnson to have 93 days of covered care rather than the 20 days her HMO had offered. For that reason the Johnson children regarded their flight from managed care as the wisest thing they could have done. As Marilyn put it, "It got us out of a very desperate situation."

As advancing years take their toll, millions of older Americans and their families will face similar situations. The diseases of old age seldom do their damage in one overwhelming assault; instead, chronic conditions wear down a person over time. Hips or knees fail. Diabetes, cancer, stroke, or congestive heart failure work in their malevolent ways. Modern medicine isn't powerless in the face of these dread diseases; it can do a great deal to slow down, stall, or even reverse the damage. But as people become older and frailer, patients and their care teams must decide how much treatment is justified. Society must determine who will pay for it.

With the rise of managed care, a new paradigm has taken hold. Doctors are encouraged to catch diseases of the elderly early, to promote better diets and exercise, and to keep older members well. That approach produces many happy, healthy 68-year-olds who feel well served by their HMO. When patients grow older and chronic diseases become more severe, however, HMOs may be tempted to shorten treatment and stop struggling so hard to retard the course of aging. Definitions of "medical necessity" become more stringent, and treatment that fails those tests isn't approved for coverage. Patients in their 70s and 80s are stunned and angry to find their medical plan backing away as their health worsens. In such cases elderly members and their families may feel abandoned in the final rounds of a hard fight with impending decline and death.

The enactment of Medicare in 1965 drastically changed the nation's approach to caring for the elderly. Until that time older Americans were regarded as largely uninsurable. Their medical needs were vast, their incomes were puny, and the few private insurance plans available were prohibitively priced. If older people got sick, they drained down their savings, pleaded with their children for financial support, or simply died in poverty. Then came government-paid health coverage for everyone age 65 and over. "No longer will older Americans be denied the healing miracle of modern medicine," declared President Lyndon

Johnson as he signed Medicare into law. "No longer will illness crush and destroy the savings that they have so carefully put away over a lifetime so that they might enjoy dignity in their later years. No longer will young families see their own incomes and their own hopes eaten away, simply because they are carrying out their deep moral obligations to their parents."

Medicare started out as a big piece of Johnson's Great Society — a $3.1 billion-a-year program covering 19 million people — and quickly grew. Today it is a $190 billion government program covering 33 million elderly people and another five million disabled. Conventional Medicare picks up most hospital bills and 80 percent of doctors' bills, provided that participants have a small amount (known as the Part B premium) deducted monthly from their Social Security checks. They have essentially unlimited freedom to pick doctors and hospitals; they also have to fill out complex forms associated with copayments, deductibles, and government-mandated fee schedules. In the past 15 years exploding health costs have led many Medicare recipients to buy supplemental private insurance as well. Those plans, known as Medigap policies, can cost as much as $300 a month. American attitudes toward the Medicare program are profoundly ambivalent; people cherish its broad coverage but chafe at its bureaucracy and cost.

In the early 1980s a managed-care version of Medicare took shape. Not many people wanted it at first. But HMOs kept pressing, and by now they can offer plans that in many ways seem like better versions of Medicare. Older Americans can opt out of conventional Medicare and join a local HMO instead. Those who do so can use only the HMO network's doctors and hospitals and must abide by the health plan's determination of how much care is medically necessary. In return the HMO offers more generous benefits packages and much less paperwork than regular Medicare. Hospital bills and lab tests are covered in full, without the sizable deductibles that have become part of regular Medicare. Prescription drugs for nonhospitalized patients are covered at least in part; regular Medicare offers no such coverage. Some HMOs even offer vision care, health-club memberships, and free annual physical exams. Members usually can get all this without having to pay a supplemental, Medigap-style premium; all they need to do is let the HMO collect the approximately $45-a-month Part B premiums that normally would go to the federal government.

To pay for all these benefits, HMOs turn to the sugar daddy of the regular Medicare program: the federal government. Under a complex formula, federal authorities give managed-care plans about $400 a month, on average, for each elderly person signed up in a Medicare HMO. Reimbursement rates vary a bit by members' county of residence, age, and a few other factors, but those variations don't fully reflect patients' medical conditions.* In this system HMOs can pocket the unspent money if members stay healthy. But if they fall sick, the health plans are expected to pay for all necessary care. They can't draw a nickel more for their sickest members, even if a patient's bills run to $50,000, $100,000, or more.

In a reprise of their tremendous success wooing corporate employers, HMOs chalked up huge enrollment gains among the elderly. Some four million older Americans belonged to Medicare HMOs in mid-1996, with membership growing 20 percent annually. Most recruiting begins with newspaper ads or mass mailings, followed by face-to-face "information seminars" at shopping malls or restaurants. In their marketing, HMOs use the same strategy that has attracted working-age members: they sell wellness. Brochures show silver-haired men and women riding mountain bikes, taking tap-dancing classes, or hauling groceries up a flight of stairs. Once senior citizens join a Medicare HMO, they can look forward to members' magazines with upbeat articles such as "How to Choose Your Cruise" and "Don't Write off Sex after Sixty." Those enticements aren't just smooth salesmanship, HMO executives maintain. They are an effort to help people 65 and over make the most of their retirement years. "Our mission is to keep people well," says William Osheroff, medical director of a leading Medicare HMO in California, the Secure Horizons division of PacifiCare.

The fact is, most people over 65 don't need a lot of medical care. In 1993 the healthiest 90 percent of the elderly incurred Medicare bills that averaged just $1,430 per person. (Their own out-of-pocket spending totaled perhaps $1,000 more.) For such people HMOs offer an appealing mix of convenience, fringe benefits, and good care. Studies show that Medicare HMO members are more likely to get timely

---

*HMO actuaries have learned to target the most profitable payment groups, such as women in their 70s in southern Florida. Federal officials have repeatedly said that their payment formula needs improvement, but they have yet to agree on a better method.

screenings for breast cancer, prostate cancer, and other malignancies. These tests can detect disease early, when cure rates are highest.

Eventually, though, almost every elderly patient confronts a medical crisis. Some of these involve high-tech rescues: replacing a worn-out knee, fixing an ailing heart in the operating room, or treating cancer through a mix of surgery, radiation, and chemotherapy. Other cases involve long hospital stays or rehabilitative care, where the goal is not so much to cure disease as it is to forestall further decline. Such care can be stunningly expensive. In 1993 the sickest 10 percent of Medicare members ran up average bills of $28,000, nearly 20 times the per-person cost of their healthier peers.

That huge schism presents Medicare HMOs with their toughest challenge: how to handle truly sick patients who become money-losers under the federal reimbursement system. Ultimately, these health plans have only three possible strategies. They can try to avoid signing up the frail elderly at all. Or they can pay for all the medical care that these patients need and absorb the financial loss with premiums from healthy members. Finally — the most alluring and most controversial choice — health plans can spend a lot less money on the very sick.

Any blatant attempt to follow the first strategy, refusing to enroll frail elders, is against federal law. Medicare HMOs do come up with ingenious ways to tilt their recruitment of new members toward the healthy. Sales representatives do most of their pitches in malls and restaurants that are hard for the infirm to get to. Orientation meetings sometimes are held in second-floor conference rooms accessible only to people who can climb a flight of stairs. Over time, though, even the most artful efforts to pack an HMO with healthy people will come undone. Aging will inevitably turn some robust members into frail patients in need of hefty care.

The second choice, spending generously on the very sick, is problematic. If HMOs pay out too much, they go broke. Most Medicare HMOs try to concentrate their big outlays on clearly lifesaving treatments with predictable costs. Harvard Pilgrim Health Care, for example, helped a 73-year-old bicycling enthusiast beat back three mortal illnesses by paying for prostate surgery, a hip replacement, and multiple angioplasties. The proud HMO put the man's story in its 1994 annual report. A few such generous payouts make an insurer look good. They also are financially sound as long as premiums from healthy members cover the expenses. But HMOs can't allow their ledgers to be overburdened with costly cases. Somewhere along the way they need to save money.

Federal authorities are supposed to watch out for evidence of managed-care skimping, though it is arguable how well this is done. The government's own watchdog agency, the General Accounting Office, concluded in an August 1995 report that "quality assurance reviews aren't comprehensive, enforcement actions are weak, and the appeals process is slow." Medicare HMO members do have the right to demand federal review of a coverage dispute. But they first must exhaust their appeals rights within the HMO, a process that can take six months or longer. Even so, about 3,000 Medicare HMO members each year formally submit their grievances to federal regulators. These complaints allege that HMOs have unjustly refused to pay for anything from a specialist consultation to a multiweek stay in a hospital. Independent reviewers at Network Design Group, a company in Pittsford, New York, rule in patients' favor about 40 percent of the time, ordering HMOs to pay out an extra $3 million to $8 million each year.

As busy as this "appeals court" is, it hears only a fraction of elderly HMO members' concerns. Federal overseers in June 1995 reported that one quarter of all Medicare HMO members didn't know they had the right to appeal. Even if members want to press a grievance, federal review applies only to coverage denials and payment disputes. It can't handle allegations of substandard care. And the long appeals process thwarts many patients whose medical decisions can't wait that long. As a result, many elderly patients unhappy with an HMO simply decide to disenroll and rejoin conventional Medicare — much as Belva Johnson did. Government rules make it easy to switch: it can be done on the first of every month with just a few days' notice. But while disenrollments solve patients' immediate problems, they don't put pressure on managed-care plans to be more responsive to their members. If anything, Medicare HMOs gain when a costly, potentially money-losing member drops out.

In Belva Johnson's case, an appeal via the Medicare review system yielded nothing. Network Design Group in 1995 ruled that the elderly woman's HMO wasn't obligated to cover her Medicare copayments, though the health plan in early 1996 finally did pick up those costs after repeated media inquiries about the case. Health Net officials generally defended their handling of the case, suggesting that the Johnson family could have pursued its appeal rights within Health Net faster if it had wanted to. "A lot of the issues in this case don't have anything to do with sound care of the patient," remarked Sylvia Seamand, a Health Net vice president in charge of the HMO's Medicare program, in a June 1996 interview.

While Medicare HMOs generally get high marks in academic studies for their quality of care, there are some disturbing gaps. In an assessment of 800 stroke patients, the health-care consulting firm Mathematica found that Medicare HMO members were discharged from hospitals quicker and sicker than a control group in fee-for-service Medicare. Hospital stays for the HMO members averaged 8.6 days, two days less than for the control group, even though the HMO patients at discharge had more trouble talking, seeing clearly, or moving their arms and legs. The HMO patients also were most likely to be sent straight home or to limited-care nursing homes instead of to rehabilitation hospitals, which cost more and work hard to help people recover. The Mathematica study, published in 1993, didn't attempt to follow patients' outcomes over the long run. In a report to federal overseers of Medicare, however, Mathematica warned that its findings raised "concern about the quality of care provided in HMOs."

In late 1995 California officials began investigating PacifiCare, the largest operator of Medicare HMOs, with about 500,000 members nationwide. PacifiCare tried to block investigators from the state's Department of Corporations from photocopying medical records pertaining to hundreds of member complaints. But a California state judge ruled that the HMO had to divulge records in 188 cases. Some of those cases soon entered the public record — and they painted a grisly picture of medical tragedies involving elderly patients with strokes, cancer, and heart disease.

Because PacifiCare contracts with independent doctors, hospitals, and nursing homes, most of the complaints centered on alleged failings of those caregivers, with the HMO's policies figuring only partly in the problems. In such cases HMOs often argue that patients' complaints should be seen as allegations of bad medicine that could arise in any setting — managed care or fee-for-service — rather than as a specific indictment of HMO policies. But California regulators weren't so sure. Any managed-care plan must decide which providers it wants in its network and which it doesn't want. When members sign up for a health plan, they count on the HMO to have selected high-quality doctors and hospitals. For such reasons, a spokesman for the Department of Corporations said, "Our overriding sense was that we needed to look at PacifiCare."

One of the most anguished complaints came from Norma Pappas of Glendora, California, regarding the treatment of her late husband, Gus. "My husband was not treated like a human being" in his final months of life, she declared. Her worst moment came in April 1995, when he was discharged from a PacifiCare-network hospital after a four-day stay for congestive heart failure. As she told state investigators, "I went to pick him up and I found him in a room all by himself. He was hooked up to a catheter, and I found he was bleeding. . . . He was a physical mess. I helped him to the bathroom. When he exited the bathroom, he was bleeding and the nurse told me I had to take him home, despite the fact that he was bleeding and still suffering from dementia." After various arguments with hospital officials, Gus Pappas was allowed to stay in the local hospital one more day and then was transferred to a Veteran's Administration hospital. Three months later he died. In her formal complaint Norma Pappas cited a host of concerns; she said her husband had not been approved for referral to a cardiologist in December 1994, and in two instances in 1994 when hospitals had admitted him, they had quickly discharged him during his losing fight with heart disease.

Other allegations of premature hospital discharge made their way into California regulators' files. One case involved Raymond Davia, a frail 84-year-old PacifiCare member with kidney disease, who underwent hip surgery in December 1993 at Antelope Valley Hospital in Lancaster, California. Three days after the operation doctors decided to transfer him to a skilled-nursing facility, a cheaper, less intensive institution where patients are sent to complete their recovery. In a formal complaint filed with the state, his daughter, Anne Breck, recalled, "I objected to the transfer of my father because his medical condition was unstable. I was told by [a managed-care case manager] that she would not authorize my father to spend one more night at Antelope Valley Hospital because it was costing $1,000 a day. . . . My father was then transferred on December 8, 1993, with my consent, only after I was assured that all medical care would continue."

Less than a month later, Davia was dead. In her complaint Breck alleged that "poor medical care . . . caused my father's death." At one stage, she asserted, nurses at the skilled-nursing facility were unable to locate the doctor who was supposed to be treating her father. At another juncture, she alleged, tests of her father's kidney function weren't performed, even though she asked that they be done. Breck later asked an independent physician, William Alton, to review the case; he declared that "Mr. Davia was allowed to deteriorate to such a degree that he was essentially nonsalvageable" when he was finally readmitted to Antelope Valley Hospital a few days before his death.

PacifiCare executives declined to talk to reporters about specific events in those cases, citing patient confidentiality. HMO officials did suggest, though, that any mistakes that might have been made weren't part of the HMO's usual treatment of elderly members. "Our philosophy is to get people the right care at the right time," explained Sam Ho, a PacifiCare medical director. "Historically, there has been overutilization in fee-for-service medicine. That means that appropriate treatment may involve less use of acute-care hospitals. But if people need to be in an acute-care hospital, that's where they will be." PacifiCare also said that it tried to ensure that sick members were sent only to high-grade facilities. If quality-of-care problems occurred, Dr. Ho said, the HMO had been known to stop using a facility or to demand corrective measures in the future. He wouldn't say whether the HMO took any action in regard to the institutions involved in the Pappas and Davia cases.

In moderation, the cost-saving strategy of trimming hospital stays for the elderly can be sound medicine. Even conventional Medicare has rejiggered its reimbursement system several times since 1983 to promote briefer hospital stays. As patients gradually recover, experts believe, they can be treated in increasingly cheaper, less intensive settings. Elderly patients might move from a $1,000-a-day acute-care hospital to a $600-a-day rehabilitation hospital, to a $400-a-day skilled-nursing facility, and then to a $150-a-day nursing home. Further steps might include home-care visits at $40 apiece or self-care at no cost at all. Done properly, this approach can wisely combine good medicine and thrift.

PacifiCare, however, has taken its crusade to shrink hospital stays to remarkable lengths. In presentations to Wall Street analysts, company executives displayed two bar charts showing annual hospital days, first for conventional Medicare, then for PacifiCare's HMOs. Groups of 1,000 elderly enrollees in conventional Medicare totaled about 2,600 days a year; PacifiCare's tallies were 1,300 and lower.

Securities analysts and big investors kept urging PacifiCare to short-
en hospital stays even more — in the belief that fewer hospital days
meant "better" medical management, at least from Wall Street's perspective.

Once elderly patients are discharged from acute-care hospitals,
HMOs aren't done trying to save money. They also take a hard look at
the amount of home care and rehabilitative services provided to those
patients. Case managers are especially likely to take a tough line in
situations where continued therapy isn't yielding much improvement.
Officially, HMOs and conventional Medicare are supposed to apply
exactly the same standards in deciding when to cover rehabilitative
services and when to disallow them. The key test involves evidence of
"steady and meaningful improvement." In actual cases, though, many
therapists believe that a double standard applies. Rules are interpreted
leniently in regular Medicare and much more strictly in HMOs.

HMOs started out with an opportunity to end some undeniably
wasteful practices. "We used to have a blank check to do what we
wanted, and to take as long as we felt was necessary," says David
Powers, head of rehabilitative services at UCLA. "Now we have to
think faster. It turns out that a lot of things that I thought patients
needed, they really don't." On the East Coast managed-care pressure
has led some intermediate-care facilities to start providing inpatient
therapy on Saturdays and Sundays so that patients can be discharged
faster. Until HMOs squawked, those centers billed insurers for seven-
day-a-week care even though therapists worked only Monday through
Friday. "It's more of a staffing challenge for us, but it's a reasonable
thing to ask," says Mel Hecht, medical director of a rehabilitation
center in Cambridge, Massachusetts.

Even so, HMOs' crackdown on waste can squeeze too hard. A
1993 survey by the Medicare Advocacy Project in Los Angeles found
that 68 percent of hospital social workers had trouble getting home
health care, durable medical equipment, or physical therapy approved
for HMO members. When coverage was allowed, the social workers
added, approval came only after a protracted fight. In Brockton, Massachusetts, physical therapist Rhonda Meyer reports that HMOs often
allow her only one course of treatment in an elderly patient's lifetime to
resolve a problem such as shoulder pain related to arthritis. That has
hampered her ability to treat ailments that flare up and then subside,
she says. In fee-for-service Medicare, she observes, patients get $900 a

year of coverage for outpatient physical therapy, allowing them to get multiple rounds of treatment for chronic ailments.

In a landmark dispute, a 71-year-old Arizona woman, Gregoria Grijalva, spent most of 1993 trying to battle both the ravages of diabetes and the coverage restrictions imposed by her health plan, FHP International. Then she and her family got mad enough to sue.

The breaking point came in the fall of 1993, after Grijalva had finished an 18-day stay in a hospital and a nursing home for complications related to a blood clot. She was discharged with a catheter in place because she didn't have urinary control. According to her suit, FHP sent her home "without making any arrangements for home care for Ms. Grijalva or instructing her family in the care of the catheter. Her family repeatedly requested home health services for Ms. Grijalva, and her physician, Dr. Gomez, attempted without success to obtain FHP approval of home health services for her." As Grijalva's son Ed later explained, "We want to care for her ourselves, but we're not skilled. We're not doctors or nurses. That's not our training."

In pressing the suit, Grijalva's attorney, Sally Wilson, chose an unexpected target. Her client's immediate complaint was with FHP. But Wilson, who has handled numerous elderly-rights cases, became convinced that the root of the problem was the slow, timid federal system for handling Medicare HMO members' grievances. Until that system worked better, Wilson believed, countless others would face delays and denials getting the care they needed. So in November 1993 Wilson filed a class-action suit against the federal government, demanding that the grievance process be speeded up. Wilson alleged that "denials of needed services by Medicare-participating HMOs are so widespread as to constitute a pattern and practice of abuse." Her claim initially was based only on examples of alleged undercare in Arizona, but other lawyers later added a dozen patient cases involving California and Oregon HMOs. Federal officials disputed the allegations and moved for dismissal of the case, known as *Grijalva v. Shalala*. Some two and a half years after the suit was filed both sides were engaged in settlement talks and other pretrial maneuverings.

In the suit Wilson told of five other FHP patients in Arizona who, she believed, hadn't received adequate care. They included a 74-year-old man trying to regain strength after knee-replacement surgery, an 83-year-old woman recovering from a broken back, an 86-year-old woman recuperating from pneumonia, and a 92-year-old woman with

Alzheimer's disease who had undergone hip surgery. In each case, Wilson contended, FHP provided less therapy, home care, or nursing-home coverage than its sick members should have received.

Wilson saved her harshest words for a case involving 68-year-old Beatrice Bennett, who had suffered a stroke that left her paralyzed and unable to speak. The woman was hospitalized for two weeks, then sent to a nursing home chosen by FHP. The suit asserted:

> During the initial phase of her nursing home stay, Ms. Bennett's daughter was forced to repeatedly demand needed services such as speech and physical therapy that FHP was not providing to her mother. . . . Although FHP eventually reimbursed Ms. Bennett for her nursing home care, she remains unable to speak or walk. If she had continued to receive speech and physical therapy following her stroke, she might have had a more complete recovery.

Such hard-luck stories carried little weight with FHP. "Families sometimes have a great deal of trouble accepting that Mom or Dad isn't going to be as good as new," remarked Jodi Horton, a spokeswoman for the HMO. "It's very easy to blame the system for a fact of life: when something is broken, it's very hard to fix it." FHP officials in March 1996 refused to answer any specific questions about the cases cited in the *Grijalva* suit because the matter was being litigated. Speaking generally, Horton said, "If the medical community believes that progress is not being made, even in a perfect world, that's what we have to go by. We would not have reached the excellent position that we hold if we were withholding care."

A government-commissioned study bolsters the theory that Medicare HMOs sometimes hew to a tighter definition of medical necessity than the rest of the geriatric-care community. The study analyzed the level of at-home therapy provided to 1,632 elderly patients after their discharge from the hospital. The analysis was conducted in 1994 by the Center for Health Policy Research in Denver at the request of the Health Care Financing Administration, the federal agency that oversees Medicare.

Researchers found that HMOs handled their home-care patients faster, cheaper — and less effectively than conventional Medicare did. HMOs on average spent $877 per case to provide patients with 12.7 home-care visits after hospitalization. Conventional Medicare spent significantly more money, $1,305 per case, and approved far more visits, 18.8 on average. Those patients ended up with "significantly more favorable outcomes," according to the study's lead researcher, Peter Shaughnessy. When treatment was finished, patients in regular Medicare were more likely to be able to feed themselves, perform toilet functions on their own, manage their medications, and carry out necessary shopping. Shaughnessy concluded, "HMOs tend to approach some aspects of home health care with more of a maintenance philosophy rather than a rehabilitative/restorative philosophy."

So far, neither HMOs nor conventional Medicare have extended much coverage for the huge costs associated with a long stay in a custodial nursing home. Conventional Medicare will pay for 100 days a year of institutionalized skilled-nursing care — but that is meant only to cover patients recovering from strokes, heart attacks, or other grave illnesses, who need considerable therapy almost every day. For the frail elderly who don't need intensive medical attention but simply aren't able to live independently anymore, regular Medicare and its HMO cousins offer little. Some private insurance companies offer long-term care insurance, but they have found few customers.* As a result, many older people must draw down their savings to pay for a prolonged stay in a nursing home. Once their assets have declined to the national poverty level, they qualify for Medicaid, the federal-state program of medical coverage for the poor, which does pay for nursing home stays. Senior citizens' lobbyists and many health economists have urged that the United States seek a more comprehensive method of funding long-term nursing care. But with such care costing more than $70 billion a year, even the most generous-minded managed-care companies haven't considered adding custodial nursing-home coverage as a benefit.

For every person, there eventually comes a point where medicine can no longer rehabilitate or even maintain life to any meaningful degree. Patients and their families hope at that stage for what surgeon/author Sherwin Nuland calls "the good death," a quick, relatively painless, dignified end to life. As Dr. Nuland observes, the good death is for many people a myth, rendered impossible by "a series of

---

*Younger people, who can afford the premiums, aren't interested. Older people, who are interested, generally can't afford the much higher premiums for their age brackets.

destructive events that involve by their very nature the disintegration of the dying person's humanity." The challenges posed for patients, family members, and doctors are immense. Even medical ethicists are hard-pressed to offer clear guidelines about when to keep trying and when to give up.

In these dilemmas, managed-care companies sometimes neglect the most important element in handling terminal illness: compassion. HMO reviewers and medical directors can analyze the costs of further care as well as the inevitable medical outcome. HMO employees can see ways to save money, either by cutting back on heroic treatment or by transferring a dying patient out of a hospital and into a nursing home or hospice. Those steps may be what families and doctors eventually want to take, if the choices are presented to them in a sensitive way. But in a situation as emotionally charged as terminal illness, doctors and family members bristle if they believe that remote bureaucrats are pulling the plug on a dying person to save money. The wisest HMO case managers meet doctors and patients halfway, with open discussions of treatment choices and a willingness to adjust coverage formulas to suit the desires of the dying person and immediate family members. But in many cases, managed-care plans have approached terminal illness with a chilly business logic that has rankled or horrified the people closest to the patient. Inevitably, there have been lawsuits and grievances.

In San Francisco, Medicare-rights attorney Lenore Gerard has challenged two HMOs about their handling of elderly patients who suffered massive, ultimately fatal strokes. In one instance an 89-year-old man was so incapacitated by a stroke in late 1993 that the local probate court had to appoint a conservator for the patient and his estate. In such cases, no amount of medical care is likely to undo the stroke's devastation. Nonetheless, Gerard became concerned that the patient's HMO was trying to provide him with far less care than he was entitled to have. HMO officials had attempted to terminate nursing-home coverage after one week. Under conventional Medicare he would have been entitled to 100 days of coverage.

In southern California, Patricia Sloan's final year of life showed how hard it can be to combine a dying person's wishes with the protocols of managed care. The 73-year-old had an advanced case of chronic obstructive pulmonary disease — a breakdown of lung function that ultimately makes breathing impossible and leads to death. As her daughter, Tricia Reis, later recounted, "We knew that my mother's condition was terminal." In October 1993, while visiting her daughter in the northern suburbs of San Diego, Sloan's disease worsened. She was hospitalized and placed on a ventilator that let her breathe. After a month's hospital stay, the case reached a crossroads: where should the patient go next?

For Sloan and her doctor, the choice was clear. They wanted a transfer to an acute rehabilitation hospital, which would try to wean the elderly woman from her ventilator so that she could once again breathe unaided. Even though Sloan's condition was incurable, she still was alert, able to communicate and to walk about somewhat. Sloan and her family wanted one more all-out try at a partial recovery, even if the gains might last for only a few weeks or months. But her HMO, Inter Valley Health Plan, had other ideas. According to a federal suit later filed in the case, "authorization for Ms. Sloan to be transferred to an acute rehabilitation facility was repeatedly denied by her HMO." Instead, the suit alleged, Inter Valley pushed for transfer to a nursing home 90 miles away. That facility would have been cheaper but, the family believed, couldn't have weaned Sloan from her ventilator.

After the fact, Inter Valley medical director Alexander Bokor acknowledged in a phone interview that "the wheels of progress sometimes work a little slowly in getting things set up in an area that's not our service area." He said the HMO considered transferring Sloan to a less intensive facility, but "when it became clear that it couldn't handle her, we backed away. We didn't deny her anything."

Sloan and her family, however, believed that a cheaper transfer was imminent, and they fought it furiously. "My mother told me, 'If I'm forced to leave San Diego, I'm going to die,'" Reis later said. Mother and daughter hired an attorney in December 1993, who threatened to go to court and seek a temporary restraining order against the attempted transfer. Sloan also filed papers to disenroll from Inter Valley as of January 1, 1994, and switch to a different managed-care plan, FHP, that she thought would provide better care.

Eventually Sloan was discharged to a rehabilitation hospital in the San Diego area, with FHP taking charge of her case. Therapists briefly weaned her off the ventilator, but a relapse after a few weeks sent the elderly woman into the hospital again. At that point Sloan and her daughter decided that high-tech medicine had reached its limits. It was time to make arrangements for Sloan to come home, get simple care to minimize her pain, and live out her remaining time surrounded by family members. It took about two months for doctors, HMO administrators, and family members to agree on exactly how to achieve that goal. Ironically, HMO administrators were the quickest to accept the family's plans; it was the treating physicians who fought hardest for further medical care.

On July 31, 1994, Patricia Sloan died peacefully after spending her last three months in her daughter's house. "It was what my mother wanted," Reis recalled. "She was able to get around in a wheelchair. We had a passive mirror valve that allowed her to talk — and she was a real talker. A nursing home never would have encouraged that." Overall, Reis said, she felt very ambivalent about her family's dealings with managed-care plans during her mother's final decline. In her opinion FHP had handled the case fairly and Inter Valley had not. "If there's one thing we learned, it is that you do have options," Reis said. "Just because an insurance company says 'I'm not paying for it' doesn't mean that you can't make them pay for it."

Nearly a decade before HMOs became a major factor in caring for the elderly, medical ethicist Daniel Callahan wrote a controversial book entitled *Setting Limits,* in which he argued for a deliberate scaling back in certain areas of medical care for the very elderly. "Beyond the point of a natural life span," he wrote, "government should provide only the means necessary for the relief of suffering, not life-extending technology." In careful, measured language, Callahan tried to craft what he believed was a morally sound response to two national crises: the runaway costs of caring for the elderly and public recognition that high-tech medicine could now preserve the last ragged edges of life in a patient when death would be a relief. In such situations, he argued, society needed a framework that would let families and doctors call for an intelligent, humane end to life-prolonging care.

But Callahan recognized that callously set limits would be worse than no limits at all. As he declared partway through the book, "I would reiterate my objection to a rationing scheme that in the name of cost containment would cut back on life-saving care to the elderly without . . . some intrinsic benefit for the elderly themselves and some rich understanding of the place of old age in human life." Embedded in that comment were the two principles that managed-care HMO officials sometimes forget as they handle hard cases. Are managed-care principles being applied with a "rich understanding of the place of old age"? And are HMO decisions of "intrinsic benefit for the elderly themselves"?

For patients and families in the midst of bureaucratic struggles with a Medicare HMO, the answers sometimes sound like a chilly no. After Patricia Sloan died, her daughter could discuss the whole case calmly — except for the brushoffs that the two women encountered in December 1993 when trying to arrange a transfer to a rehabilitation hospital. As Tricia Reis put it, "You expect some compassion. You expect people to realize 'This is somebody's mother. It could be one of my parents.' But then you get these business people who simply say, 'We don't have to do this.' It's a shocker."

11

Poor Patients,
Shoddy Care

EVERY SUMMER RESEARCHERS from the University of Tennessee, Nashville, gather up their clipboards and fan out across the state, asking poor people how they view their health coverage. That survey took on special significance in 1994, the year that Tennessee first required poor people to sign up for managed care. Some 1.1 million people — one in every five Tennesseans — were steered overnight into HMOs or other managed-care organizations. Another 300,000 followed within a few months. The audacious new program, known as TennCare, superseded traditional Medicaid, the long-time federal-state program of free health care for the indigent. It also covered many thousands of low-paid workers who previously lacked any form of insurance.

The researchers expected to find some "adjustment problems" with the state's new system and the dozen private-sector HMOs that provided care under its umbrella. But the intensity of public anger and distrust surprised them. More than half the people who joined TennCare after being on traditional Medicaid thought their health care had deteriorated. Even among the previously uninsured, 10 percent said TennCare was worse than having no health coverage at all and relying on charity care offered by doctors and hospitals.

Nobody in state government ever asked Carrie Zotter to explain those results. She didn't have a master's degree in public health; she hadn't even finished high school. She was simply a 20-year-old rural mother on TennCare, trying to keep her baby daughter, Savanna, healthy during a brutally cold winter. But the Zotters' experiences in early 1996 encapsulated some of TennCare's most exasperating failings.

Trouble started in late January when Savanna Zotter was four days old and briefly stopped breathing. Frightened, Carrie Zotter called the local hospital's emergency room, identified herself as a TennCare member, and asked if she should bring in the baby. By that time Tennessee hospitals had learned the hard way that managed-care plans often didn't pay for noncrisis emergency visits. So, Carrie Zotter recalled, she was told to keep her baby at home and not worry: breathing cessation was "normal." A few minutes later, after talking with her husband and mother, Zotter decided she had been given dangerously bad advice. She and her husband bundled up the infant and drove to the hospital they had consulted earlier in the day, Athens General, a small-town facility about eight miles from their home. A doctor examined the baby and decided that she had a bladder infection; she was admitted for a weeklong stay. Savanna's infection could be devastating if ignored but would be easily treatable with intravenous antibiotics three times a day for the next 10 days.

Once the baby's condition had stabilized, pediatrician Iris Snider wanted to arrange for a home-care nurse to visit the Zotters' home and inject the final four days' doses of antibiotics. Such an arrangement would have been standard under traditional Medicaid. But TennCare didn't work that way. It required the Zotters to drive into town for each injection, saving the state money while moving more of the burden of care onto the family. The Zotters and their doctor weren't thrilled, but so far, at least, they could see the state's rationale.

Then it began to snow. Tennessee's back roads became so icy and treacherous that as the Zotters returned one evening from getting Savanna's 10 P.M. injection, their car couldn't climb the final hill back to their house. The parents had no choice but to bundle up their 10-day-old girl and carry her the last quarter mile home in a blizzard. The next morning they had to repeat the ordeal, walking down to the bottom of the hill, unlocking their abandoned car, and driving into town. The Zotters tried to find someone at their managed-care company who could bend the rules and approve some home nursing visits. But rules were rules. Relief didn't come until the Zotters' pediatrician, Dr. Snider, heard about the family's problems, got angry — and wrote her own rules. The doctor arranged for an ambulance to take

Savanna to Athens General so that the baby could be admitted for a further overnight stay. That guaranteed the baby a warm, dry place in which to battle her illness. A few days later the life-threatening infection cleared up.

As Carrie Zotter and her pediatrician saw it, the baby survived a scary infection not because of TennCare but in spite of it. Managed care hadn't improved the baby's initial care and early diagnosis; it had nearly blocked timely treatment in the emergency room. Managed care hadn't promoted safe treatment; its rules put a sick infant at risk during a snowstorm. Managed care hadn't even been cost-effective. Because of the health plan's refusal to pay for home nursing visits in a crisis — at about $80 apiece — the cost had mushroomed to nearly $1,000 for hospital and ambulance. There was only one way that TennCare's architects could claim victory. The state system didn't have to pay any of the baby's major bills because the Zotters' managed-care plan had denied coverage. The ambulance ride and hospital stay would become ad hoc donations of services by Tennessee's medical community, unless the Zotters could scrape up the money themselves.

"We never had these kinds of problems with Medicaid," a peeved Carrie Zotter said when her baby finally was well again. She and her 23-year-old husband were trying to work their way out of poverty; he had taken double shifts at a carpet warehouse, hoping to save enough money to buy a small house. His job didn't provide any health insurance, so TennCare filled the gap. The state managed-care program was meant to take care of low-income working families. But to Carrie Zotter — and the doctors who treated her baby — the state's promises were a mirage.

"With TennCare, you have a problem finding a hospital that will see your kids," Carrie remarked. "You have a problem finding a doctor or a nurse that will see them. It is a real pain."

If managed care hadn't already existed, state governors would have wanted to invent it. By the early 1990s they faced intense budget pressures related to Medicaid. What had started as a small poverty-relief program in the mid-1960s — an afterthought to Lyndon Johnson's Great Society program — had turned into a $100 billion-a-year behemoth, growing nearly 20 percent a year. Unlike almost every other government health program, care for the poor wasn't fully funded by federal authorities. The *rules* for Medicaid were set in Washington:

how many people were entitled to coverage and what benefits they would get. But only part of the *money* for Medicaid was provided by federal authorities; states typically were liable for a third to half of the total costs. To their dismay, state budget analysts in the early 1990s discovered that traditional Medicaid — with almost no limits on patients' ability to get services — was about to overtake public education as the states' biggest expense. Something needed to be done. As former Tennessee finance commissioner David Manning said: "When you've got a tiny program growing 20 percent a year, that's a problem. When you've got a program that's one fifth of your budget growing 20 percent a year, that's a disaster."

From the lofty vantage of a governor's office, a managed-care solution looked enchanting. The escalating cost of Medicaid wasn't just bad government; it was a political liability. Middle-class voters wanted schools, roads, and police forces; they fumed at the fact that their state tax dollars were being consumed by Medicaid (particularly by unpopular items such as neonatal care for premature babies of drug-addicted mothers). Until 1993 managed care had been largely off-limits as a way to fix Medicaid, because regulators wanted to allow poor people a wide choice of doctors. Only Arizona and a handful of cities had won permission to put HMOs in charge of local Medicaid. The federal stance changed dramatically, however, when Bill Clinton, a former governor himself, became president in January 1993. Governors were invited to submit plans for statewide Medicaid HMOs; federal bureaucrats quickly waived traditional Medicaid rules to permit greater use of managed-care plans.

A stampede ensued. States, led by New York, California, Florida, Tennessee, and Oregon, moved 200,000 people a month into Medicaid managed-care plans. Expectations were that overall Medicaid spending growth would slacken to just 6 percent to 9 percent a year; per-capita outlays might actually drop. In the midst of this euphoria, state officials seldom questioned the money-saving tactics that the HMOs planned to use. There was a sunny assumption that any cost abatement would come from greater efficiency, with no curtailment of essential care. Health plans naturally encouraged this belief.

Too often, however, states have opened the door to managed neglect instead of managed care. Bureaucracy and profiteering have thrived, as have marketing scams and incompetent or just plain mean medical management. One small Medicaid HMO in Florida paid its top executives more than $1 million a year, yet seemed unable to keep track of how many children it immunized. Door-to-door marketers of Medicaid HMOs have been arrested or sued in a half-dozen states for alleged offenses ranging from intimidation of customers to forgery and bribery. Two tightfisted Tennessee HMOs ruled against the use of so many costly antibiotics that their doctors couldn't stop a small epidemic of a bowel infection; the physicians knew what drug to prescribe but — much like Peace Corps volunteers in a remote Third World village — they couldn't get it.

Managed care should be able to do a lot of good for the Medicaid population. Preventive medicine and preassigned personal physicians can greatly improve poor people's health while cutting down on expensive services such as emergency-room visits. Some of the best-run Medicaid HMOs, in fact, have delivered on that promise. These health plans have identified high-risk pregnant women and helped them bring healthy babies to term rather than delivering tiny "preemies" that can cost $100,000 or more to nurse to health. Leading Medicaid HMOs also have done a lot to improve the management of asthma, a common childhood illness. By giving parents cheap monitoring equipment that can readily detect breathing problems, HMOs have kept asthmatic children healthier and made it more likely that they will use basic medicine in a timely manner. That can greatly reduce the number of out-of-control episodes that lead to emergency-room visits and hospital stays.

Such bright spots are overshadowed by two chronic failings of Medicaid HMOs. The first is a tendency to bog down patient care in a web of rules and procedures that ultimately make it harder — not easier — for doctors and hospitals to practice good medicine. New members' HMO enrollment cards aren't processed on time. Their assignments to primary-care doctors are bungled. Calls to member-services phone lines are met with the tiresome *bonk, bonk, bonk* of busy signals. Those bureaucratic snafus may be simply the result of trying to cover too many new members too fast. Many Medicaid HMOs, however, are not rushing to fix these problems. Most Medicaid recipients don't have the poise and white-collar savvy to press complaints effectively; some don't even know that they are allowed to file complaints. Gridlock becomes a potent way to keep managed care's costs down, even if it does infuriate members.

Many Medicaid HMOs are also willing to take advantage of doctors and hospitals. When states put in managed-care programs for the poor, they typically cut medical pay scales but promise to pay more promptly and reliably. In practice, many Medicaid HMOs seize these discounts — and then look for ways to dodge the bills. Coverage approvals become so byzantine that doctors in a complicated case simply give up, deciding it is easier to finish treating the patient for free. Such tactics help squeeze more care out of a tight managed-care budget. But doctors feel exploited for their compassion, convinced that the health plans are pumping up their own earnings by selectively failing to honor payment contracts.

Some of the worst scandals have arisen in Florida. "Medicaid HMOs have made obscene profits and have not delivered the services they offered," state fraud investigator Mark Schlein testified at a legislative hearing in the Fort Lauderdale area in March 1995. Later that year Florida officials levied fines for rule violations against 12 of the 29 Medicaid HMOs operating in the state; some were unable even to produce records showing that essential care was delivered. "Everything is not great," remarked Doug Cook, head of the Florida Agency for Health Care Administration. "There are significant problems."

One Florida plan operating in the early 1990s became a legendary example of how not to serve the public interest. As investigative reporters for the *Fort Lauderdale Sun-Sentinel* found out, Better Health Plan in 1991 paid for its top executives to rent boats, visit Las Vegas, spend $6,000 on meals and entertainment, and lease two Mercedes-Benzes. Each of the Medicaid HMO's top executives earned more than $1 million that year, even though Better Health was a small plan with just 48,000 members and $38 million in revenue. The HMO members weren't nearly so lucky. When Medicaid auditors interviewed 360 plan members, they found that 55 percent were unhappy with the plan or didn't understand how it worked. A state auditor wrote, "With a few exceptions, it looks like the [Better Health] providers in the Tampa Bay area stink." The Medicaid HMO was sold to a bigger rival in early 1992 for $8.3 million; executives of the original plan have repeatedly declined to discuss their business practices.

Many other states have encountered problems nearly as bad. In the summer of 1995 New York health investigators posed as patients and called 18 of their state's largest Medicaid HMOs, asking for doctors' appointments. At 13 plans the investigators had such difficulties getting scheduled for prenatal care, babies' immunizations, or other services that those plans were officially rebuked for providing substandard care. HMO officials contended that the problems weren't as severe as they appeared and that steps were being taken to fix them. Nonetheless, the state's commissioner of health, Barbara DeBuono, a long-time fan of managed care, declared, "This industry has grown largely outside of a lot of oversight. It's time to look at the HMOs."

In Dayton, Ohio, Medicaid HMOs failed to provide adequate prenatal care for as many as 45 percent of women who gave birth in 1993. That rate was nearly four times worse than HMOs reported for their regular commercial members. Adults and children often didn't get the regular checkups that are a mainstay of good managed care; 15 percent of one Medicaid HMO's enrollees in the Dayton area hadn't seen a doctor in three years. In San Francisco a group of Vietnamese-Americans sued Foundation Health in state superior court in 1994, alleging that they were "misleadingly induced into enrolling" in a managed-care Medicaid plan. In two instances, the patients' lawyers alleged, Foundation's door-to-door marketers held up a tape recorder, asked questions in English that the Vietnamese-Americans didn't understand, and told them to respond "Yes" after each question. Foundation Health disputed the charges but later agreed to stop marketing its Medicaid HMOs in San Francisco.

Tennessee's story is a poignant mix of big promises, chaos, hard work, and grievous mistakes. Some of those who created TennCare insist that its successes eventually will outweigh the failures. Most observers, though, regard Tennessee's rush into Medicaid managed care as a classic case of too much too soon. During the bumpy first year of Tenn-Care, state planners created a medical quagmire stretching from the operating suites of Memphis's chief public hospital to the exam rooms of dozens of beleaguered country doctors in east Tennessee. Young children and their pediatricians were buffeted especially badly. Birth rates in Tennessee are highest among low-income women, so nearly half of all babies born in the state now receive their medical coverage through TennCare.

In perhaps the worst blunder, Tennessee officials naively assumed that a dozen new health plans wouldn't need much regulation because they would compete to deliver the best possible service. Only after a year of turmoil and outright fraud did the state start telling health plans more clearly what money-making tactics were allowed and which weren't.

Tennessee's push to do *something* about Medicaid was driven by budget numbers. When Democratic Governor Ned McWherter took office in 1987, Medicaid was a $1 billion-a-year program covering 507,000 people. By 1993 enrollment had doubled, and spending had nearly tripled. Dwindling federal support meant that Tennessee faced a fiscal crisis if Medicaid spending trends continued. During the winter of 1992–93 McWherter kept inviting a few key aides to the governor's mansion. They huddled in a dining nook next to his kitchen and asked, "What are we going to do?" Managed care looked like the answer. Tennessee already had moved 200,000 of its state employees into PPOs; that program was saving money and was palatable to workers. Besides, McWherter and his aides liked the idea of a market-driven health-care solution. They saw themselves as New Democrats, interested in the public good but skeptical of government programs. The governor's team expected that doctors wouldn't like the switch to managed care, but that didn't bother the political insiders. Most physicians voted Republican anyway; they weren't a key constituency.

In early April 1993, Governor McWherter pounced. Knowing that the state legislature was about to wrap up business in a few weeks, he rolled out the plan for TennCare in a stirring, dramatic speech to a joint session of the senate and house. Then he exhorted legislators to pass the bill — fast. "If we are brave enough to abandon a Medicaid system that has run its course," McWherter declared, "I offer you a Tennessee without limits."

McWherter's vision of TennCare was hugely ambitious. It aimed to cover not just 1,000,000 Medicaid recipients, but also as many as 700,000 working poor people who had no health insurance. While that second group wouldn't get free care, their premiums would be alluringly low, thanks to heavy state subsidies. The wide embrace of TennCare would halve the number of poor people who could not pay their medical bills and had to depend on charity care. Yet the firm discipline of managed care would hold spending growth to just 8.3 percent a year, an amount Tennessee could live with. McWherter's bill sped through the legislature in record time; TennCare quickly was written into law with a start-up date of January 1, 1994. McWherter was thrilled at his ability to ram through bold legislation — even as the

Clinton administration was involved in its long and ultimately futile effort to guide a national health plan through the U.S. Congress.

McWherter's triumph quickly turned into mass confusion. Mailings to Tennessee's Medicaid members in the autumn of 1993 tried to explain the new program, informing people about the 12 new managed-care plans they could join and asking them to choose one. But the mailings lacked the most important facts: lists of participating doctors. Physician contracts hadn't been signed yet, pending final approval of TennCare by federal authorities. Health plans weren't even sure which parts of the sprawling state they would serve.

Some 500,000 people tried to pick a health plan anyway, only to discover that their HMO might not have any doctors in their town. Many TennCare-eligible people among the working poor didn't join, waiting to see how it would work. Meanwhile 600,000 former Medicaid recipients who hadn't picked a managed-care plan were randomly assigned to one by the state. In TennCare's hands "random" took on grotesque new meanings. Mark Gaylord, a neonatologist in Knoxville, treated a woman with newborn twins just as TennCare began. State officials assigned each twin to a different health plan — and put the mother in a third.

State officials were so eager to enroll people in TennCare that they allowed the HMOs almost total latitude in their marketing pitches. In theory salesmen were supposed to explain the plans fully, allow all Medicaid-eligible people to join, practice no discrimination on the basis of health status, and avoid signing up ineligible people. But enforcement was spotty. And in some areas those rules were taken about as seriously as a "Don't Walk" sign in midtown Manhattan.

In the Memphis area OmniCare signed up 69,000 members with much better than average health. Much of its door-to-door marketing was guided by Coby Smith, a veteran political campaign worker, who coached OmniCare's sales representatives on how to canvass the city's public housing projects. As Smith later told the *New York Times,* his tips went as follows: "Knock on their doors. Be observant. If you see a physical problem, you don't need to sign those people. If you see someone who's very pregnant, you don't need to sign those people. If you see someone with eyes dilating, you don't need to sign those people. Do not create a risk situation for the company if you can help it."

Managed-care plans in general pursued healthy people, offering them free turkeys, credit cards, life insurance deals, and other perks.

TennCare officials originally regarded such gimmicks as benign. But critics pointed out that these giveaways amounted to a diversion of money meant for health care. In January 1995 — after 1.4 million people had joined TennCare — the state finally published marketing guidelines that barred such enticements.

In the anything-goes climate of TennCare's launch, HMOs were allowed to pay "per-head" commissions to door-to-door sales workers. That led one man to sign up prison inmates, who were already getting free health care through the correctional system. The marketer, a gym coach at Shelby County Correctional Facility, eventually was found guilty of mail fraud in connection with his submission of new-member lists to OmniCare. He was sent to jail for 14 months. He also was ordered to surrender $3,600 in commission checks from Omni-Care, which had paid him $18 per enrollee. OmniCare officials tried to dissociate themselves from the incident. Yet with the state paying HMOs an average of $106 per month for each new TennCare member enrolled, it was easy to see why the behind-bars crowd — who needed no care — looked alluring.

Such abuses happened in part because of the priorities set by state officials, who were concerned that the new system wouldn't attract enough managed-care companies. In 1992 Tennessee had only one Medicaid HMO, Access MedPlus, a well-regarded small plan serving 35,000 people in the Memphis area. State officials in early 1993 persuaded the largest commercial health insurer in Tennessee, Blue Cross/Blue Shield, to launch a Medicaid managed-care plan. "But we felt we needed competition," recalled David Manning, the state's finance director in 1993–94. Thus, the state went out of its way to make the $2.8 billion-a-year TennCare program appealing to health plans rather than maximizing consumer protection. Tennessee decided, for example, that it wouldn't require Medicaid plans to be federally certified. "We looked at it, but we felt we had to get that requirement removed," Manning later said. "All the hoops and restrictions involved would have severely limited the competition we wanted."

TennCare attracted a remarkable grab bag of managed-care plans. John Deere, the tractor company, created a Medicaid HMO; it won 38,000 members in its first year and was modestly profitable. Three university health systems tried to launch health plans but didn't do nearly so well. Those plans became magnets for hemophiliacs and other very sick people who used university hospitals; TennCare's reimbursement system didn't begin to cover the patients' costs, which in one instance reached $300,000 in a single month. Access MedPlus, Tennessee's pioneer in Medicaid managed care, made a strategic error: it tried to expand statewide without being well enough organized to keep track of its members' records and their bills. At its peak in early 1995, Access MedPlus had 300,000 members — and a mountain of complaints. Members couldn't get assigned to the right doctor; physicians weren't being paid. At the first opportunity to switch plans, more than 20,000 Access MedPlus members quit. In early 1996 the HMO's financial position became perilous; it won some breathing room only by negotiating a loan guarantee from a major Memphis hospital, which took seats on the HMO's board of directors.

Though Tennessee officials liked their cornucopia of health plans, federal overseers weren't nearly as impressed. Bruce Vladeck, head of the Health Care Financing Administration in Washington, gave TennCare the final go-ahead in November 1993, but expressed some doubts about the program, including concern that its budget wasn't sufficient. Without enough money in such a program, health experts say, there are only two ways to make ends meet. Managed-care plans will shortchange members on necessary care — or they will refuse to pay the doctors and hospitals who do the work. TennCare's health plans ultimately did a bit of both.

In dollar terms Tennessee's hospitals took the hardest blows. They were powerless to negotiate prices with the Medicaid HMOs, which controlled such a huge chunk of the population that they could set prices at will. Hospitals had no choice but to accept whatever discounts the HMOs decided were "fair," even if those prices didn't cover costs. A study by the consulting firm Ernst & Young found that TennCare's health plans typically covered only 45 percent of hospitals' charges, down from 85 percent in traditional Medicaid. That quickly translated into closures of multibed units within hospitals, layoffs of nurses, and deterioration in hospitals' credit ratings. "I'm worried," remarked a typical hospital chief executive, Ruckhard Welch of Claiborne County Hospital, in May 1995. "Anyone would be when they see their reimbursement base almost evaporate."

Particularly controversial was TennCare's impact on Tennessee's landmark public hospital, the 165-year-old Regional Medical Center in Memphis, known as the Med. State officials had expected TennCare to squeeze the Med's $200 million-a-year budget, and they originally regarded that as a good thing. Throughout the early 1990s, indigent care at the Med kept consuming an ever-larger share of state resources, with some huge bills for late-stage heroic treatment of people whose illnesses should have been caught and cured far sooner and more cheaply.

But if state officials expected that TennCare could gracefully shrink the Med's budget, they guessed wrong. As managed care took hold, hospital doctors invited journalists in to see how hard they worked, how desperately in need of care their patients were, and how hard it was to make ends meet under TennCare. "You add up the bureaucracies and the profits and you don't have to be a genius to see that they are taking money away from care at the bedside," trauma doctor Timothy Fabian told the *Dallas Morning News*. When the Med was forced to close two 20-bed units, its officials blamed TennCare for hurting patients' well-being. In early 1995 the Med sued Access Med-Plus, alleging that the Medicaid HMO had failed to pay for $39 million of care. A year later that case was still working its way through the courts.

Doctors' frustrations with TennCare were every bit as intense. The main doctors' group, the Tennessee Medical Association, filed suit in state court in late 1993, trying unsuccessfully to block implementation of TennCare on the grounds that it imposed unduly harsh payment terms on doctors. At the same time Felicito Fernando, a pediatrician in rural east Tennessee, began writing anguished letters to state legislators once the pay scales of managed-care companies were known. "TennCare threatens to cut my salary in half," Dr. Fernando wrote. "I have gone deeply into debt for the privilege of serving medically where I am needed. Sir, I cannot repay my student loans with a salary of $34,000 a year."

Once TennCare got started, doctors found that low pay scales were only half of the problem. Many managed-care plans fell badly behind in their claims processing, leaving physicians with unpaid bills for months. Access MedPlus at one point mailed out "interim" checks, with an apologetic note saying that its payments didn't cover the full amount of services owed but might help doctors with cash-flow problems. One physician with dozens of Access MedPlus patients got a check in mid-1994 for $3.94. "I don't know whether to cash it and spend it all at McDonald's or frame it on my wall," he wryly told colleagues.

Other doctors floundered in the face of coverage rules that required the HMO's preapproval of many costly treatments. The health plans promised quick reviews of doctors' requests, but often that didn't happen. Internal confusion at the managed-care plans made it hard for doctors to find out if an MRI, a specialist consultation, or even a simple surgery would be approved — or who might make that decision. Faced with sick patients who needed treatment fast, doctors sometimes gave up waiting for the HMO go-ahead. They simply treated the patient and wrote off the case as charity care. Phil Campbell, a hospital administrator in Etowah, a small Tennessee town near the North Carolina border, watched with sadness as local pediatricians kept helping children for free while TennCare plans dithered. "Pediatricians are very compassionate," he observed. "And it's hard to win in managed care if you're compassionate."

Consider Iris Snider, a pediatrician practicing in Athens, population 14,000. She grew up in Tennessee farm country; when she finished her medical training in Knoxville in 1971, she and her obstetrician husband eschewed the high-paying city jobs that attracted many of their classmates. Instead, they headed home to a peaceful Bible Belt district. Their county has more than 100 churches and no liquor stores or flashy restaurants. The tallest building in Athens is the three-story courthouse; once a year town officials thrill rural schoolchildren by letting them ride its elevator. In this bucolic setting Dr. Snider practices medicine the way her heart tells her: first treat the patient, then worry about payment.

"I don't do anything but pediatrics," explains Dr. Snider, a short, energetic woman in her early 50s with an abundance of mahogany red curls. "But if a sick mother brings her child in, I'll treat momma's throat too. Some of my patients need their ears washed out. Why pay $90 to go to a specialist? I'll fit them in for a fraction of what a specialist would charge."

In the eyes of the Medicaid managed-care plans, a soft-hearted physician like Dr. Snider might as well wear a sign that says "Exploit Me." During the first 24 months of TennCare's operation, she calculates, her two-doctor practice provided more than $100,000 of unpaid care. That wasn't deliberate. TennCare companies were supposed to reimburse her practice for almost all office visits, prescription drugs, and vaccines. But payments never showed up. Sometimes the managed-care companies couldn't match patients' records with their computer files. Other times they denied coverage for reasons that Dr. Snider couldn't fathom. On the van that she drives to work, Dr. Snider sports a bumper sticker that sums up her frustrations. It shows the official TennCare logo with a small word inserted in the middle, so that the sticker reads "Tenn *don't* Care."

While doctors grumbled, state officials tolerated a level of dishevelment in Medicaid HMOs that would have been deemed grossly unacceptable in the employer-funded market. The biggest TennCare plan, run by Blue Cross–Blue Shield, refused to pay for pediatric care of newborns until the infants had Social Security numbers — a process that can take months. Two of the HMOs that served Clarksville, about 30 miles northwest of Nashville, set up shop without having any network doctors in common specialties such as pediatric orthopedics. When children needed bone or joint surgery, their HMOs told them to look for a suitable doctor in the phone book.

TennCare officials asserted that the chaos was the result of starting a big managed-care system and would be short-lived. But that explanation didn't carry much weight with Rufus Clifford, Jr., a pediatrician working about 40 miles south of Nashville. Three Medicaid HMOs operated in his town, but two existed in name only; they lacked contracts with the local hospital or his pediatric clinic, the only one in the area. Yet TennCare kept assigning newborns to those HMOs. Parents didn't know where to turn for care; they implored local doctors to see their babies for free, outside the formal TennCare system. Doctors often relented, providing care that didn't cost the state a penny. But in Dr. Clifford's eyes, the clumsy workings of TennCare bureaucracy hurt his pocketbook and jeopardized the health of his town's little children.

When state officials enacted TennCare, they thought managed care would be most controversial in the rare cases of very sick patients wanting expensive, desperate treatments, where fiscal prudence said no and emotional arguments said yes. Those dilemmas did occur as expected, with TennCare plans having to decide whether to pay for liver transplants, extended physical therapy for children with cerebral palsy, and the like. Mixed in with those tough judgment calls, however, were outright blunders by health plans handling simple cases. In those instances badly thought-out HMO administration translated into substandard care.

TennCare's record on immunizations, for example, included some ugly steps backward. The state's overall immunization rate inched up slightly in TennCare's first year, to 80.8%, as more poor children began seeing doctors. That overall statistic masked some sizable drops in areas where managed-care plans failed to cover the cost of vaccinating infants against measles, mumps, rubella, diphtheria, pertussis, tetanus, and polio. State officials didn't aggressively police such problems; they simply assumed that pediatricians would dip into their own incomes to provide poor children with the full battery of vaccines regardless of payment tussles with managed-care plans. Some doctors did just that. Other pediatricians, however, cut back. After years of priding themselves on immunizing every child they could, these physicians started telling TennCare mothers that if they wanted their children vaccinated, they should find a federally funded public health clinic that would do it for free. Some parents made that extra trip; some never got their children immunized on schedule.

Pediatrician Douglas Cobble struggled for nearly a year to do the right thing before giving up. Practicing on the edge of the Cherokee National Forest in east Tennessee, Dr. Cobble had no wealthy patients who could pay high rates and give him an economic cushion to cover his expenses for poor children. The solvency of his practice depended almost entirely on what TennCare's health plans paid him. In February 1994 he wrote Access MedPlus, explaining that immunizations already were a money-losing proposition for his practice and asking for help. The situation didn't get better. Two years later Dr. Cobble reluctantly admitted, "We've quit giving immunizations because they're so expensive. We've cut back on personnel; we've even stopped phonebook advertising. We've cut everything we can."

When young children don't get prompt care, including immunization, epidemics can break out. Diseases such as diphtheria — which once was a major childhood killer but since has been tamed in the developed world — once again can wreak deadly damage. Health scares of nineteenth-century proportions may return, with diseases festering in poor, unsanitary parts of town, then spreading rapidly in schools and playgrounds to strike children of all backgrounds. By and large, the risk of renewed epidemics remained unrealized in TennCare's first two years, with one striking exception.

In March 1994 an acute bacterial bowel infection known as shigellosis swept through Sweetwater, a small town about 60 miles northeast of Chattanooga. Over a three-week span what started as an illness involving a few children expanded throughout Sweetwater and the surrounding farm communities, spread by flies, contaminated food, and ordinary human contact. Shigellosis passed from sibling to sibling, from classmate to classmate, even from school to school. Some 150 children eventually came down with the disease, which is marked by bouts of bloody diarrhea, sometimes more than 20 episodes a day. Several children became so dehydrated they needed to be hospitalized.

Paulus Zee, the only pediatrician in town at the time, knew exactly how he wanted to treat the disease. First he tried a combination of two cheap antibiotics that often works: trimethoprim and sulfamethoxazole. When the bacteria proved resistant to those drugs, Dr. Zee stepped up his attack. He began prescribing Suprax, a brand-name antibiotic that cost about $35 for a six-day course of treatment. When parents took those prescriptions to the local pharmacy, they received an unpleasant surprise: the two main TennCare plans in town wouldn't cover the medicine. Suprax wasn't on their list of approved drugs; months earlier they had deemed it too costly. Without insurance coverage, many poor families couldn't afford the medicine. Dr. Zee pounded out angry letters to the managed-care plans, to no avail. "An epidemic is running its course," he wrote. Only after county public health authorities stepped in, demanding that the HMOs make a special exception to their formularies, did Dr. Zee's patients get insurance coverage for the drug they needed. That finally squashed the epidemic. Until then Sweetwater dealt with the epidemic the same way that Americans did 50 years earlier: closing schools, boiling the clothes of infected children, and promoting endless hand-washing in an attempt to slow the spread of the disease.

John Morgan, a cardiologist in Chattanooga, ran into other bureaucratic problems trying to help a TennCare patient with an artificial heart valve. To help prevent dangerous clots that could trigger a heart attack or stroke, Dr. Morgan prescribed 6 milligrams a day of Coumadin, a low-cost anticoagulant. (The active ingredient of the drug is used in much higher doses in rat poison.) To get the dosage just right, Dr. Morgan told his patient to take one five-milligram tablet and half of a two-milligram tablet each day. But the TennCare plan, Access MedPlus, refused to approve the full prescription, saying it would only pay for the five-milligram dosage. Dr. Morgan protested. With Coumadin, dosage is crucial, he wrote Access MedPlus. Too little of the medicine doesn't prevent clots; too much leads to uncontrolled bleeding. "I do not know how you decided that a 5 mg. tablet was more important than a 2 mg. tablet," Dr. Morgan wrote.

As the Coumadin example suggests, Tennessee's version of low-income managed care could lead to especially grave mistreatment of the seriously ill. Health plans, in theory, were supposed to help patients with cancer, heart disease, or other serious ailments get good continuity of care. That meant ensuring that patients were sent to the right hospital for the right procedure, stayed for an appropriate time, and then were intelligently guided through therapy, home care, and other stages of treatment. That nice model, however, often hasn't worked in Tennessee.

Access MedPlus, for example, spent more than $30,000 to provide a day-old baby with heart-valve surgery, but it clamped down on recovery-related expenses afterward. The baby, David Owens, Jr., was born in Knoxville in October 1994 and was quickly diagnosed as having a faulty heart valve. He was transported by helicopter to Vanderbilt University Hospital in Nashville, where top pediatric surgeons operated on his heart. His parents brought him home after a weeklong stay, at which point their disappointments with their HMO began.

The boy's mother, Teresa Owens, said she asked for home care and didn't get it. She and her husband also asked the HMO to teach them cardiopulmonary resuscitation in case the baby's heart stopped. But because the parents had requested at Vanderbilt that extreme measures not be used to prolong the baby's life, Access MedPlus refused to provide CPR training. The parents asked for equipment to monitor the baby's breathing day and night; the HMO provided a night monitor only after the Owenses made a fuss, Teresa recalled. And instead of agreeing to cover regular follow-up visits to pediatric cardiologists in Nashville, Access MedPlus directed the Owenses to take their baby to a general pediatrician near their home for most care. Frustrated with the HMO's attitude, Teresa Owens switched her baby's coverage to a different managed-care plan, Blue Cross–Blue Shield, in February 1996. Now, at last, she could be sure her son was seen regularly by a pediatric cardiologist. To the parents' delight doctors said the little boy, at 16 months, was developing normally. Teresa Owens gave all credit to the surgeons at Vanderbilt and the prayers of family members; she was relieved no longer to be dependent on her first HMO for follow-up care.

Another weak spot in TennCare involved emotionally disturbed children. Therapist Brenda Hartgrove shuddered more than a year later when she recalled the case of a destructive boy not yet 10 years old. The child had already tried to throw himself out of a moving car and had once pursued his foster mother with a knife. Hartgrove regarded the child as homicidal and wanted to treat him in a psychiatric hospital unit, especially when the boy's foster mother pleaded for help one afternoon. In traditional Medicaid, Hartgrove could have made the hospitalization decision herself. But in TennCare, coverage depended on approval by case managers who had never met the child. As Hartgrove later recounted, a case manager and a doctor at the boy's HMO analyzed the case over the phone, deciding not to approve a hospital stay because they thought it inconceivable that such a young child could be homicidal. That night the boy tried to attack his foster mother with a pair of scissors. Only because she wasn't sleeping well could the woman fend him off.

Eventually Tennessee acknowledged that emotionally disturbed children posed challenges that TennCare couldn't handle well. The state created a separate program to provide health care for more than 1,000 such children. Specially trained psychiatrists and psychologists were given key roles in making coverage decisions; per-patient budgets for care were increased well beyond the customary $106 per month in TennCare.

In the fall of 1994 TennCare's performance became a major political issue in the state gubernatorial race. Democratic Governor Ned McWherter, the chief architect of TennCare, wasn't seeking reelection; he had already served the maximum two terms allowed by the state constitution. But his party's candidate, Phil Bredeson, a former HMO executive himself, tried to portray TennCare as a well-run, wise program with only a few small flaws. The Republican candidate, Don Sundquist, took a much more combative stance. He declared that TennCare needed major changes, and he championed several proposals made by doctors' groups. Tennessee voters elected Sundquist by a 150,000-vote margin out of 1.6 million ballots cast.

Throughout 1995 state officials tinkered with TennCare, generally increasing regulation to protect members' interests and relieve doctors' complaints of unfair treatment. Managed-care plans were subject to stricter marketing rules. A quality-review committee began taking a closer look at HMO practices. Extra money was set aside to take care of the sickest patients, who otherwise might be neglected under TennCare's strict per-patient monthly payment formulas.

David Manning, the aide to McWherter who helped launch Tenn-Care, left state government in late 1994 to become a vice president at Columbia/HCA, the nation's largest for-profit hospital chain. In a later interview Manning insisted that his laissez-faire approach had been the right way to start TennCare. "We knew there were going to be market-ing problems for a program growing this fast," he said. "The question was, should we be overly regulative at the start, or should we let the market work, see where the problems were, and then go in and investi-gate?" In Manning's view the second approach had worked well. Oth-ers, however, saw it as an invitation to chaos, putting many thousands of residents at risk for many months until state officials stepped in to clean things up.

"You have to be certain that your contract with the managed-care organization contains everything you want done," remarked Yvonne Wood, who headed Tennessee's Medicaid fraud unit until she retired in February 1996. It was such a simple lesson, she observed. But Tennes-see for some reason hadn't demanded much of its managed-care plans for the poor. Only in 1995 did the state start requiring the TennCare health plans to tell government authorities about any suspected fraud by members or doctors. "You'd just assume they'd do that," Wood said. "But they didn't."

Many doctors and patients gradually made peace with TennCare. It wasn't as good a health system as they wanted, and its hasty implemen-tation brought back horrid memories. Donald Lighter, a Knoxville physician who briefly helped run a TennCare HMO, likened the entire program to "emergency surgery on Medicaid," when a slower ap-proach — "elective surgery," as he put it — would have been wiser. Nonetheless, doctors who jousted with HMO managers and state offi-cials did make headway. Under pressure from doctors or patients, plans started making better drug-formulary decisions, speeding up re-imbursements, and paying more attention to continuity of care.

Some physicians, however, regarded the traditional approach of providing free care to the indigent, at a doctor's discretion, as a bet-ter and more humane approach. Surgeon Charles Cox reminisced fondly about the days when patients who couldn't pay for an operation would offer him goods in return: a truckload of wood or gravel for the driveway.

In other cases, doctors got so disgusted by Tennessee's version of managed care that they stopped trying to work with the system. Among them was Donald Swietzer, a reconstructive surgeon in Bristol, in the far northeastern tip of Tennessee. In August 1994 he wrote a blistering resignation letter to Blue Cross–Blue Shield, which had just paid him barely 10 percent of his $3,740 bill for repairing a young child's cleft palate and cleft lip.

"I prefer to donate my services to indigent patients," Dr. Swietzer wrote, "rather than participate in this sham."

12

The Best Lobbyists
in America

WHEN CONSERVATIVE POLITICIANS want an extra edge in a campaign, they hire the pollsters at American Viewpoint. Dozens of times a year the firm, based in Alexandria, Virginia, surveys voters' moods and then shares confidential insights with its clients. What issues are troubling people the most? What new tactics or campaign slogans might impress voters? Newt Gingrich used the firm in 1994 when he faced a tough reelection battle for his Georgia congressional seat. Richard Lugar signed on in 1996 during his short-lived bid for the presidency. In political circles the firm is famous for three-page reports that begin with polling data, then launch into blunt "action recommendations" that tell a candidate how to move up in the polls.

So in early 1995, when more than 25 states began debating bills that would regulate HMOs more tightly, the national Blue Cross and Blue Shield Association decided that American Viewpoint was the right firm to call for advice. Like most big insurers, Blue Cross loathed the legislative proposals. But Blue Cross officials weren't sure how to combat bills that had substantial support from the American Medical Association, from local doctors in each state, and from some leading consumer groups. They needed a strategy. Pollster Gary Ferguson, a senior executive at American Viewpoint, showed them the way.

"All the subtle arguments we tested were ineffective," Ferguson wrote in a three-page memo dated March 28, 1995. He and his aides had chatted for hours with focus groups of consumers and employers in Boston, Atlanta, and Las Vegas. Those people believed that fee-for-service medicine, not managed care, did the best job of protecting their medical choices. People also doubted the claims made by managed-care companies that greater regulation might drive them out of business. A highly technical, fact-based campaign against the proposed new laws would lose, Ferguson warned. "As a result, visceral direct attacks against this legislation and its sponsors — and government involvement in general — are necessary."

"Go after the AMA through surrogates," Ferguson advised. "Surrogates from the business community could carry the message even more effectively than a direct attack from insurers." He identified the Chamber of Commerce and the National Federation of Independent Business as ideally suited for the task. Recommended tactics included a fax campaign by small businesses. Most important, Ferguson asserted, insurers needed to define the battle on their own terms. Opponents of the bills should hammer out simple messages such as "government involvement . . . higher costs . . . bad for business . . . rich doctors versus consumers and employees . . . matters that should be decided in the marketplace, not the legislature."

Gary Ferguson's advice proved astute. Blue Cross paid close attention to his words, as did many of its peers in the health insurance and managed-care industries. Those companies broadened their lobbying beyond the old-fashioned approach of making big campaign contributions to state and national candidates. HMOs still paid high-profile lobbyists as much as $300,000 a year to buzz around state capitols, take legislators to lunch, and relentlessly promote the managed-care cause. But often efforts to sway government officials became much more subtle. Managed-care plans adroitly got other people upset about pending legislation, then used those stand-ins to argue their case.

Mass mailings, phone calls, and rallies became favorite ways for health plans to cement a natural alliance with corporate customers. Fear became the dominant message. Again and again managed-care companies raised the specter that new regulations would jack up health premiums and invite a return to the medical inflation of the 1980s. Even mild measures of extra supervision of HMOs were portrayed to employers as brazen attempts to "sabotage" the cost-effectiveness of managed care. Once such alarmist messages were spread about, HMO lobbyists could sit back and enjoy the results. Health-benefits managers of big companies swarmed into legislative hearings to testify that bills regulating managed-care were bad news. Small business owners bombarded legislators with letters and faxes, opposing whatever bills their health plans didn't like. When such campaigns were well orchestrated, the original sponsor's fingerprints were almost impossible to detect.

With such tactics, health insurance companies hope to achieve their second decisive lobbying win of the 1990s. In 1993–94 insurers converged on Washington to denounce President Clinton's version of health reform. They helped ensure that the flawed White House proposals ultimately went nowhere. Now the battle to reshape America's medical coverage system has moved to individual states. Doctors and patient groups are pushing for state laws to curb the excesses of managed care. The crusaders have scored some superficial victories, particularly with new laws requiring HMOs to pay for full two-day maternity stays. Yet insurers often find ways to dodge the full implications of those laws. And in a surprising number of cases, seemingly popular proposals for managed-care reform have run out of steam partway through the legislative process. Lawmakers' enthusiasm has dwindled. Widely supported bills never quite make it to a final vote. And even when state assemblies and senates have approved managed-care reform, governors sometimes have vetoed the bills.

Knowing how to set up such roadblocks is a big part of any political battle. As authors Donald Barlett and James Steele observed, "Successful lobbies are measured by the legislation that they stop, not by the laws they get passed." Some veteran politicians who challenge the managed-care industry come away bruised and dispirited. As those lawmakers discover, they have taken on a savvy, relentless force in American politics.

In mid-May 1995 hostile phone calls began coming into the hometown office of Texas state senator Jim Turner, a proponent of the managed-care curbs in House Bill 2766. "Don't tax my health care," callers told Turner's office manager, Patricia Lucas. "I want to go on record as anti–H.B. 2766," they added, in tones that ranged from matter-of-fact to highly abusive. Every time Lucas looked up, the red light on her desk phone was blinking again. The usual calm of her office in Crockett, a ranching and steel town 120 miles north of Houston, was turning into pandemonium. All she could do was log in each call, tell people that she would pass along their concerns to the senator, and wonder what was going on.

Gradually a fuller picture emerged. Many of the callers hadn't set out to phone Turner's office at all. They had been called a few minutes earlier by a lobbying firm that told them why H.B. 2766 was bad for business and then offered them a free phone connection to Turner's office. As many as 33 calls a day were being patched to Crockett this way. "We asked callers who was behind all this," office manager Lucas later recalled. "They never seemed to know." Senator Turner soon formed his own conclusions. The Texas chapter of an advocacy group called Citizens for a Sound Economy — which welcomed insurance-company donations — was running radio ads in Turner's district, claiming that his proposed managed-care curbs would amount to a $1 billion tax on Texans' health care. That claim was ludicrous, Turner believed. But it closely paralleled what callers were being prompted to say. Opponents of his bill, he decided, were using conduit groups such as Citizens for a Sound Economy to undermine his standing with his own constituents.

In an angry speech a few days later on the floor of the Texas senate, Turner accused insurers of "Astroturf lobbying" — setting up a front organization to create the appearance of grassroots opposition to his bill. The normal code of political lobbying had been breached, he declared; insurers were distorting the issues and trying to smear him. "We've done everything we can to be fair," Turner asserted. "If we're going to restore trust in government, those who have interests in this body are going to have to stop doing the kinds of advertising and misleading, false media campaigns with Astroturf organizations that are taking place on this bill."

Fellow Texas senators cheered Turner's outburst. But his opponents saw no reason to apologize. Hours after Turner spoke, the head of Texas Citizens for a Sound Economy, Peggy Venable, told the *Dallas Morning News:* "It's amazing to me that he doesn't want to hear from his constituents, especially if they disagree with him on an issue. If you can't stand the heat, get out of the Senate."

Like most players in the U.S. economy, the HMO industry lobbies through its main trade organization in Washington, the American Association of Health Plans (AAHP). Old-timers remember a funky, idealistic feeling to the trade group in the 1970s, when it was known as the Group Health Association of America. HMOs were small and little noticed then; members of the trade group saw themselves as participants in a social movement rather than as profit-minded executives with business interests to protect. At the trade group's annual meetings in the early years, HMO officials "would show up with guitars and sit in hotel rooms in the evening, drinking whiskey and singing old union songs," recalled Kennett Simmons, a pioneer of Prudential Insurance's move into managed care in the 1970s. By the early 1980s, however, the guitars had disappeared. The lobbyists had taken over.

During the 1993–94 national debate about health-care reform, the HMO association and its largest members contributed more than $2 million to candidates for the U.S. Senate and House of Representatives. Overall, the insurance industry in 1994 became the largest corporate bankroller of political campaigns, ahead of traditional leaders such as the banking industry, telecommunications companies, and the Wall Street securities houses. During the first two years of Clinton's presidency, the HMO association channeled two thirds of its donations to Democrats. When the Republican Party won control of Congress in the 1994 midterm elections, managed-care companies quickly changed loyalties. Some 80 percent of their campaign donations in the first half of 1995 went to the newly powerful Republican politicians.

Managed-care plans showed their clout when congressional Republicans in late 1995 tried to reduce Medicare's spending growth by $270 billion over a five-year span. As legislatures drafted retrenchment measures, health-plan lobbyists successfully protected one of their industry's most important money streams: payments to Medicare HMOs. Congressional leaders eventually penciled in an 8 percent rate increase for Medicare HMOs, more than two percentage points higher than earlier proposals. HMOs laid claim to some Medicare money set aside for subsidizing patient care at teaching hospitals — even though HMOs seldom send members to teaching hospitals because those facilities are too expensive. The lobbying victory ultimately proved unnecessary, because President Clinton vetoed the Republican-sponsored budget package. Still, the HMO industry's vigorous protection of its interests earned it an "A" for lobbying effectiveness in a year-end rating by the editors of *Modern HealthCare* magazine. The AMA and the American Hospital Association, by contrast, received only "C" ratings.

HMO executives kept looking for fresh ways to extend their political influence. At one of its annual meetings, the HMO association briefed 50 executives for nearly three hours on the topic "Using the Power of Grassroots to Achieve Legislative and Policy Goals." The session opened with sunny advice. Melinda Ferris, a one-time adviser to First Lady Barbara Bush, explained how HMOs could befriend legislators during campaign season. (Among her tips: set up tours of medical clinics in which politicians can get what they really want — media coverage of themselves, sitting at a coffee table, talking to voters.) After her talk the session became spicier. Executives from five managed-care plans, including Cigna, FHP, and United HealthCare, gave firsthand summaries of their roles in recent lobbying victories. In a panel discussion they laid out strategy and tactics much the way a West Point military instructor might review a wartime battle. As the executives started sharing their adventures, a journalist in attendance was evicted from the room on the grounds that press coverage of the HMOs' ploys would be "inappropriate."

Some of the nerviest maneuvers have been at the state level. In Pennsylvania managed-care plans for years chafed at delays in getting state approval to expand into new geographic regions. The top state regulator in charge of HMOs, Steve Male, generally supported managed care but was a stickler for consumer protection. With Pennsylvania about to elect a new governor in 1994, the state's biggest HMO, U.S. Healthcare, decided to flex its muscles. Usually the chairman, Leonard Abramson, supported Democratic candidates. But this time he switched sides and personally contributed $25,000 to the successful campaign of Republican Tom Ridge. Another U.S. Healthcare executive, David Simon, pitched in a further $2,600 and became chairman of Ridge's health-care transition team after the election. In March 1995, Male was told that he would be reassigned. Pennsylvania officials denied acting at the request of U.S. Healthcare. But in a statement to local newspapers, David Simon suggested that his health plan's interests shouldn't be overlooked. As Simon observed, "It is essential that Mr. Male's replacement understands the proper role of government in regulating the health system through this period of dynamic change."

In other cases managed-care lobbyists have artfully derailed bills they don't like. Florida, for example, appeared nearly certain in early 1995 to crack down on marketing abuses by Medicaid HMOs. The Florida house passed a bill that would have banned door-to-door marketing and other forms of mischief, while budgeting $2.3 million so that 49 new state inspectors could enforce the laws. HMO lobbyists never fought the bill head on; they simply professed to want a different approach, involving much more self-policing by the industry. After much debate, state senators in early April approved a bill combining government oversight with self-regulation. That bill was passed in the final hours of the legislative session, leaving no time for the senate and house to reconcile their versions. So both bills died.

As it happened, a leading supporter of self-regulation for HMOs in Florida was Alberto Gutman, chairman of the powerful Health Care Committee of the Florida senate. Two months after the legislature adjourned, journalists discovered that Senator Gutman had collected a $500,000 fee in 1994 for consulting work with a Florida HMO. Editorialists at most big Florida newspapers expressed shock that Gutman could earn so much money from the industry he was supposed to oversee. State officials, however, took a more lenient view. Gutman eventually signed an agreement with Florida's Department of Business and Professional Regulation in which he admitted no wrongdoing but agreed not to engage in similar deals in the future.

Occasionally HMO lobbyists have been caught flat-footed. In early 1995 the Arkansas legislature voted, 120 to 2, to force HMOs to accept into their networks any doctor who wanted to join. If HMOs aren't allowed to exclude wasteful, substandard, or surplus MDs, they say they can't run efficient managed-care networks. But Arkansas doctors fought hard for the bill, viewing it as essential job protection. Even though HMOs hadn't made much headway in Arkansas, anxiety about their future impact was running high. Lynn Zeno, director of government affairs for the Arkansas Medical Association, later credited his side's success to a single newspaper ad, which ran in most major Arkansas papers. "We showed two guys in business suits reading the *Wall Street Journal*," Zeno recalled. "The ad said: 'These men don't know you. They've never been to your home town. They want to pick your doctor.'" As much as anything, Zeno said, that image spooked legislators into enacting the managed-care restrictions.

In many states, however, HMO lobbying has slowed or stalled the reformers. In New York, Lieutenant Governor Elizabeth McCaughey in April 1995 tried to require HMOs to disclose contracts that reward doctors who give less care or that punish them financially for providing more care. Her bill won overwhelming approval in the state assembly, but it was bottled up in the senate until the legislative session ended. In an angry letter to the *New York Times,* McCaughey in October 1995 fumed — to no avail — about HMOs' fierce resistance to regulation. She seethed at the industry's contention that further disclosure of contract terms would only "confuse" consumers. Still, her only recourse was to reintroduce the bill a year later and hope it would pass then.

To understand how the managed-care lobbying machine works, it helps to look at a single regulatory battle in detail. One of the best case studies unfolded in Texas in the first half of 1995 over the bill known as H.B. 2766, the Patient Protection Act.

The Texas saga had its moments of farce, including an official state senate tribute to television doctor Marcus Welby. One lobbyist kept threatening to unleash an "atomic death ray"; angry doctors referred to HMOs as "a concoction of the devil." Fundamentally, though, the battle over the Patient Protection Act was a giant tug of war involving doctors and patients on one side, HMOs and employers on the other. Physicians at first believed that they couldn't lose. They had strong lobbyists, close ties to key legislators — and a bill that they regarded as a well-drafted, appealing way to fix most of the perceived excesses of managed care. Then HMOs and their employer allies stepped in. At crucial junctures this side proved stronger and smarter than the doctors' lobby in working the political system to its advantage. When the legislative battle was over, the Patient Protection Act had collapsed into dust.

Texas doctors got things rolling in late 1994 by drafting a model bill to "fix" everything that bothered them and their patients about managed care. One HMO had recently dumped more than 30 Houston doctors from its managed-care network without providing much explanation; doctors decided they wanted much better guarantees of due process before they could be fired from HMO networks. Patients were having a hard time getting approval to see specialists, so doctors drew up a provision allowing HMO members much freer access to medical "centers of excellence." The plans weren't paying for many emergency-room visits; doctors wanted HMOs to be required to approve coverage within 60 minutes of being contacted on an emergency case. A fourth section of the model bill required HMOs to disclose far more about their payments to doctors and the quality of care they provided; doctors and consumer groups figured that the glare of publicity would prevent HMOs from using pay schemes that encouraged undercare.

Finally, doctors in the Texas Medical Association proposed that large employers be required to offer more than just an HMO to their workers. At the very least, the doctors proposed, employers should offer a "point of service" alternative, which would let workers join an HMO but sometimes go outside the health plan's network if they paid a sizable part of the medical costs themselves. "Perhaps we were naive, but we thought we could win with this," recalled Joe Cunningham, an internist from rural East Texas, who helped draft the model bill. "We saw ourselves as the good guys. This wasn't about doctors' pocketbooks; this was about trying to build a better health-care system."

In a moment of giddy optimism the TMA briefly tried to enlist the HMO industry as a fellow supporter of reform. Physicians and managed-care executives met at an Austin hotel for three hours in January 1995 to discuss legislative ideas. The session was a disaster. Doctors complained about the arrogance of managed care and "sleazy" HMO practices. Managed-care executives charged that the meeting was a sham; the doctors already knew exactly what sort of bill they wanted and thus weren't interested in negotiating. A few weeks later Republican Representative John Smithee and Democratic Senator Jim Turner introduced a close approximation of the doctors' model bill into the Texas legislature.

HMO lobbyists shuddered at the bill's implications. "It was pretty darned ugly," recalled Jeffrey Kloster, a lobbyist for PCA Health Plans of Texas. "The bill was completely out of line." At first, though, the lobbyists had a hard time figuring out how to fight it. Donald Gessler, president of the Texas HMO Association, sounded stiff and defensive in early newspaper interviews. Mostly he tried to deflect doctors' accounts of patient mistreatment in managed care, calling such reports "anecdotal."

After a few weeks the HMO lobbyists hit their stride. Rather than defending the way health plans handled patients, they portrayed doctors as fat cats trying to protect their incomes. Earthy images worked best. Tom Bond, an Austin attorney who lobbied part-time for HMOs, explained at one point, "Hospitals and doctors are like big oil refineries running low on crude oil. The only way you can be certain to keep the machine running is access to patients." Asked later about his tactics, Bond explained, "You need to demonize the enemy. In the legislature you need a sharp sword. You can't make it in rational, analytic arguments."

Jeffrey Kloster, the lobbyist for PCA, also sharpened his attack. Early in the lobbying battle he complained to a reporter, "Our opponents go after us with anecdotal plays on emotions. The way we defend ourselves is to get into the facts, and there's not always time." Then Kloster began to master the sound-bite game. Even if legislators allowed him only 30 seconds in their offices, he did his best to quickly undermine the populist appeal of the anti-HMO bill. "We have a new nickname for the bill," Kloster would say, "the Physician Protection Act." Check the actual language of the bill, he would add slyly. He himself had reviewed an early draft of the bill; the word "physician" showed up 50 times, while the word "patient" appeared just six times. Even if legislators shooed him away after that fleeting message, he still considered the visits a success.

Meanwhile doctors, consumer groups, and their lobbyists buzzed through the Texas legislature, trying to build a case for the bill. Connie Barron, a lobbyist for the Texas Medical Association, argued that the bill would merely "codify into law what already are best practices among HMOs." But with health plans aggressively disputing that view, legislators found her position hard to accept. Another TMA lobbyist, Kim Ross, sketched out elaborate decoys and counterattacks that were supposed to benefit his side. At one point he welcomed the appearance of a dozen lesser bills on managed care — including some that had no chance of passing — because he thought they would distract the opposition. At other stages he threatened to unleash an "atomic bomb" of heart-wrenching stories involving bad patient care by HMOs.

When hearings began on the Patient Protection Act, however, the head of the House Insurance Committee, John Smithee, made clear that he didn't want a parade of anguished patients testifying before his committee. It would distract from the main issues, he told lobbyists from both sides. Texas doctors tried to put a few aggrieved people on the record anyway, going so far as to pay travel costs and overnight lodging for some. But when one star witness, Brenda Walberg of Houston, testified on April 12, 1995, about her HMO's shortcomings in treating a stomach disease, legislators weren't swayed. Walberg wasn't allowed to testify until shortly before midnight, in a hearing that began at 4 P.M. After she recounted her troubles, state representatives asked why she had chosen an HMO in the first place. When Walberg explained that her condition, Crohn's disease, made it hard to get insurance and that the HMO offered better coverage than a traditional indemnity plan, the managed-care lobbyists regarded her as an unwitting supporter of their side. Lobbyists for the Patient Protection Act were left wondering if they had made the beginner's mistake of bringing in a witness without fully knowing whether her testimony would help or hurt their cause.

Then employers started weighing in on the HMOs' side. Houston city officials said they didn't want more regulation of managed care; they were hard-pressed as it was to pay for workers' health benefits and dreaded any state action that might jack up their costs. Health-benefits managers from Marathon Oil and several business federations voiced similar concerns. The most vocal of the bunch was Nancy Sims, a lobbyist for the Texas Business Group on Health, an employers' coalition that included American Airlines and Compaq Computer. "We think managed-care plans are good, not bad," Sims told legislators and reporters. "HMOs have provided tremendous cost savings for employers."

In protracted bargaining sessions that ran well into the night, Texas representatives pressed the doctors and HMOs to find some middle ground. Representative Smithee, who wanted to design a fair bill that wasn't beholden to either side, paid close attention to input from Sims, the business coalition official. Lobbyists for Texas doctors repeatedly tried — and failed — to have her kicked out of negotiating sessions. In early May the house insurance committee completed its work. It weakened language on several provisions of the Patient Protection Act, including approval of emergency-room coverage and access to centers of excellence. The house panel also deleted the point-of-service provision entirely. The full Texas house passed the bill by voice vote on May 10, sending the legislation on to the state senate.

At this stage managed-care lobbyists developed their most lethal attack, asserting that the Patient Protection Act would send health insurance costs soaring 18 percent or more. If such a figure were true — or even if it could be taken semiseriously as a worst-case scenario — HMOs would have no trouble mobilizing angry business executives to denounce this costly new attempt at government regulation.

Such a high number, it turned out, could be justified only by the most imaginative calculations. The statistical model underlying the 18 percent claim assumed that health plans would be swamped with inefficient doctors, thanks to the bill's due-process and point-of-service provisions, and that patients would flock to the most extravagant of these physicians. The number crunchers also assumed that health plans would be liable for all extra costs, rather than members picking up a greater share of out-of-network expenses. In the real world none of those assumptions was likely to hold. Even the main employers' coalition, the Texas Business Group on Health, told members in May 1995 that it expected the Patient Protection Act would boost premiums just 1 to $1\frac{1}{2}$ percent.

During the lobbying battle, however, HMO partisans decided to make the Patient Protection Act look as bad as possible. A full-page ad in the *Austin American-Statesman* screamed: "Watch Your Wallet: Special interest groups want you to pay millions for health care." The ad showed a pickpocket in action; it told readers to call their state legislator and demand a no vote on any bill that might make health coverage costlier. The ad was sponsored by an entity calling itself Texans for Quality Health Care; reporters soon discovered that it was an insurer-funded lobbying group formed only a few months earlier.

From out of state, the Health Insurance Association of America weighed in as well. Bill Gradison, president of the Washington trade group and a former U.S. congressman, sent a mass mailing to 500 small business owners in Texas, telling them that costs would "rise dramatically" if the Patient Protection Act were passed. In an artful blurring of issues, Gradison lumped the bill with more extreme anti-managed-care measures — and then attacked this grouping of bills by citing estimates of how much the extreme proposals would jack up costs. He concluded with a plea that legislators be told to vote no on all the bills. Leaving nothing to chance, Gradison included five "writing points" that Texans could invoke in letters to their legislators. All five of Gradison's points hit on the HMO industry's favorite themes: no government intervention, no cost increases.

Even shriller denunciations of the Patient Protection Act followed. On May 15, 1995, two HMO allies — the Texas Association of Business and Chambers of Commerce, along with Texas Citizens for a Sound Economy — ran a full-page ad in the *Austin American-Statesman,* labeling the initiative "a true tax bill." The ad declared: "Under this House bill, over the next five years Texas taxpayers will pay over $1 billion dollars in new health care costs and taxes because of government-required regulation and bureaucracy. . . . Tell your Texas state senator to vote 'No.'"

That ad, senators decided, stretched the facts too far to be condoned. The Patient Protection Act had no tax provisions at all. It did propose that HMOs follow new rules, along the lines of auto safety requirements or food purity standards, but those could hardly be deemed taxes. The lobbyists were overreaching, concluded David Sibley, chairman of the Senate Economic Development Committee. To drive home that point, Sibley's committee publicly upbraided one overzealous advocate, Chamber of Commerce president Dane Harris. Asked at a committee hearing about his group's tactics, Harris at first said, "I have not personally used the term 'tax.'" When he was shown his group's newspaper ad, he claimed not to remember it. So a senator read the ad to him. "I stand corrected," Harris finally said. "Since my organization is quoted there and I'm the president, I accept that responsibility."

Nonetheless, HMO lobbyists greatly advanced their cause by creating the brouhaha about costs. One of the state's main newspapers, the *Houston Chronicle*, editorialized against the Patient Protection Act, saying that patients would not be able to benefit from the savings achieved by managed-care plans. More big employers spoke out against the bill, including Houston's mayor, Bob Lanier. He branded the bill an unfunded mandate, adding, "Cities must maintain flexibility to address the needs of employees within available tax dollars." The physicians' lobby was forced to run defensive television and radio ads contending that its champion, Senator Turner, was under attack "because he stands up for what's right."

As senators deliberated, pressure from lobbyists on both sides led to further tinkering with the language of the bill. The controversial point-of-service requirement was reinserted. The provision allowing patients wide access to centers of excellence was rewritten so it applied to only one medical center in the state, the renowned M. D. Anderson Cancer Center in Houston. The original provision for detailed disclosure of HMOs' physician contracts was rejiggered too. Regular mailings to HMO members would have to discuss physician pay in only the broadest possible language. If members wanted more details, they could write a letter asking for them.

On May 23 the Texas senate passed this modified version of the Patient Protection Act, 26 to 3. That large majority, however, masked growing doubts about the bill. One of its outright opponents in the senate, Jerry Patterson, said he simply wasn't that sympathetic to complaints about managed care. "Most of the horror stories associated with HMOs come from people who joined because they liked the idea of a $5 office visit but didn't want to read the fine print," he told a reporter. Even David Sibley, chairman of the senate committee that did the most work on the bill, came away irritated at the intransigence of both sides. The unending hearings on the bill were "my idea of what hell was like," he later said. Only debates on abortion policy were as shrill and interminable. "Everyone kept saying the same damn thing over and over again. You never changed anyone's mind."

After the senate vote, the Patient Protection Act remained one crucial signature away from being law. The state's Republican governor, George W. Bush, son of the former president, needed to decide whether to sign the bill or veto it. Lobbyists from both sides strained to catch his attention. The Texas chapter of Consumers Union had endorsed the bill in late May, but it had little access to the governor's mansion. Its political ties had been to the previous Democratic governor, Ann Richards. Officials of the Texas Medical Association thought it had a friend in Governor Bush, for it had contributed to his successful campaign in 1994. But major corporate opponents of the bill also believed they could claim the governor's loyalty.

In such situations the side with the best slogans usually wins. Throughout the spring of 1995 opponents of the Patient Protection Act had been perfecting their rhetoric. They likened the proposal to any-willing-provider bills, which would require HMOs to abandon most efforts to screen doctors in their networks and simply take all who applied. Even though the Patient Protection Act didn't go that far, opponents of the bill kept arguing to Governor Bush that he should view the legislation as government intrusion into the business choices of HMOs. Limiting HMOs' ability to choose or discard doctors made about as much sense, they argued, as telling a major league baseball team that it had to hire "any willing shortstop." That analogy became a favorite of HMO lobbyists; it was catchy and it played to Bush's previous job as managing general partner of the Texas Rangers. One lobbying group spent $5,600 for a newspaper ad that reveled in the baseball/health-care analogy, complete with a photo of a clumsy infielder about to miss a ground ball. "We've got a baseball-literate governor," explained Tammi Cotten, a lobbyist who helped underwrite that ad. "We felt that if we could get just one reader, and it was the governor, the ad would go a long way."

On June 16 HMOs and employers got what they had hoped for. Governor Bush vetoed the Patient Protection Act, citing "my core philosophy of local control and limited government." In a stinging

denunciation of the bill, Bush labeled it "too little protection for patients and much too much protection for special interests."

Managed-care officials and their allies broke into loud, boisterous
cheers. The president of the national HMO trade group, the Group
Health Association of America, Karen Ignagni, hailed the veto as "a
true act of patient protection." One of her aides, in San Diego for a
policy meeting, began calling East Coast reporters and telling them,
"The mood here is very elated and optimistic. This was an important
one for the HMO world." Meanwhile doctors, consumer groups, and
their allies saw the veto as a slap in the face. Senator Turner called the
governor's decision "a big win for large insurance companies and a big
loss for patients." Mark Kubala, president of the Texas Medical Association, gloomily predicted, "The trend toward patient abuses and
corporate control of medical decisions will accelerate."

But politics in Texas is never simple. Beneath his blistering rhetoric,
Governor Bush wasn't nearly as opposed to regulation of HMOs as it
appeared. The doctors' arguments hadn't been totally lost on him; the
anguish of some patients' frustrations with managed care had made an
impression as well. Within two weeks of vetoing the Patient Protection
Act, Bush asked the state insurance commissioner to take a fresh look
at HMO oversight. Maybe the commissioner could patrol managed
care from the executive branch by drafting new state regulations that
would accomplish many of the goals of the Patient Protection Act
without infuriating HMOs and their business allies as much as the
doctors' bill had done.

Over the next six months insurance commissioner Elton Bomer
took command. He drafted new HMO regulations in the summer of
1995 and invited public comment before they took effect. His new
rules called for faster determination of emergency coverage; further
disclosure of HMO business practices; and special rules that would
let pregnant women, cancer patients, and other people in continuing
treatment keep seeing a favorite doctor even if an HMO wanted to
eliminate that physician from a managed-care network. In a shrewd
tactical move, Bomer left out the provision of the Patient Protection
Act that had bothered HMOs the most: requiring health plans to offer
members a point-of-service alternative. Doctors hailed Bomer's proposals as a big step forward. Consumer groups — which had spoken
up only belatedly in the debate about the Patient Protection Act —
became early and loud champions of the proposals. HMO lobbyists

grumbled a bit about the initiatives but decided their industry could live with them. On January 1, 1996, the first half of Bomer's regulations took effect, with more to follow.

Ultimately the Texas tussle carries lessons about both the extent of the HMOs' lobbying power and its limits. Managed-care advocates were most effective when they could whip up business anxieties about a big regulatory bill, portraying it as too far-reaching and too costly. But these lobbyists weren't nearly so formidable when faced with a more carefully drawn package that omitted strident attacks on managed-care methods. The HMO lobbyists eventually yielded in the face of steady, focused pressure from regulators, doctors, and consumers.

Those lessons have national implications. During the feverish 1995 legislative cycle, various states debated some 100 proposals to regulate managed-care companies. Health-plan lobbyists beat back at least two thirds of those bills, according to a tally by the AAHP. But a meaningful number of less ambitious, precisely targeted reforms made it through the gauntlet. California enacted a new law requiring HMOs to speed up their handling of members' grievances, while making it much easier for members to take their troubles to state authorities if they felt a health plan was dragging its feet. Arizona required HMOs to disclose far more about their financial contracts with doctors and hospitals. When the Los Angeles–based Center for Health Care Rights at the end of the year surveyed all 50 states' HMO laws, it found consumer protection rules in a half-dozen states that it said could become model statutes for the rest of the country.

In an ironic tribute to HMOs' clever tactics, some managed-care opponents borrowed a page from the insurance industry's playbook and began using "surrogates" to argue their case. Well-financed doctors' groups and drug companies began building ties to patient-advocacy groups, which had collected the most compelling examples of managed-care failures, but which were strapped for cash and had little lobbying expertise. California doctors helped bankroll Citizens for the Right to Know, a doctor-patient lobbying group concerned about managed-care practices. The Ohio State Medical Association similarly joined hands with patient groups to form Health Advocacy Network. And Pfizer, a giant pharmaceutical company concerned about managed-care drug formularies that were hurting its sales, allied itself with groups of black ministers in Tennessee in a joint expression of concern about poor people's medical choices.

Both patient advocates and medical lobbyists squirmed a bit in their new relationship. But they grudgingly acknowledged that the only way to challenge the breadth and strength of the HMO-employer lobby was to band together. "This is not a contrived alliance," insisted Steve Thompson, a top lobbyist for the California Medical Association. "Doctors may be unhappy with the plans' bureaucracy and reimbursement. But the people who really suffer from those decisions are patients. We believe that from an ethical, plus a practical, political context, we need to advocate for patients."

13

A Question of Quality

ASK NEW YORK CITY cardiologist Lonnie Riesman what he
thinks about today's managed care, and he will tick off a list of perceived flaws. "We're creating this massive industry devoted only to
customer service, wellness, and prevention," he says. "The tragedy is
that some people are quite ill and don't get referred to specialists."

As a practicing physician, Dr. Riesman can't do much about those
concerns. But he is more than a front-line doctor. He has a second job
as a managed-care detective, working for the health-care consulting
firm of William M. Mercer on behalf of some of the largest U.S. corporations. Companies such as American Express, IBM, Sears, Marriott,
and ITT hire him to investigate the quality of care delivered to their
HMO employees. Other people may savor the cheerful marketing images of health-plan members riding bicycles, playing with their dogs, or
jogging on the beach. Dr. Riesman is the one who inspects full medical
charts on costly cases at each HMO that have gone awry. Then he asks
the hard questions.

Why wasn't a six-year-old's growing brain tumor detected for a
year, Dr. Riesman demands of one plan, even though the boy kept
bumping into walls and his parents repeatedly asked their HMO pediatrician what was wrong? In another review session Dr. Riesman
turns the clock back on a $150,000 heart-transplant case to look at the
patient's medical condition two or three years before. Why didn't the
patient's HMO doctors notice signs of a failing heart valve earlier, he
asks, when simple valve surgery, at $35,000, could have prevented
further deterioration?

"I've seen horrendous mismanagement," Dr. Riesman says. "There are always four to five cases that show that these health plans are not delivering what they're marketing." Primary-care doctors don't recognize crucial symptoms. Specialists aren't consulted in time, and patients' well-being spirals downward while HMOs and their doctors fritter away chances for a timely rescue. As a result, problems that could have been cured in good time with an astute diagnosis turn into calamities. While such mistakes are hardly unique to managed care, they are especially galling in a system that is supposed to coordinate medical care and catch diseases early. In many cases, Dr. Riesman finds, managed-care plans simply aren't providing the smart medical guidance and oversight that they espouse.

Dr. Riesman's work is one of many signs of an emerging power struggle over how to monitor and police the quality of HMOs. It is easy for everyone concerned — employers, consumers, doctors, health plans, and regulators — to say that they favor high-quality care. But the various parties emphasize drastically different things when talking about "quality." After nearly two decades of letting HMOs define the quality debate on their terms, the people who use or pay for HMOs are finally starting to speak up. They are focusing attention on a long-overlooked area: managed-care companies' failings in taking care of the very sick.

Some of the most intense questioning is coming from giant companies that now see themselves as stewards for their employees' well-being. Accounts of HMO blunders unnerve health-benefits managers at those companies. Equally troubling is the notion that these major corporations each spend $200 million or more a year on employee health care, without really knowing what they are buying. As Fran Bastien, head of health benefits at Digital Equipment, puts it, "We have a responsibility to our employees, now that we have them in managed care, to show them how the plans are performing."

State and federal regulators also are taking a keener look at managed care. In one renowned case California in late 1994 announced a $500,000 fine against TakeCare, an HMO that had wanted a urologist, not a pediatric cancer specialist, to operate on Carlee Christie, a nine-year-old girl with a rare form of kidney cancer known as Wilms tumor. The girl's parents, Harry and Katherine Christie, paid for the top surgeon themselves but filed a protest with state authorities. California regulators ordered the plan to pay the family's bills as well as the fine. In an accompanying statement, California's HMO regulator, Gary

Mendoza, accused TakeCare of "failure to provide appropriate access to quality medical care, putting in jeopardy the life of a young patient."

Other pressures are mounting as well. A federal court ruling in early 1995 suggested that HMO members ought to have more freedom to press lawsuits against their health plans over allegations of negligence or bad care. Many suits had been impossible to pursue because of complex, intertwined laws regarding jurisdiction over health benefits. Meanwhile journalists from mid-1995 onward have focused much more aggressively on perceived quality problems at managed-care plans. Magazines tell of "Death by HMO." Television talk-show hosts regularly invite critics of managed care on the air. Some reports are more lurid than informative. But many accounts of health-plan tragedies point out avoidable errors and thus serve a valuable teaching purpose.

Some HMOs don't like this new attention one bit. A Florida plan got a court order to block state regulators from disclosing data on any HMO's performance. A California plan that flunked an accreditation review announced that it would sue the accrediting agency, seeking to block publication of the news. And when medical directors at several plans have come up with costly but effective ways to improve members' health, they have been told by the marketing and finance specialists to slow down or abandon their initiatives. The apparent reason: profits matter more than patient care.

There are signs, though, that the customers' campaign to improve crisis care may be making headway. At HMOs such as Kaiser, Health Net, and United HealthCare, officials have absorbed painful lessons from cases that went wrong. Then they have begun building safer systems for handling emergencies, breast cancer, mental illness, and other diseases. The high-efficiency discipline of Total Quality Management — which has worked so well in boosting the use of simple preventive measures such as mammograms — is being adapted to the harder issues of managing chronic diseases such as asthma and diabetes. In the trickiest cases HMO officials sometimes put aside cost considerations and let themselves be guided by principles from the pre-managed-care era: compassion and a willingness to do the most they can for each patient.

When Congress passed the HMO Act of 1973, it knew that someone needed to police the quality of health plans. Lawmakers expected a new federal agency to do the job, much as the Food and Drug Administration oversees pharmaceutical companies and the Federal Aviation Administration watches the airlines. The logical candidate was the Department of Health, Education and Welfare, where Congress had just created the Office of HMOs. But managed-care companies had other ideas. "The industry made a very strong case that it ought to oversee quality itself," recalled Howard Viet, head of the Office of HMOs during the Carter administration. Managed-care executives contended that their industry was so distinctive that outsiders couldn't fathom it properly. Even doctors might be biased by concern about managed care's tendency to shrink their incomes and autonomy.

To head off government supervision, the two main HMO trade groups in the late 1970s set up their own oversight body, naming it the National Committee for Quality Assurance. "There were the obvious concerns about the fox guarding the chicken coop," Viet recalled. Yet his doubts were ignored. Deregulation was in vogue. Senior Carter administration officials were vying with Republican challengers to get government out of the day-to-day supervision of business. Free-market thinking reigned supreme.

For the next 12 years NCQA specialized in doing very little. Until 1983 it had a contract from the government to review HMOs — and passed every plan it saw. Those with "deficiencies" were allowed to stay in business and avoid sanctions by developing "programs of corrective action." As a result, no health plan reviewed by NCQA ever flunked. After 1983 even the pretense of doing government audits was dropped. NCQA on its own inspected 73 health plans and once again decided that they all passed. Its budget was less than $1 million a year. The group was so strapped for cash that at one board meeting, the group's then-chairman, Gail Warden of Henry Ford Health System, warned that if new funds weren't found, the group might have to disband.

Most state regulators were equally languid. Many states felt that their role was to promote HMOs so as to rein in hospital and physician costs. State bureaucrats were more likely to organize conferences telling entrepreneurs how to set up an HMO than to police the ones in existence. A few states, such as Louisiana, had no requirements for starting a managed-care plan. Most states regulated HMOs through their insurance departments, which focused on financial solvency rather than medical quality. California tucked HMO regulation into the Department of Corporations, which oversaw everything from penny-stock promoters to the paperwork associated with setting up a new business. In its leanest years California put only two full-time employees in charge of reviewing HMO member complaints. Delays in responding to members were so long that few people bothered complaining to the state.

For most HMOs, lax supervision was just fine. Most managed-care plans claimed the care they provided was at least as good as traditional fee-for-service medicine, but few wanted that assertion strenuously tested. In particular the health plans didn't want to be held legally accountable for any failings of care. And none wanted to be branded "below average." Many HMOs found it easier to compete on an unmarked playing field, where they could sign up members, expand briskly, and make whatever claims they wanted about medical quality.

The first stirrings of change occurred in 1989. A half-dozen northeastern companies wanted data on their HMOs' performance. The health plans were willing to oblige but said they would rather answer one standardized request than have to recalculate data for each company. That posture led a small group of employers and HMOs to meet in Stamford, Connecticut, at the behest of Howard Viet and Daniel Wolfson, head of an HMO trade group. (By this time Viet had become a health-benefits consultant, advising Xerox, GTE, Digital Equipment, and a handful of other companies.) After nearly a year's work, negotiators for the two sides settled on a few standard items that HMOs would report on to the companies: immunization rates, mammograms, and other preventive services. The initial yardsticks were rudimentary and played to HMOs' strengths. The proponents of these standards represented only a handful of health plans and employers. But drafters of the standards, known as HEDIS 1.0, hoped they could be refined and win wider acceptance.

In 1992 Wolfson, Viet, and their clients realized that they needed national sponsorship for their standards — and a neutral, national organization that could develop them further. Otherwise the HMO industry and the benefits-consulting business would split into pro-HEDIS and anti-HEDIS factions, and further progress would be impossible. Casting about for a national sponsor, Wolfson and Viet proposed that future work be led by the little-known National Committee for Quality Assurance. NCQA had recently received a $400,000 grant from the Robert Wood Johnson Foundation, which was meant to let the organization widen its original charter. NCQA at the time operated in a few leased rooms in a downtown Washington building and had a staff of less than 20 people. No matter. That blandness and obscurity were seen as advantages. NCQA appeared to be a blank slate, ready to take on whatever characteristics health plans and employers wanted. And both sides had big ambitions.

Suddenly prominent was Margaret O'Kane, a former respiratory therapist who had become president of NCQA in 1990, when no one else wanted the job. From 1992 onward she would play her own version of shuttle diplomacy, pressing HMOs to upgrade quality one moment, then asking employers not to bombard the HMO industry with burdensome record-keeping requirements. Her defenders praised her as a pioneer in a perilous field, advancing managed-care quality about as quickly as anyone could. Her critics contended that HMOs had such a strong grip on her organization that it was practically impossible for O'Kane and her staff to move any faster than the managed-care industry wanted.

O'Kane's résumé was a striver's success story. Born in Brooklyn, she had a bachelor's degree (with a major in French) from Fordham University in the Bronx. She had taught second grade for a while, but later said she rejected it as "such a traditional women's job." Respiratory therapy had seemed like a good career switch. But working at a top Boston teaching hospital gave her a jaded view of medical practice in the fee-for-service era. "I did a lot of unnecessary procedures," she later recalled. In the early 1980s she moved to Baltimore, where she got a master's degree in public health from Johns Hopkins University. That one-year program was the career catalyst she had been seeking. One of her professors, Samuel Shapiro, was a lifelong champion of greater efficiency in medicine, using rigorous mathematical techniques to study patient outcomes. From that point onward O'Kane worked in the managed-care industry, looking for ways to apply Shapiro's techniques. She later said, "I fell in love with the field."

Under O'Kane's leadership NCQA became the epitome of a by-the-numbers quality-monitoring shop. Staff members approvingly quoted industrial quality experts such as W. Edwards Deming. NCQA officials threw new muscle into health-plan accreditation. They visited HMOs at length and made sure that each one had processes for checking doctors' credentials, for handling members' complaints, for encouraging physicians to meet new quality targets. By February 1996 NCQA had reviewed 218 HMOs and awarded three-year, one-year, or conditional accreditations to 191 of them. Another 27 health plans flunked the review. In the eyes of O'Kane and many HMO officials, those reviews showed that the organization was serious about holding managed-care plans to very high standards.

The problem was, few outsiders could see much difference among the health plans that won high, middling, or low marks from NCQA. When *Consumers' Checkbook* magazine in late 1994 surveyed 90,000 federal employees regarding their HMOs, the editors were surprised to find that members rated health plans with provisional or one-year accreditations from NCQA just as highly as those with three-year accreditations. An even more awkward moment arose for Xerox in mid-1995 when NCQA flunked a major Washington-area health plan, Mid-Atlantic Medical Services. Xerox's policy was to stop offering its members HMOs that hadn't won NCQA accreditation. But Mid-Atlantic had the most positive ratings in its area from Xerox employees in an internal survey. Eventually Xerox decided to keep Mid-Atlantic in its roster and give the HMO a second chance at passing NCQA's review.

NCQA accreditation became enough of a marketing badge that health plans jockeyed for the organization's seal of approval. In candid moments, though, some HMO managers questioned whether accreditors really did much to judge true medical quality. Most of NCQA's reviews focused on paperwork and procedural issues rather than on what actually happened inside a doctor's office. Humana's south Florida HMO, for example, flunked the accreditation review in 1993, but took the test a second time in 1996 and passed with high marks. In the interim the HMO had asked consultants for advice on how to win accreditation. They helped the health plan install all the trappings of TQM, including 22 paper charts on the walls of its offices in Plantation, Florida. Those charts were packed with red trend lines, yellow control lines, and other such ornaments. "A lot of the foundation [to win NCQA approval] had been laid previously," the HMO's top Florida official, Christy Bell, said in March 1996. "But we didn't know how to present it," deputy Joe Burdell added.

NCQA liked to portray itself as an "independent" organization, separate from the managed-care industry that it patrolled. But NCQA's finances and board membership told a different story. A hefty 78 percent of NCQA's operating budget in 1993, for example, came directly from HMOs in the form of accreditation fees. Those contributions dwarfed the organization's other two revenue sources: grants and publication fees. Similarly, six of the organization's 17 directors in the mid-1990s worked directly for HMOs — and another three board members had links to the managed-care industry. As NCQA grew bigger, it became somewhat less dependent on HMO money. But its financial arrangements nonetheless belied its claims of independence.

Eventually large employers began holding HMOs to higher standards. In a June 1995 interview Margaret Jordan, the benefits manager of southern California's largest utility, Edison International, complained, "We don't have enough quality measures to tell when we cut into muscle. You don't want to be in some hospitals. They've got non-nurses doing things they shouldn't. I expect plans to stay on top of that. Are they?" She and other California employers banded together in a business coalition that began pressing HMOs for more data about their treatment of the seriously ill.

In New York, American Express installed a medical ombudsman to review employees' disputes with their HMOs. If the facts warranted, the ombudsman had the power to order health plans to provide more coverage. American Express also tested the quality of its HMOs' referral networks by conducting what it called "live case probes." Prompted by American Express, doctors would phone health plans with a simulated case involving a patient with AIDS or another grave disease. They would ask for permission to send the patient to a specialist, then take notes on the HMO's response. Those spot checks became "a good way to find out if health plans were referring cases properly or just trying to minimize utilization," explained LuAnn Cash, head of employee benefits at American Express.

American Express had moved 70 percent of its work force into HMOs from 1992 to 1995, Cash observed. The switch saved the company money and had the potential to provide high-quality care. But Cash and her colleagues were determined to police these health plans to make sure they were delivering the full range of necessary care. "It's nice to keep everyone healthy and to focus on prevention," Cash remarked. "But when you ask employees what matters most, they don't care about cholesterol or mammograms. Their fear is that when they get sick, HMOs won't take care of them."

Of particular concern to many overseers was whether HMO members could visit a specialist when they needed to. On their own, corporate benefits managers hardly knew enough to judge whether managed-care plans were handling this issue well or not. They might suspect that gatekeepers were limiting referrals too severely. To probe further, however, corporate employers needed expert advisers. That created a niche for physician-consultants like Dr. Riesman, the New York cardiologist who regularly probed HMO case records.

After two years of reviewing managed-care cases, Dr. Riesman found plenty of evidence that access to specialists could be problematic. "Specialists are still anathema to the managed-care industry," he explained in an interview. "The attitude is, they have access to high-cost technology, which they will use indiscriminately. That's true. But behind the technology is extra knowledge. Primary-care doctors just don't realize when they are in over their heads."

In face-to-face meetings with HMO officials, Dr. Riesman would first establish that there was a problem, then set out ways to fix it. HMO medical directors didn't always welcome his criticisms. But as they reviewed clinical charts together, their opposition crumbled. One memorable case involved a woman considered for a small-bowel transplant, a $200,000 procedure. Her medical history for the previous two years included a 60-pound weight loss, which treating doctors had mistakenly attributed to depression. If a gastroenterologist had been consulted earlier, Dr. Riesman observed, the woman's intestinal problems could have been addressed with minor surgery. The opportunity was lost; no consultation had been ordered.

In another case Dr. Riesman zeroed in on a patient who had been hospitalized for weeks with meningitis. The medical chart showed that the patient had been examined earlier by his regular HMO doctor, who noted the symptoms of a 102-degree fever and a stiff neck but didn't order a spinal tap to check for possible meningitis. "Why not?" Dr. Riesman asked. That question provoked a flurry of indignation and embarrassment on the part of the HMO's medical director. As Dr. Riesman recalled, "He said, 'We just got a three-year NCQA accreditation. No one has ever asked these questions before. Now we're going to lose 10 corporate clients.'"

Nasty as such confrontations could be, they paved the way for HMOs to improve care. Health plans could manage care cost-effectively and still avoid many poor outcomes by making smarter use of specialists, Dr. Riesman pointed out. In many cases HMOs could ask a specialist for expert advice without automatically commissioning

$3,000 worth of tests. A brief consultation might be enough to rule out a possible serious illness — or suggest that the case did warrant more tests. Once tempers cooled, Dr. Riesman found, several HMOs invited him back to talk further about improving the way they handled their toughest cases.

Such concerns weren't lost on the formal overseers of HMO quality at NCQA. In mid-1995 the organization began an 18-month effort to draft better measures of HMO performance that finally would look at treatment of serious diseases. NCQA president O'Kane readily acknowledged flaws in her group's earlier work but promised improvements. "This is a first-generation project," she told a media briefing in December 1995. "We're painfully aware of its shortcomings. But this is a story of progress."

Outsiders stepped up pressure on O'Kane and her colleagues to tackle the hard questions with alacrity. At one NCQA strategy session, particularly challenging questions came from Mark Smith, a practicing California internist who was also an executive vice president of the Kaiser Family Foundation. "It would be a shame if all this quality work resulted in a health-care system that works great as long as you don't really need it," he remarked. "If you're elderly with arthritis, the fact that a health plan works well for people who square-dance twice a week may not be important for you." He urged quality-monitoring officials to focus less on common minor services for the healthy and more on how well HMOs were treating people when serious illness struck. NCQA officials gulped a bit and said yes, they would try harder to do so.

In some circles sentiment grew that NCQA lacked either the speed or the willpower to probe deeply into the performance of HMOs. A new organization and a fresh start, these critics believed, would be necessary to ensure that consumers and employers get good data on how HMOs handled the real work of medicine. Without such information, consumers and employers couldn't hope to pick good HMOs or goad them to try harder.

Leading this line of attack was Paul Ellwood, one of the grand old men of the HMO movement. Trained as a pediatric neurologist in the early 1950s, he had been an outspoken crusader for health-care reform from the mid-1960s onward. The very term "health maintenance organization" was his coinage, thought up during a 1970 brainstorming session with health-care officials in the Nixon administration. In the

1970s Dr. Ellwood had bubbled over with optimism about the prospects for HMOs, convinced that they would readily disseminate information about clinical outcomes, allowing consumers to make smarter medical choices. When that didn't happen, Dr. Ellwood became increasingly irritated at the evolution of the HMO industry. "People who run these plans aren't clinically oriented; they're financially oriented," he complained in a 1995 interview. "If they're to be held accountable for people's health, that's not something they know about."

Hoping to shake things up, Dr. Ellwood invited health-benefits managers for federal employees and approximately 20 major companies to a June 1995 strategy session at his Jackson Hole, Wyoming, estate. He barbecued chicken for them, arranged a rafting trip, and tirelessly talked up the idea that only big employers could hold HMOs accountable. "The driving force in reshaping the health system is clearly business," Dr. Ellwood declared. "It wasn't until the purchasers got serious that the system changed. Businesses more or less feel they've got the cost side knocked. You are now ready to focus much more on quality."

Dr. Ellwood's courtship of the employers worked as planned. A few months later, those who had been guests at the Jackson Hole retreat announced that they were forming the Foundation for Accountability (FAcct). It would develop in-depth measures of medical quality for 10 major illnesses, ranging from depression and low back pain to breast cancer and heart disease. An Oregon health researcher, David Lansky, took command of the day-to-day workings of the project, lining up leading doctors and medical researchers to set appropriate standards for each disease. American Express announced that it would apply the FAcct standards to its HMOs from 1997 onward, and the 9.4 million-member federal employees' health plan said it was considering doing the same. "This is going to lead to a different kind of medicine," Dr. Ellwood predicted in April 1996.

Meanwhile federal courts began to chip away at a major shield that HMOs had used to protect themselves against lawsuits by members alleging bad care. The HMOs' defense was known among lawyers as the "ERISA exemption," because it related to a 1974 federal law governing employee benefits, the Employee Retirement and Income Security Act (ERISA). Drafters of that bill hadn't intended for it to govern HMO negligence cases. But certain provisions of ERISA exempted corporate employee benefit plans from state laws. When HMO members who belonged to such corporate plans filed negligence suits in state courts, HMOs swiftly moved to have the cases transferred to federal court. Then the health plans argued that ERISA provisions required that any claims for punitive damages be dismissed. Judges generally agreed, holding that ERISA plans could be sued only for the cost of disputed medical services. As a result, most of the landmark lawsuits by patients against HMOs were brought by federal employees or schoolteachers, who weren't covered by the ERISA provisions. The majority of HMO members, who worked for corporations, didn't have such legal recourse if things went wrong.

But some federal judges began taking a fresh look at the ERISA exemption. Two such cases came before federal appellate judge Walter Stapleton in early 1995. One involved the death of a Pennsylvania man, Darryl Dukes, after ear surgery, amid allegations that diabetes-related complications weren't detected because of delays in ordering blood tests. The other involved a woman, Linda Visconti, who alleged that complications in her pregnancy were ignored and led to the stillbirth of her baby daughter. Both plaintiffs sued the treating doctors and their HMO, U.S. Healthcare, in state court, alleging negligence. The cases were transferred to federal district courts which dismissed the negligence claims against U.S. Healthcare, citing the ERISA exemption. In the appeals case, however, Judge Stapleton disagreed. In a June 19, 1995, ruling, he held that the Dukes and Visconti allegations against the HMO should proceed in state court. "Patients enjoy the right to be free from medical malpractice regardless of whether or not their medical care is provided through an ERISA plan," Judge Stapleton wrote.

State regulators, meanwhile, turned greater attention to HMO members' concerns about medical quality. California in October 1995 installed an "800" number that HMO subscribers could phone if they were having problems with their health plan. In the hotline's first month of operation, the state received 450 calls — twice as many complaints as in its previous system of having HMO subscribers submit complaints in writing and then wait weeks or months for a response. By March 1996 complaints had surged to 4,000 a month — a 20-fold increase from the rate a year earlier. California officials were somewhat flabbergasted at the increase, but accepted it as evidence that many dissatisfied HMO members hadn't been able to bring their concerns to the state's attention through the previous system.

In Florida the state's Medicare peer-review organization in 1994 and 1995 asked several of the state's leading HMOs with elderly members to change their criteria for cataract surgery. Traditionally the review group had focused mostly on problems with individual doctors rather than systemic problems with an entire HMO. But after a primary-care doctor complained that he couldn't get approval for cataract surgery in a patient with deteriorating vision, the Medicare review group examined health plans' policies in this area. It found that "HMO beneficiaries did not have equal access to evaluation for cataract surgery." As the review group put pressure on the health plans, three of them, representing 250,000 Medicare members, agreed to bring their cataract-surgery standards in line with national norms.

For most regulators and health policy researchers, HMO quality was an abstract topic best measured by statistics. But for some patients and their doctors, managed-care quality — or the lack of it — took on intensely personal overtones. They had emotional, sometimes heart-rending stories to tell. They brought human faces and drama to health care, a subject that Americans widely believed was important but often found too complicated or ethereal to follow. It took a while for journalists to understand the importance of stories about personal medical experiences in the age of the HMO. But from mid-1995 onward the travails of individual health-plan members became a hot topic for newspapers, magazines, and television shows.

The most thorough media reports were remarkable case studies of managed care gone wrong. In February 1996 *Glamour* magazine published a 4,000-word account of the death of Karin Smith, a 29-year-old Milwaukee woman, from cervical cancer. Starting six years before her death, Smith had repeatedly asked her HMO gynecologist for an explanation of her heavy menstrual bleeding. Her doctor had ordered a Pap test in 1988, a Pap test in 1989, and biopsies in 1989 and 1990 to look for the possibility of cervical cancer. Each time the lab affiliated with the HMO reported that nothing had shown up in the samples. Only when Smith's cancer began to spread irretrievably did doctors finally make the correct diagnosis. At that point she was beyond help. "I am only 28 years old and suffer from advanced cervical cancer, which is the direct result of a three-year misdiagnosis by my HMO," Smith told a congressional committee in July 1994. "I am the victim of unmanaged care, and its inherent abuses have cost me my life."

Glamour's account, and a subsequent ABC-TV news report on the case, focused in large part on the personal tragedy of Smith's death. But both the magazine and the television show also questioned whether her cancer could have been caught much earlier, when it would have been easily treatable. ABC-TV producer Joann Breen said she tried to build in a broader warning in her program, along the following lines: "People are happy with HMOs if they're healthy. But the people we focus on are very sick. They were treated as if they were healthy all the way through, until past the point of no return. The system is rife with opportunities for failure."

In the *Glamour* article, writer Edward Dolnick pinpointed a systemic failure that wasn't obvious — but could put millions of people at risk if their HMOs or health insurers didn't watch carefully. The Milwaukee lab that did the Pap tests reinspected one in every 10 slides for quality control, Dolnick reported, as is standard practice in the industry. But a technician testified in a sworn deposition that the lab double-checked only those slides whose code number ended with a 2 and that this system was known among the technicians. As a result the quality-control system was practically useless. As Dolnick wrote, "A technician could race along to her heart's content so long as she remembered to slow down and pay extra attention to those special slides."

Managed-care executives who looked closely at the Smith case found a lot of lessons in it. Before the Milwaukee woman's death hit the headlines, though, some large health plans had appeared far less concerned with the quality of work done by subcontracting medical laboratories. Price seemed to be the main concern. "I marvel at the kinds of deals we're able to get" from medical labs, the chief actuary of a major California HMO remarked in late 1994. "It's literally impossible for labs to make money at the rates we're getting." Despite that puzzlement his company decided to do business with the low-priced lab in its main market.

Some media accounts of managed-care problems didn't try nearly so hard to explain why mistakes happened — and how they could be avoided. Television talk shows often reduced complex medical issues to slogans. Guests on the *Donahue* show appeared with seven- or eight-word labels in front of their images, such as "5-Year-Old Son Victim of HMO Policy," and "Says Husband Died Because of HMO Policy."

In such situations HMO executives contended that they were being unfairly blamed for medical accidents that could have happened in any health-care system. "There are people who have a vested interest in undermining us," declared HMO industry spokeswoman Susan Pisano. "There has been an aggressive attempt on their part to do so." Indignant HMO executives collected evidence that trial lawyers or physicians' lobbying groups were trying to generate negative publicity about managed care. One target of their wrath was a personal-injury lawyer who conducted "media auctions" of his cases, asking various television programs to compete for the right to interview clients with tragic stories. HMO executives also seethed at notices in medical-specialty newsletters that asked doctors to submit examples of managed-care injustices so that the publications could share them with legislators or the general media.

But the notion that HMOs were simply victims of a plot to discredit managed care was hard to take seriously. The health plans were on display every day, and some jarring examples of their handiwork were impossible to dismiss. Some of the best-known critiques of HMO quality, in fact, evolved from unsettling medical experiences in the lives of writers and legislators. Pulitzer Prize–winning journalist William Sherman had been interested in HMO issues when one of his tennis partners, a physician, began telling him about managed-care abuses. From that casual conversation, Sherman began months of research that led to a five-part investigative series in the *New York Post*. Several California state legislators took a keen interest in managed-care issues after family members had trouble getting approval to keep seeing a trusted medical specialist when they switched health insurers. And Florida cartoonist Don Wright took aim at HMOs after a plan tried to discharge his ailing mother-in-law from a hospital hours before a hurricane was due to hit. "She wasn't capable of sustaining herself," a family member angrily recalled. "We really had to fight them to keep her in."

After that debacle Wright began a series of devastating portrayals of managed-care mischief. His best-known sketch for the *Palm Beach Post* showed a phone clerk at "KuddlyCare HMO" telling a distraught caller that her husband didn't qualify for emergency coverage. "Gasping, writhing, eyes rolled back in his head?" she declared. "Doesn't sound all that serious to me . . . He's dead? Then he certainly doesn't need treatment, does he?" That cartoon became widely reprinted throughout the United States and was used by emergency physicians as a rallying cry for legislation that would require HMOs to relax emergency-coverage rules. The dialogue was invented, Wright readily admitted. But it drew from his family's own anger at being shunted by an insensitive system. "I really wanted to create someone who was terribly efficient and terribly cruel at the same time," Wright later explained. "It sums up what happens to people."

Periodic reports of HMO patients' anguish have led some people to wonder whether the public champions of managed care trust their system enough to use it for their own family's care. In most cases the answer is yes. Top executives at Kaiser, Health Net, and other managed-care companies all say that they belong to their HMOs. Care to date has been superb, they add. Every now and then, though, a prominent HMO supporter tells a quite different story concerning personal or family medical coverage.

One such example involves Jeffrey Harris, head of the Office of Managed Care at the Centers for Disease Control in Atlanta. In June 1995, at the inaugural meeting of the Foundation for Accountability, Harris argued vehemently for using broad statistical methods to evaluate and improve health-plan quality. It just wasn't productive to dwell on the implications of unusual individual cases, known as outliers, he asserted. But when he was asked after the meeting which HMO he and his family used, there was an awkward pause. He and his wife weren't in a managed-care plan, Harris explained. His wife had a chronic condition and her favorite specialist at Emory University didn't belong to any of the HMOs available to the couple. They were outliers. So they got their own medical care through a traditional fee-for-service plan.

For the NCQA's O'Kane, a medical crisis involving her daughter brought home how little managed-care plans have done to eliminate guesswork in picking doctors and hospitals for the very sick. In 1991 the nine-year-old needed surgery to repair an atrial septal defect in her heart. The family's HMO told the O'Kanes to use its standard local facility for complex cases, Georgetown University Hospital. For the next few weeks O'Kane used all her own medical contacts to gather information on Georgetown's pediatric heart-surgery program. Most of the answers were reassuring, so after some agonizing, O'Kane decided to stay with Georgetown rather than push to have her daughter treated at Boston's renowned Children's Hospital.

The heart surgery was a complete success, yet whenever O'Kane talked about the case afterward, she cited it as an example of how much more work had to be done before patients and HMOs could make smart choices in a medical crisis. After three weeks of research, she knew much more about Georgetown's heart program than her HMO had when it signed a contract with the hospital. Even so, she felt she was taking a gamble without really knowing the odds. "I'm probably as good a consumer as you can get," O'Kane said, "but it was hard for me to get information. Ultimately it was a matter of faith."

Such cases point out the great need for fresh voices in the debate about how to measure and improve HMO quality. Managed-care plans see all patients as essentially alike. They are units of production in a medical/insurance factory, to be handled cost-effectively as they move through various treatments. That view has dominated managed-care quality analysis for the past decade. It has yielded rapid progress in the parts of medicine that can be standardized, and indifference or careless cost cutting in the rest.

When serious illness strikes, though, we want to be treated as someone special. Managed-care plans haven't always been able to do that. At times the executives running HMOs appear blinded by statistics. They are so busy watching means and variances in the easy-to-measure areas of medicine that they lose track of what is happening in the essence of patient care, the parts that can't fit on a graph. Now that customers and users of HMOs have begun to speak out, the great challenge will be to fix this failing.

14

Building a Better System

F ASTER THAN ALMOST ANYONE expected, managed care has become the de facto national health policy of the United States. This takeover happened without a single public referendum or a congressional vote. There was never a launch date, a nationally televised speech, or a managed-care manifesto explaining why this change was occurring. Yet the percentage of the population covered by HMOs and PPOs keeps climbing every year. By the year 2000, managed-care plans will probably cover four out of every five Americans with health insurance — whether employer-funded, Medicare, or Medicaid. As this juggernaut rolls onward, crucial questions about medical quality remain unresolved. Will managed care become more than just a ruthless way to cut costs? Will this new system ever fulfill its potential to make U.S. medicine better? And who will decide how far managed care's restrictions will extend?

Unless changes are made, important aspects of the health-care system may be in peril. Parts of the HMO industry operate under their own version of Gresham's law, in which bad plans drive out the good. Cost cutting predominates, even if it means denying care and trying to keep sick people off membership rolls. Profiteering becomes the norm; quality-improvement programs are scrapped if they don't yield quick financial payoffs. Meanwhile the people writing checks for this coverage — corporate employers and government administrators overseeing Medicare and Medicaid — often don't seem to care. They channel workers and beneficiaries into the cheapest managed-care programs they can find, with little regard for medical quality.

Yet much better results are within reach. The theoretical appeal of managed care remains immense: a well-planned system that will steer patients to the appropriate level of care whether they are healthy or sick, instead of leaving them to grope randomly for medical help in a crisis. Public understanding of the potential and the pitfalls of managed care is growing rapidly. All that is missing is a mechanism to bring better human judgment into the system.

To fix managed care, power must be shared beyond the confines of an HMO's headquarters. Consumers, doctors, employers, and regulators all have important roles to play. They can ensure that the trade-offs between saving money and taking good care of patients are handled fairly and intelligently. They can challenge overly stingy treatment guidelines and push for wiser standards. As we have seen, lessons for improvement are embedded in many of managed care's worst mistakes. If participants in the system are willing to speak up, dangerous flaws can be detected quickly and remedied before they impair members' health. That cooperative approach will promote better medicine faster than anything the managed-care industry can design by itself. Specifically:

Consumers can become much more savvy and assertive about managed care. Health plans' rules about what doctors to see, what pills to take, and what facilities to use may seem formidable. Nonetheless, some HMO members and their families are mastering the art of negotiating for better treatment. Consider the case of Tricia Reis, the daughter of a Medicare HMO member described in Chapter 10. During a yearlong tussle with two HMOs, Reis and her mother won four separate battles to give the elderly woman treatment that went beyond what her health plans initially wanted to cover. As Reis remarked, "If there's one thing we learned, it is that you do have options. Just because an insurance company says 'I'm not paying for it' doesn't mean that you can't make them pay for it."

Doctors, nurses, and hospital managers can speak up too. Managed care's crusade against medical extravagance and inefficiency should be weighed against the professional judgment of people on the front lines of medical care. Some managed-care efficiency programs are wisely conceived and should be accepted by all. At other times, though, HMOs cut into necessary care or pursue false economies. In those cases doctors and other providers can and ought to fight for better care. Pediatric cardiologist Stuart Kaufman provided a model example of how to do so in Chapter 6: he identified the heart surgeon with the best outcomes and pushed hard to have managed-care plans refer sick children to that doctor. The plans fought him for years. Then in early 1996 one of the biggest HMOs in Dr. Kaufman's region, U.S. Healthcare, finally relented and began approving some of the referrals he wanted.

Employers have a special role to play. They write the checks that finance managed care; they control the purse strings. Many corporations remain fixated on cost containment, echoing the concerns of Allied Signal described in Chapter 2. Such employers don't assume responsibility for the quality of care they are buying. There are encouraging signs, though, that some large companies are demanding more. Chapter 13 cited some of the most promising initiatives in this area, including the push by LuAnn Cash, benefits manager at American Express, for concrete information on how HMOs handle care of the sick. Also encouraging are the attempts by several business alliances to gather data on medical outcomes of HMOs' treatment of breast cancer, heart disease, and other serious illnesses. As those data emerge, they should be a powerful force for improved care.

Finally, regulators can do much more to hold HMOs to high standards. A light regulatory touch may be appropriate for many other industries, which thrive in unfettered competition. But health care is different. Without clear coverage rules, competing health plans will engage in a race to the bottom, devising audacious ways to avoid treating the sick. In many jurisdictions health insurance regulations haven't kept pace with the growing power of managed-care plans to decide what is medically necessary and what isn't. To ensure that health-plan members don't get shortchanged, state and federal regulators must examine what is being promised versus what is being delivered. Then the regulators must help define acceptable standards of coverage — and enforce those rules. As was shown in Chapter 9, those issues arose in Rhode Island when regulators cracked down on a mental-health plan that, they believed, was regularly denying necessary care to its members. Similar abuses are likely to need tighter policing by regulators across the United States.

To achieve these goals, here are 10 specific steps that will improve managed care as it is practiced today.

1. Consumers need to make the managed-care system work for their own interests.

Even the HMO industry acknowledges that new members are most likely to be unhappy with the strictures of managed care. Suddenly subscribers confront a gatekeeper system, limits on their ability to see specialists, and tight controls on their usage of medical services. Most HMO members gradually learn how to get the care they want within the system. But that can be a long process of trial and error. Millions of newcomers to HMOs and PPOs need pragmatic written guides to managed care, with candid tips and advice beyond what is provided in the health plans' own brochures. Like any complex administrative system, managed care is full of bureaucratic snags and informal short-cuts. People who master these "unwritten rules" fare much better than those who don't.

Over the next few years various "Underground Guides to Managed Care" are likely to emerge, either as full-fledged books or as magazine articles, pamphlets, or television programs. Among the most valuable points that such guides could make:

- If there is a potential bias in managed care, it is toward undertreat-ment. HMO doctors and case managers aren't likely to commit the sins of fee-for-service medicine: ordering nonessential tests and sending too many patients into surgery to jack up revenue. The pressure is in the opposite direction, toward conservative treat-ment with few interventions. Often that may be the wisest medical choice. But as patients seek care, they should no longer ask "Do I really need this?" Instead, the key question to ask doctors and plans is "Is this sufficient?"

- If members ask a managed-care plan to approve more care, it may yield. Many HMOs like to portray themselves as infallible judges of what is medically necessary and what is not. In fact, some requests for care fall into a gray zone. Continuing physical therapy for a sports injury, for example, may fall far short of a life-and-death necessity yet be more than a frivolous request. The same often applies to an extra day in the hospital after surgery. More care isn't always necessary and in many cases HMO restrictions may result in optimal care. But if patients believe they need more treatment, speaking out about it will sometimes cause an HMO to be more lenient.

- People with chronic medical conditions should seek allies within the health plan who can help fight red tape. The HMO's official rules may amount to a rationing system, making it hard to get as much physical therapy, high-cost maintenance medications, or other services as patients desire. Patients whose doctors or case managers take an intense personal interest in their well-being may be able to break through those barriers. Robert Brook, the head of health policy research at Rand Corporation, mischievously wonders how far patients should go to gain an edge. "If this were China, you would send your doctor a gift," Dr. Brook says. "You would find a way to play the bureaucracy so that you would become special." His imagery is extreme, but his point is intriguing: extra care will go to patients who can persuade an HMO insider to lobby for them.

The emergence of truly well-informed consumers will be a threat to badly run health plans and a boon to well-run ones. HMOs won't find it nearly as easy to shunt members' medical needs and preferences aside. But the chances of achieving managed care's oft-stated goal — delivering appropriate care at all times — should actually be improved. Knowledgeable consumers will seek out preventive-care programs offered by HMOs, such as diet counseling and stop-smoking programs, which can reduce the risks of cancer and heart disease. Most of all, well-informed consumers will become partners with their doctors and health plans in making medical decisions, rather than waiting passively to see what the HMO will do for them.

2. Doctors need to accept the principles of cost-effective medicine but be able to challenge specific managed-care rules without fear.

Most doctors acknowledge the need for wiser control of medical spending. Yet many of them find the rules of managed care exasperating. They clash and battle so often with HMOs that they have insufficient time to practice good medicine. Other physicians grow so dispirited or indifferent that they may shirk their obligations to difficult patients in favor of keeping a "clean record" with HMO administrators. Both approaches are troubling.

If managed care is to succeed, doctors and other medical providers must find a comfort zone between those two extremes. They must find ways to hold down costs yet provide the right care to their patients. Chapter 5 showed in detail how a small pediatric practice is trying to find that middle ground. Its experience is instructive. Pediatrician

Brian Greenberg generally adhered to HMO drug formularies but insisted on exceptions when he felt a child's comfort and well-being were at stake. Dr. Greenberg also found some ways to extend a maternity stay beyond an HMO's formal guidelines without getting mired in benefits denials and appeals. Pediatrician Victoria Millet pressed hard to have a young girl with leukemia seen by the right cancer specialist even when her managed-care plan balked.

Doctors traditionally are so independent and strong-willed that almost any intrusion into their practice habits can evoke indignation. But unfocused anger isn't likely to produce victories for physicians — or better health care. Managed-care companies believe they must make rules about almost every area of medical practice: the length of office visits, the choice of drugs to prescribe, the number of specialist consultations and tests, even the selection of hospitals. In the age of HMOs, the most effective physicians will be those who abide by rules that are tolerable — and save their anger for rules that impede good care. HMOs came under heavy fire, for example, when they insisted on "gag clauses" in physicians' contracts that limited doctors' freedom to talk with patients about medical choices or the financial bias of managed care. When doctors protested, several states made such clauses illegal. The other states should follow.

Patients, meanwhile, ought to seek out doctors who can best maneuver the managed-care maze. Something as simple as a 10-minute chat with a physician or a medical office manager can help patients discover which doctors make the HMO work for their patients and which ones don't. If consumers spend at least as much time picking a doctor as picking a health plan, they will begin to reassert their uniqueness. Then it will be harder for HMOs to treat 500,000 or so members as production units flowing through a medical factory. And patients' odds of being treated as special when illness strikes will also be improved.

3. Doctors, employers, regulators, and HMOs need to combine forces to develop treatment guidelines that people can trust.

One of the most alluring — and potentially troubling — aspects of managed care is the notion that the treatment of many common diseases can be standardized. If medical experts can agree on the right way to treat low back pain, asthma, and so on, the thinking goes, HMOs can then install those methods in thousands of hospitals and doctors' offices around the country. That approach could improve the lives of many thousands of patients and save money if the experts pick the right approach. The danger is that the experts may get it wrong. The original treatment model itself could be flawed. Or the transfer to bedside practice could overlook important variations in the ways that real patients present themselves to real doctors.

To make these decisions properly, medicine needs more extensive reliable data on treatment outcomes. Fields such as cardiovascular care have been guided for years by well-regarded studies that show what types of patients respond best to the two main forms of treatment: CABG surgery and angioplasty. Academic researchers are trying to develop similar guidelines for conditions ranging from stroke to schizophrenia. A handful of nonprofit HMOs, notably Kaiser Permanente and Group Health Co-operative of Puget Sound, have long been active in gathering and using their own outcomes data to improve treatment standards. But they are in a dwindling minority. As the managed-care industry becomes dominated by publicly traded for-profit companies, objective research within the industry is becoming rarer.

In the future, leadership in outcomes research and the development of treatment guidelines will need to come from outside the HMO industry. Health plans themselves can assist in studies, chiefly by providing raw data on patients' histories. But for-profit HMOs aren't likely to be the best stewards of honest medical inquiry. If HMOs are left in charge, some potentially costly diseases won't be studied. Definitions of successful treatment may be manipulated in favor of what is cheap as opposed to what is effective. A hint of that danger appeared in the breast cancer controversy, as HMOs "went shopping" for an academic study that would support their business interests in denying bone marrow transplants.

The more promising initiatives in outcomes research and treatment guidelines involve wide-ranging collaborative efforts. Academic researchers ought to take the lead, working together with payers, health plans, doctors, and hospitals. As already noted, corporate employers are moving into this area, thanks to initiatives by the Foundation for Accountability and the National Committee for Quality Assurance. These organizations alone can't find all the answers, but they can help refocus attention on how HMOs treat serious diseases such as breast cancer, heart disease, diabetes, and depression.

One further approach would be to deduct a tiny amount from

health-plan premiums — perhaps as little as five cents per member per month — to pay for outcomes studies and development of trustworthy treatment guidelines. Independent researchers could then determine which therapies and which centers have the best survival rates or long-term positive outcomes. This research would be best coordinated through a government-related entity that could uphold high standards of objectivity and thoroughness. A small arm of the federal Department of Health and Human Services, the Agency for Health Care Policy and Research, tried to play this role for a few years but found itself hard-pressed to ward off political attacks. Other government agencies, however, may have more clout and staying power. Handled properly, such research could do a great deal to improve patient care. Handled badly or left unsupervised, it will become a tool for misuse.

4. Regulators need to patrol the ways that HMOs pay doctors.

Managed care is based on the idea that the payment system in traditional, unsupervised fee-for-service medicine is deeply flawed. In critics' eyes, overtreatment is inevitable if doctors and hospitals are paid a fee for each exam, test, or surgery. To fix this problem, HMOs have created new pay systems that range from the well-conceived to the dangerous. The common feature in most managed-care pay systems is that incentives tilt in the other direction. Doctors and hospitals get a flat-rate payment per member in the system known as capitation. Providers thrive if they can keep patients healthy; they share in financial losses if sickness and costly cases abound. In moderation this new system can encourage good, cost-effective medicine. But dosage is everything.

If capitation's penalties for all-out care are too steep, or if the rewards for undercare are too great, doctors can no longer act as patients' advocates. An extreme version of such problems surfaced in Tennessee, where some pediatricians stopped immunizing poor children in Medicaid HMOs because bare-bones capitation rates turned even basic care into a money-losing proposition.

The only logical remedy involves stricter regulation. HMOs like to contend that their contracts with doctors and hospitals are proprietary business dealings — no more suited to government regulation than the terms by which Microsoft hires its computer programmers. But that argument ignores the deep public interest in making sure that people receive good health care. It also ignores the changing balance of medical power. In many regions a few giant health plans dominate the market to such an extent that they can dictate terms to individual physicians on a "take-it-or-go-out-of-business" basis. In such situations members' only hope is that the HMOs themselves will watch for signs of undercare and will take steps against doctors who neglect patients in order to keep a greater share of capitation payments. That isn't sufficient protection.

By focusing on ill-thought-out or poorly monitored contracts, state and federal regulators can decide what terms are fair and what aren't. The basic concept of giving providers financial incentives can be preserved. But health plans would need to demonstrate that monthly capitation systems don't tempt (or force) doctors to skimp on care. Financial provisions for high-cost patients also would deserve a close look. Some managed-care systems use reinsurance and special risk pools to ensure that doctors with very sick patients won't run up severe financial losses under capitation. Other payment schemes leave individual physicians shouldering most of the financial risk associated with sick patients — an unwise state of affairs that regulators should police. Otherwise providers will end up viewing their sickest patients as financial disasters to be dodged by whatever ruses can be devised.

Some states already have begun to regulate managed-care contracts to this degree of detail, and others are looking at doing so. Interestingly, in early 1996 the federal overseers of Medicare proposed contracting rules designed to limit the amount of financial risk that HMOs could load onto small medical groups seeing elderly patients. It may take some time to figure out what blend of incentives, penalties, and safeguards in doctors' contracts can best promote efficiency while protecting patients. That is all the more reason why this search should not take place behind closed doors at HMO headquarters.

5. Regulators, doctors, and HMOs need to improve the rules for deciding tough cases.

When sick patients are candidates for costly treatment at research hospitals, they may not expect great charity from their health plan. But patients should feel confident that coverage decisions will be governed by prevailing medical norms. That isn't always true. Such cases put the two main missions of an HMO in conflict. As an insurance company, an HMO may want to avoid paying costly claims. Yet as a supervisor of medical care, the HMO must decide which treatments fall within the boundaries of appropriate, necessary care and which ones don't. As much as HMO officials insist that sound medical judgment guides their thinking, judges, juries, and arbitrators don't always agree. In the wrenching breast cancer cases of the early 1990s, Health Net repeatedly came under fire for denying coverage for a costly treatment that it deemed experimental, even though some prominent community doctors argued otherwise.

Fortunately, the Health Net debacles point the way toward a better solution. When HMOs are faced with a rare, perplexing case, it is good medicine — and perhaps even good business — to call in an impartial panel of experts. Even if HMO medical directors don't feel business pressures tugging at them to deny care, their own training generally isn't sufficient for them to make precise judgments on the frontiers of cancer therapy, organ transplantation, or other specialized fields. Turning to a panel of specialists in that field will produce a wiser decision.

In setting up such advisory panels, HMOs must allow experts enough room to be experts. Health Net stumbled in 1993 when it called in cancer specialists from UCLA and asked them to review cases according to a stricter standard than the doctors applied in selecting their own patients. That inevitably led to the anguish of the deMeurers case, described in Chapter 7, where UCLA's dual role left it arguing both for and against a bone marrow transplant for a breast cancer patient. Such mistakes can be avoided if experts have room to offer the same judgment to the HMO that they would provide to their own patients. Other countries, notably Germany, go one step further and let government authorities and medical experts define the entire sweep of health-benefits packages. Insurers administer plans set up entirely by others, a smaller but still profitable role that avoids all such conflicts of interest.

Efficient, American-style managed care may still require HMOs to keep control of coverage decisions in routine cases. For the hardest cases, though, outside advisers could play a useful and much more prominent role. One such proposal was put forth by California physicians Martin Shapiro and Neil Wenger in late 1995. In an editorial in the *New England Journal of Medicine,* they recommended the creation of independent review boards for each HMO, staffed partly by HMO members, that would keep an eye on the health plans' utilization-review decisions and agitate for changes when necessary. "Plan members may lack medical sophistication," the UCLA doctors wrote, "but they should be expected to ask tough questions and observe patterns of care-giving behavior." If things go wrong, Drs. Shapiro and Wenger added, a public outcry by those reviewers might be the fastest way to get problems redressed.

6. Regulators and HMOs need to open up the emergency room.

Of all the judgment calls made by managed-care plans, the ones that go most painfully awry involve medical emergencies. A feverish baby with a life-threatening infection is sent on a 42-mile drive to a remote hospital. A man with searing chest pains isn't approved for coverage at the hospital his family selects. A dangerously dehydrated woman and her husband delay getting care during an out-of-state trip because they believe they must use only HMO-approved hospitals. Many such cases end in tragedies; others are near misses.

Such misjudgments are the ugly consequences of HMOs' efforts to second-guess their members about what constitutes a true emergency and what doesn't. Academic studies have found that 50 percent of emergency-room visits aren't essential and that as much as $7 billion a year could be saved if all those nonessential visits were directed to a primary-care doctor's office or self-care instead. But what HMOs fail to realize is that many true emergencies can't easily be distinguished from false alarms until after the fact. A system that cracks down too aggressively on "wasteful" use of the emergency room is all too likely to maroon some gravely ill people as well.

How can this problem be fixed? The most drastic solution is to rewrite state health insurance laws so that HMOs would be obligated to provide fuller emergency coverage. One such proposal, known as the "prudent layperson" rule, comes from the American College of Emergency Physicians. It would define an emergency as "acute symptoms of sufficient severity such that the absence of prompt medical attention could reasonably be expected to result in: placing an individual's health in serious jeopardy, serious impairment to bodily function, or serious disfunction of any body part or organ." That rule would allow the person with chest pains to head straight for the emergency room without fearing that the HMO will deny payment if those symptoms do not signal a heart attack. Such a definition would make it harder for HMOs to squeeze emergency-room costs. Some cost savings over unmanaged care could still be realized, while patient care would be protected. California, Maryland, and several other states have told HMOs to widen their coverage of emergency care; other states are likely to follow.

More tempered approaches involve stricter rules on how HMOs explain emergency-care policies and provide after-hours care. Many plans don't inform members that they are allowed to call 911 in an extreme crisis and get full HMO coverage of subsequent medical bills; that message should be spelled out. Many HMOs also require members to seek approval for emergency services beforehand from their primary-care doctor, yet they don't make sure that the physician or a backup is available for advice around the clock. Such gaps ought to be fixed. Otherwise HMOs are administering draconian policies on emergency coverage without attempting to meet patients' real needs.

7. Lawmakers and the courts need to make HMOs accountable for their mistakes.

The 1974 federal law governing employee pension benefits was intended to do many things — but shielding HMOs from many lawsuits wasn't among its missions. Nonetheless, that law has taken on a second life as a mechanism by which managed-care plans often can avoid state-court jurisdiction when members sue. Health plans insist that these suits alleging negligent medical care be transferred to federal court. Once that transfer occurs, federal judges generally rule that the pension law exempts both corporate employers and health plans from being sued for negligence.

That legal maneuver has saved HMOs a lot of money in potential damage awards or settlements. But it has left them essentially blameless for odious mistakes made within their networks of doctors and hospitals. Recently some judges have begun to question whether the pension law is being applied appropriately or whether it is being stretched unduly.

Both Congress and the federal courts have it within their powers to clarify this issue. If they change or reinterpret the law, HMOs will become much more accountable for bad care delivered within their medical networks. Some of those cases might be classic malpractice disputes in which HMOs would be only peripheral defendants; there would be little reason to examine their role. But in other cases HMO policies on specialist referrals, the ordering of expensive tests, and other medical services might figure at the heart of the dispute. The public interest would be well served by putting HMO practices under the spotlight. Undercare would be more severely penalized. HMOs — like doctors, auditors, amusement-park operators, and car makers — would have a powerful new incentive to avoid business practices that might put them on the losing end of a multimillion-dollar civil judgment.

8. Consumers need to know how to file effective complaints.

When something goes disastrously wrong in managed care, a lawsuit may be the answer. Most member complaints, however, involve small to medium irritants. A specialist referral is delayed. An asthma inhaler or a wheelchair isn't covered. Drug-formulary decisions appear onerous. Such situations hardly call for a trip to the courthouse. Yet annoyed health-plan members may want to do more than simply grumble to themselves.

Patients' rights attorneys recommend the following tactics. First, ask the treating physician in person, or the HMO's member-services department over the telephone, if either one can intercede. Some doctors and HMO administrators try hard to resolve such disputes while they are small; others simply hope that they go away. If those gentle initial approaches don't work, send a written complaint to the plan's medical director and member-services department. If the issue is sufficiently serious, send a copy to state regulators — and let the HMO know you are doing so. In the complaint letter, lay out the problem and propose a remedy. Look for an ally within the system — a treating physician, a therapist, or a hospital manager — to help make the case. If the wrong is truly egregious, consider seeking press coverage of the dispute or asking a lawyer to file further complaint letters.

Such tactics aren't meant to turn every small difference of opinion into a protracted battle between member and HMO. But they are designed to help members press for the coverage they believe they are entitled to. In states such as California that have made it easier for managed-care participants to file grievances, the volume of complaints has increased tremendously. That suggests that health plans to date have bottled up more complaints than they have resolved.

9. *Regulators need to keep the profit motive in check.*

Managed-care executives like to judge themselves by the standards applied to most other for-profit industries. They believe their mission is to achieve corporate revenue and earnings targets, make money for shareholders, and then allow senior management to be rewarded accordingly. As one HMO chairman put it, "If you want to regulate that, you take away what's great in this country: the free enterprise system." But that view is incomplete. As noted in Chapter 4, managed care is fundamentally different from other industries in that its goal is to impose austerity on others. Managed care's good years are ones in which doctors, hospitals, and patients get by with less. If HMO executives and their shareholders can grow rich by denying care, there is potential for abuse. That concern is intensified by the fact that investors repeatedly have rushed to sell shares in an HMO that indicated it was about to spend more money on patient care — news that members might welcome but that Wall Street dreads.

As wealth piles up in the HMO industry, some intriguing ideas have emerged about how to restrain avarice. A bill introduced in the Florida legislature in early 1996 proposed that HMOs be required to spend at least 80 percent of premium income on patient care. (Some plans currently spend 70 percent or less.) In California nonprofit HMOs that want to become for-profit are required to use the proceeds of any stock sale to set up public-interest foundations that will uphold the health plan's original, non-money-making goals, such as promoting wellness. In a few states, such as Minnesota, all HMOs are required to be not-for-profit — a rule relaxed in the early 1980s in most other states. If for-profit HMOs became greedier, all such countermeasures deserve a closer look.

A simple way to help for-profit HMOs keep their priorities straight is to insist on greater public disclosure. Currently HMOs' financial results are reported only to shareholders and insurance-industry regulators; they aren't widely circulated. But regulators could require HMOs to spell out their patient-care outlays on the front page of any marketing material in bold black letters, along with the industry norms. Car companies must disclose fuel-efficiency ratings; cereal makers must provide nutritional information. If those industries can live with prominent public disclosure of vital facts, HMOs can too. Customers could choose as efficient or inefficient a health plan as they wanted. But they would do so with clear knowledge of important facts.

10. Employers, doctors, and regulators need to establish better report cards on the quality of health plans.

"Which HMO is best?" "Which one is right for me?" The numerous health-plan report cards that appear in consumer magazines or employee-benefits brochures purport to answer those questions. Most of these assessments are dominated by two types of statistics: how reliably HMOs provide cholesterol checks and other preventive care and how each plan rated in a quick survey of member satisfaction. That data may be better than nothing, but it suffers from glaring defects and omissions. And in some cases, ostensibly independent report cards are nothing more than marketing gimmicks underwritten by the plans themselves. As one HMO surveyor confessed, "Our primary business is to sell to the Kaisers and Aetnas and Cignas of the world. We don't want anything in print that would get them irritated."

So far, managed-care assessments have sidestepped the public's most important question: "If I get really sick, will this plan take care of me?" That omission should be fixed as soon as possible. Reviewers must gather data on HMOs' performance in treating serious diseases. They also should pay close attention to what chronically ill people say about their HMOs. After all, these frequent users best know the health plan's strengths and weaknesses. And surveys should probe the underbelly of managed care by asking members how easy it is to see a specialist or to get coverage for an emergency-room visit. Leading health-care researchers such as Robert Blendon at Harvard and Eve Kerr at UCLA say such questions can better gauge members' true attitudes than the gentle query, "Are you satisfied with your health plan?" which almost always elicits a positive answer.

The HMO industry's main current overseer, the National Committee for Quality Assurance, has periodically been criticized for being too close to the business that it is supposed to monitor. NCQA officials have taken some steps in recent years to achieve partial independence from the HMO industry. As of mid-1996, however, NCQA still got 40 percent of its funding from HMOs, which control at least one third of the organization's board of directors. Those percentages are too high to allow NCQA to be fully independent of the industry that it ostensibly monitors. As long as the managed-care industry plays a major role in funding its assessors, the public report cards are likely to highlight only the information that HMOs want to present.

The easiest way to get independent oversight would be to reconstitute NCQA, either with consumer, business, and foundation funding or with a federal charter. NCQA's recent moves toward greater independence suggest that the first approach may work. But if it falters, direct government oversight would be called for. That would parallel the approach to financial markets (overseen by the Securities and Exchange Commission), air travel (overseen by the Federal Aviation Administration), and a host of other industries dependent on public trust.

None of these ideas is likely to be embraced willingly by the HMO industry. Leading managed-care companies have prospered greatly under the status quo, and they will portray most changes as tampering with the free market. But that misrepresents where we are today. HMOs compete in what is, unfortunately, a rigged market. Customers know little about the health insurance they buy until it is far too late to switch. Managed-care contracts are packed with ambiguities and rubbery definitions that customers wouldn't tolerate if they were buying a home, a car, or even a box of breakfast cereal. HMOs enjoy wide latitude to concoct upbeat marketing campaigns, yet keep secret how they pay doctors, how they treat serious illnesses, how they decide what is medically necessary. No industry graced with such advantages would surrender them without a fight.

Even so, the HMO industry's current supremacy is built on a surprisingly fragile base. Managed-care companies climbed to prominence not because their methods were universally admired but because national frustration with steeply rising medical bills became so intense that almost any form of restraint seemed worth trying. Now, with medical inflation having slowed greatly, much of that urgency has disappeared. There is time to take a calmer look at how medicine and health insurance ought to be organized. Few people are entirely happy with managed care as it functions today. Doctors, consumers, and employers question whether health plans really know how to handle the full complexities of patient care. Liberals are unhappy with many HMOs' open pursuit of profits. Conservatives dislike the way that these plans narrow patients' choice of doctors far more than fee-for-service plans and subject physicians to too much outside supervision.

To maintain this present power, HMO executives must continue to position themselves as the great middlemen of medicine. They must find more employers who desperately want to hold down medical costs but aren't sure how to do it. And they must find doctors and hospitals that won't practice cost-effective medicine on their own but that can be persuaded by HMO contracts to change their ways. If HMOs can connect those two groups — and be seen as the only cost-effective way to unite medical payers and providers — then they can skirt their critics' objections. That strategy may still work for a few more years, but its days are numbered.

Over the next few years employers and doctors will be asking the question that changes everything: "Do we really need HMOs standing between us?"

The answer may well be "No, we don't."

Expertise about the most worthwhile parts of managed care is developing among doctors, employers, and patients' rights groups, rather than remaining the secret preserve of HMOs. Many companies are building prevention and wellness programs into their benefits packages without help from HMOs. Pitney Bowes is teaming up with a major drug company to counsel diabetic employees on how to keep their blood-sugar levels under control. A host of companies, including Johnson & Johnson, U-Haul, and Honeywell, are using financial incentives to encourage employees who smoke to enroll in stop-smoking programs. Other companies are requiring morbidly obese workers to sign up for weight-loss programs and rewarding them when they shed pounds and keep them off. As employers acquire the confidence and skill to improve the well-being of workers themselves, HMOs no longer can claim a monopoly on effective ways to deliver simple preventive care.

Changes are taking place even faster in the medical community. While a minority of doctors still fight managed care in any form, far more physicians are building its best aspects into their own practices, thereby serving patients better and becoming less dependent on HMOs to tell them how to practice cost-effectively. Doctors' groups around the country are finally gathering data on themselves, trying to identify the best practices and learn from one another. Obstetricians talk openly about their cesarean section rates and agree that, within reason, lower rates are better. Medical journals every week publish major articles on the cost-effectiveness of various treatments for back pain, prostate cancer, and hundreds of other illnesses. Such research is doing a great deal to restrain overtreatment and is encouraging doctors to make each health-care dollar stretch a bit farther.

The most intriguing development is the consolidation of doctors into large group practices, consisting of at least 50 M.D.s — and sometimes as many as 500 — in a wide range of specialties. By virtue of their sheer size, these groups can take over many HMO functions on their own: setting up drug formularies, deciding when to approve hospital stays, and keeping an eye on doctors who may be overtreating or undertreating patients.

This medical-group version of managed care will need to be closely watched and answerable to outside authorities. As recent history has shown, the mere appearance of an "M.D." after a person's name doesn't guarantee exemplary conduct. Yet physician-initiated managed care has considerable promise. In contrast to a remote HMO, key decisions can be made by people who treat patients every day and keep a close eye on one another. Managed-care decisions needn't be based solely on statistical data that can fit onto a computer spreadsheet; there is more room for human judgment and attention to the complexity of individual patients' needs. Large group practices such as the Mayo Clinic and Cleveland Clinic often are praised for their ability to combine very high quality and cost-effectiveness. In southern California, big physician groups are rapidly becoming an important way of delivering care. Other parts of the United States also may find that clusters of doctors can put a more human face on managed care.

If these trends are taken one step further, employers may negotiate managed-care contracts directly with doctors' groups and hospitals, bypassing the HMO middlemen entirely. This approach would end medical providers' dependence on HMOs for access to patients. That could be appealing in several ways. It would cut overhead costs, ensure that a bigger share of premiums went to patient care, and put economically responsible doctors more directly in charge of health care. Such contracts will work only if doctors' groups show a sure hand at administration and learn enough about risk management to price their services properly — neither of which will be easy. If doctors fail to master those two challenges, internal squabbles and badly negotiated contracts will wreck even the most medically skillful groups. But these issues should be surmountable. A business coalition in Minneapolis that represents 100,000 workers has said it will try direct contracts with doctors' groups starting in 1997. The coalition's director, Steve Wetzell, views such contracts as having great promise. Currently, he complains, HMOs are jousting over acquisitions, marketing slogans, and exclusive contracts to freeze out rivals. "We think competition is on the wrong level. What employees care about is doctors, nurses, and specialists — not health plans."

So how will history treat the HMO industry? The whole field is young enough that the verdict isn't likely to be clear for another decade or two. On the positive side of the ledger, HMOs undeniably will receive credit for getting a grip on medical costs and for bringing modern, efficient business methods to the very fragmented world of medicine. But HMOs will get much harsher marks for gaps in care when patients most need their services. And away from Wall Street, HMOs' success at earning big profits for middlemen — and outfitting executives with 75-foot yachts, Rolls-Royces, and other trappings of luxury — will be seen as uncomfortable hypocrisy for an industry that publicly preaches the virtues of austerity.

Eventually the pioneers of the HMO industry may be viewed much like the corporate raiders of the 1980s. That is, they will be seen as intensely provocative "change agents" who briefly seized control of a big piece of the economy but faded from the scene as society found a more palatable way of carrying out that mission. We are only partway through that cycle; HMOs continue to lambaste doctors and hospitals for wasteful ways, just as raiders stormed into corporations in the mid-1980s, accusing long-time executives of running bloated empires that didn't serve shareholders' interests. But if the analogy holds, at some point doctors will figure out how to run a cost-effective medical system without abandoning compassion — just as corporate executives figured out how to satisfy shareholders without ripping apart businesses so drastically. And at that point the swashbuckling middlemen will be left with much less to do.

Notes

Each chapter of this book draws heavily on personal interviews and firsthand observation of medicine as it is practiced in the age of managed care. Those examples have been augmented by clinical records, legal documents, and financial filings. In addition, secondary sources have provided important context for many medical and business issues. The most frequently cited publications are the *New England Journal of Medicine* (*NEJM*), the *Journal of the American Medical Association* (*JAMA*), the *Wall Street Journal* (*WSJ*) and the *New York Times* (*NYT*). Also valuable have been various articles in *Health Affairs, Modern HealthCare, BusinessWeek, Fortune,* the *Fort Lauderdale Sun-Sentinel,* the *Washington Post,* and the *Los Angeles Times.*

In-person interviews are cited by day, month, and year. Telephone interviews are cited by month and year. Chapters 11 and 12 benefited greatly from additional research by Elizabeth Corcoran and Nina Youngstrom. Their interviews are denoted by (EC) and (NY), respectively. All other primary-source interviews are by the author.

Where dialogue has been reconstructed, the notes that follow identify the principal sources for each exchange, as well as any significant variances in participants' accounts. No additional dialogue has been invented or synthesized.

1. A Baby's Struggle

PAGE

1 Resting her infant son and subsequent details: interview with Lamona and James Adams Jr., 22 February 1995; Lamona Adams deposition 24 March 1994 in *James Jr. and Lamona Adams v. Kaiser Foundation Health Plan of*

Georgia Inc., filed in Fulton County state court, Georgia, 1993; Lamona Adams court testimony in *Adams v. Kaiser,* 25 January 1995.

2 Exchanges between Lamona Adams and the hotline nurse, Esther Nesbitt: Adams remembered Nesbitt's specific quotes in her 24 March 1994 deposition. Nesbitt did not reconstruct dialogue but said in her 18 February 1994 deposition in *Adams v. Kaiser:* "I gave her the direct number to the emergency room at Scottish Rite in order — I don't feel comfortable telling people how to get to places, especially if they need to get to a hospital and it's the middle of the night."

2 Details of the drive to Scottish Rite: interview with James Adams Jr., 22 February 1995.

4 A nurse grabbed the infant and subsequent details: as cited in medical chart of James Don Adams III, Kennestone Hospital, 27 March 1993.

5 "He's following the bear!": Dr. Jose's quote was recalled by Lamona Adams in an interview, 22 February 1995. On the medical chart for James Don Adams III at Scottish Rite Children's Medical Center, 6 April 1993, Dr. Jose wrote: "Child follows my face (I have to open eyelids) side to side & Teddy Bear side to side."

5 Details of Adamses' life after baby's discharge from hospital: interview with Lamona and James Adams, Jr., 22 February 1995.

7 "Since acute bacterial . . ." Robert Berkow M.D., ed., *The Merck Manual of Diagnosis and Therapy* (Rahway, N.J.: Merck Research Laboratories, 1992), p. 1467.

7 Dr. Juster's exam: described in Lamona Adams's deposition in *Adams v. Kaiser.*

8 Kaiser's cost-containment briefing: deposition of Carol Herrmann in *Adams v. Kaiser,* 8 March 1994.

8 Lamona Adams's sense of obligation to Kaiser: In her 24 March 1994 deposition in *Adams v. Kaiser,* Lamona Adams said, "The materials provided indicated that you should know that you are in an emergency situation before you run to an emergency room."

9 Esther Nesbitt's background: Nesbitt's deposition in *Adams v. Kaiser.*

9 Kaiser's fever guidelines: The three-page tip sheet was introduced as evidence in *Adams v. Kaiser.*

9 "I had no indication . . .": Nesbitt's deposition in *Adams v. Kaiser.*

9 Conversation between Nesbitt and Dr. Herrmann: The two accounts appear in the two women's depositions in *Adams v. Kaiser.*

10 Kaiser's discount at Scottish Rite: as specified in "Agreement for Hospital Services," a 20-page contract between Kaiser and Scottish Rite Children's Medical Center, signed by Edgar Carlson on behalf of Kaiser, 4 December 1990.

11 Malone's damage estimates and rationale: interview with Malone, 22 February 1995.

11 Jury award of $45.5 million: *Atlanta Constitution,* 4 February 1995.

11 Jurors' reaction: *American Lawyer's Daily Report,* 6 February 1995; interview with Lamona Adams, 22 February 1995.

11 Helping her son grow up: Description is based on a personal visit to the Adamses' home, 22 February 1995.

12 "Is there anything . . .": Kaiser's policy switch was described by Ann Beech, a Kaiser physician and quality manager in Georgia, in a telephone interview, April 1996.

12 She gave her home number: telephone interview with Dr. Herrmann, March 1995.

13 "We don't need": interview with Lamona Adams, 22 February 1995.

13 HMO membership: statistics from the American Association of Health Plans, the main HMO industry trade group.

14 "Anytime health benefits . . .": Margaret Jordan, head of employee benefits at Edison International.

15 Adams–Dr. Herrmann exchange: Precise quotes were recalled by Lamona Adams in interview, 22 February 1995. Dr. Herrmann confirmed the substance of the conversation in a phone interview, March 1995.

2. Dismantling the Old System

16 Edward Hennessy's indignation and subsequent details: separate phone interviews with Hennessy, Ted Halkyard, and pension consultant Joseph Martingale, August 1995. Hennessy recounted the review of high-cost bills; Martingale recalled the reference to Boone Pickens; Halkyard reconstructed the budget meeting.

19 "We can afford to spend more . . .": as quoted in Paul Starr, *The Social Transformation of American Medicine* (New York: Basic Books, 1982), p. 281.

20 "Growing confidence . . .": ibid., p. 288.

20 Extent of private insurance: as cited in *Source Book of Health Insurance Data* (Washington: Health Insurance Association of America, 1994), p. xx.

20 Growth of General Motors plan: Joseph A. Califano Jr., *America's Health Care Revolution* (New York: Random House, 1986), pp. 13–14.

20 "Chrysler opened its treasury door . . .": ibid., p. 14.

20 Hospital costs: Rosemary Stevens, *In Sickness and in Wealth* (New York: Basic Books, 1989), p. 263.

21 "Halfway technology": Lewis Thomas, *The Lives of a Cell* (New York: Viking, 1974), p. 39

21 Chrysler and psychiatric benefits: Califano, p. 19.

22 Number of open-heart-surgery units: Dale A. Rublee, "Medical Technology in Canada, Germany, and the United States," *Health Affairs*, fall 1989.

22 American leadership in medical technology: The ambivalent implications of the high-tech buildup in health care are discussed in Henry Aaron, *Serious and Unstable Condition* (Washington: Brookings Institution, 1991).

22 People with private insurance: *Source Book*, p. 37.

23 Strikes over health benefits: *Newsday*, 1 December 1991.

23 Admonition to Blue Cross insurers: as quoted in Abraham Ribicoff, *The American Medical Machine* (New York: Saturday Review Press, 1972), p. 96.

23 Evidence of regional variation: A landmark report is John Wennberg and Alan Gittelsohn, "Variations in Medical Care among Small Areas," *Scientific American*, April 1982.

23 Rand's estimate of unnecessary surgery: interview with Robert Brook, 7 June 1995.

24 "It's awful . . .": Leslie Aun, "Helping Doctors Boost Revenue Turns Into an Industry," *Washington Business Journal,* 30 July 1990.

24 "I'll be back . . .": as quoted in Lani Luciano, "A Cure Your Doctor Won't Like," *Money,* 22 September 1990.

25 "We were the ones . . .": phone interview with Halkyard, August 1995.

27 Elk City health plan: as described in Kennett Lynn Simmons, *Managed Health Care: Right Idea — Wrong Rules* (Austin: University of Texas, 1992), pp. 79–83.

27 Formation and growth of the Kaiser health plan: John G. Smillie, *Can Physicians Manage the Quality and Costs of Health Care?* (New York: McGraw-Hill, 1991).

28 Passage of the 1973 HMO Act and aftermath: Joseph L. Falkson, *HMOs and the Politics of Health System Reform* (Chicago: American Hospital Association, 1980).

30 Allied Signal's contract with Cigna: separate phone interviews with Hennessy, Halkyard, and Martingale, August 1995; *Newsday,* 2 December 1991; *Newark Star-Ledger,* 16 March 1990; testimony by Hennessy before the Senate Finance Committee, 16 April 1991.

31 "It was emotional . . .": phone interview with James Bronson, August 1995.

32 Smith's lobbying on heart center: *WSJ,* 24 May 1993.

32 The Ninja Turtle comparison: cited in testimony by Kenneth Macke before the Senate Finance Committee, 16 April 1991.

32 "I used to hate . . .": phone interview with Steve Enna, July 1995.

32 "Flow from a surreal world": Janice Castro, "Condition: Critical," *Time,* 25 November 1991.

33 "We'd like to think . . .": phone interview with John Erb, July 1995.

33 "Health care costs have created": *Time,* 25 November 1991.

34 "Health care is our single largest . . .": phone interview with Russell Hawkins, July 1995.

3. The New Mandarins

35 Letters from Tufts: described in separate telephone interviews with Barry Levine and Paul Shellito, March 1994.

35 The Tufts evening conference: described in separate phone interviews with Dr. Levine, Dr. Shellito, and Joe Gerstein, March 1994. Tufts managers referred to these meetings as "jury duty" for recalcitrant doctors.

38 Forty doctors work for U.S. Healthcare: The figure is from interview with Leonard Abramson, 28 June 1995, who at the time was chairman of U.S. Healthcare.

38 "Most people work . . .": interview with Jay Rosan, 14 January 1993.

39 Charts with orange and red dots: cited in Chuck Appleby, "The Measure of Medical Services," *Hospitals & Health Networks,* 20 June 1995.

39 "It's beautiful . . .": ibid.

40 Berwick's speech: as reprinted in *Medical Care,* December 1991.

41 "We'll reap 10 times . . .": as quoted in Maria Kassberg, "Managed Care Report Cards: How Will You Rate?" *Managed Care,* June 1993.

41 Harvard Community Health Plan's interest: telephone interview with Kathryn Coltin, August 1995.

41 "If we needed expertise . . .": telephone interview with Janet Corrigan, August 1995.

42 "It has changed . . .": telephone interview with Dr. Shellito, March 1994.

42 Dr. Gerstein's concerns: multiple telephone interviews with Dr. Gerstein, February and March 1994.

43 "There's been a history . . .": interview with Tom Rosenthal, 6 June 1995.

43 Exchange between Malik Hasan and Edward Cadman: Dr. Hasan provided the fullest account, including the line "I wouldn't send my dog to your hospital," in an interview, 30 August 1995. Dr. Cadman in a September 1995 telephone interview confirmed the tone of the conversation and the canine allusion, but he didn't remember precise language.

44 Qual-Med's clash with Swedish Medical Center: *Seattle Times,* 26 August 1991.

45 Dr. Hasan's visit to UCLA: The remarks "It's a Darwinian world . . ." and "When I was at Rush . . ." were recalled by Francine Chapman, UCLA's head of managed-care contracting, in an interview, 6 June 1995. Dr. Hasan in an interview 30 August 1995 didn't recall precise language but confirmed the overall tone of his remarks. Dr. Hasan said he brought out Medicare cost data to bolster his points.

47 "Our core values . . .": interview with William Speck, 12 May 1995.

47 Peter Slavin's concerns: phone interview with Dr. Slavin, June 1995.

48 President Clinton's remarks: Gannett News Service, 12 February 1993.

49 "With very few exceptions . . .": *WSJ,* 10 September 1993.

50 "We got ripped . . .": interview with Bill Elliot, 18 June 1995.

52 Linda Peeno's career: interview with Dr. Peeno, 17 November 1995.

53 "I sat at my desk . . .": personal essay by Dr. Peeno, "Going Beyond the Requirements," spring 1994.

54 "There is no code . . .": testimony by Dr. Peeno before the House Committee on the District of Columbia, 14 September 1993.

54 "The whole system . . .": phone interview with Dr. Peeno, April 1996.

4. *The Barons of Austerity*

55 Purchase price of Dr. Hasan's Beaver Creek home: county records, Eagle County, Colorado.

55 Description and background of Dr. Hasan's house: various sources, including Connie Knight, "The Story of a Castle in Paradise," *Vail Valley Magazine,* spring 1995; telephone interview in January 1996 with Charles Sink, an original architect of the house; telephone interview in March 1996 with Don Dethlefs, the other original architect of the house. Dr. Hasan, in a phone interview in March 1996, confirmed that he had bought the house at a "good price"; he declined to discuss it further.

56 Sink's visit to Beaver Creek: telephone interview with Sink, January 1996.

57 Garrey Carruthers's interest in HMOs: telephone interview, July 1994; *WSJ*, 20 July 1994.

57 David Jones's private jet: Ownership of a jet is disclosed in Humana Inc.'s "Proxy Statement for Annual Meeting of Stockholders," 11 May 1995, p. 13. A Federal Aviation Administration spokesman specified in a March 1996 telephone interview that the plane is a Cessna 560. Jones's payments to Humana are disclosed in the company's proxy.

58 Richard Burke's purchase of a hockey team: various stories in the *Minneapolis Star-Tribune*, with the most notable appearing 4 May 1995 and 20 October 1995. The quote: "This is not . . ." comes from the 20 October 1995 article.

58 Leonard Abramson's early background: The fullest account appears in Mary Beth Grover "Poverty Pays," *Forbes*, 23 December 1991. Abramson confirmed his cab-driving stint in an interview, 28 June 1995.

58 Abramson's taste for luxury: The three-hole golf course was shown on *CBS Evening News*, 25 July 1995. Family members on the payroll were disclosed in U.S. Healthcare's "Proxy Statement for Annual Meeting of Shareholders," 27 April 1995, p. 15. The yacht is registered with the U.S. Coast Guard.

59 "This is a phenomenal company . . .": interview with Abramson, 28 June 1995.

61 "I never made much money . . .": Interview with Robert Gumbiner, 1 September 1995.

61 Financial goals in annual reports: "Providing the highest return on investment" was cited in the 1991 annual report of United Wisconsin Services. "Enhancing the value of your investment" appeared in the 1994 annual report of Health Systems International. "Our record-breaking financial performance" was mentioned in the 1992 annual report of U.S. Healthcare.

62 Industry medical-loss ratios for 1993 and 1994: as computed by Sherlock Company, a financial advisory firm based in Gwynedd, Pennsylvania, that specializes in the HMO industry.

62 HMO cash positions: *WSJ*, 21 December 1994. The text of the article refers to nine HMOs with $9.5 billion in cash; more complete information on the 10 largest HMOs appears in an accompanying table.

63 "Our problem is what to do . . .": *WSJ*, 21 December 1994.

64 Executive pay packages: Robert Gumbiner's salary in the 1970s cited in an oral history of FHP published by Dr. Gumbiner; Leonard Abramson's 1982 salary cited in "Prospectus," United States Health Care Systems Inc., p. 23; Dan Crowley's pay package disclosed in "Proxy Statement," Foundation Health Corporation, 10 October 1994, pp. 10–11.

64 Tom Elkin's indignation: phone interview with Elkin, June 1995.

64 "It's doggone piggy . . .": *Sacramento Bee*, 24 June 1995.

65 Value of Steve Wiggins's options: as disclosed in a Form 10-K filing with the Securities and Exchange Commission by Oxford Health Plans Inc. for 1994, p. 25.

65 Norman Payson's pay package: as disclosed in "Proxy Statement: 1995 Annual Meeting of Shareholders," HealthSource Inc., 9 May 1995, p. 8.

66 "We're losing competition . . .": *WSJ*, 30 March 1995.

66 "We at the AMA . . .": phone interview with James Todd, December 1994.

67 Dr. Hasan's background: *Denver Post,* 31 January 1993.

68 "I wanted to go . . .": interview with Dr. Hasan, 30 August 1995.

68 Dr. Hasan and medical equipment: Dun & Bradstreet business directories list Dr. Hasan as a partner in C.T. Scan Lab of Parkview and as a partner of Neurological Neurosurgical, both based in Pueblo, Colorado. Other partners in those ventures identified Dr. Hasan as the lead investor in buying a CAT scanner and an MRI for use by Pueblo neurologists, including himself. Dr. Hasan in an interview 30 August 1995 confirmed investing in scanning machines, explaining that local hospitals lacked the capital to do so and that he believed the machines would improve the local standard of care.

68 "Malik always knew . . .": phone interview with Michael Pugh, former administrator of Parkview Hospital in Pueblo, August 1995. In a May 1996 phone interview, Dr. Hasan said, "I can imagine someone looking at my work and saying, 'He orders a lot of tests.' But I was seeing an awful lot of patients, and I was doing work in a concentrated fashion." Medicare reviewers who watched for overuse of tests "questioned very few of my cases," he added.

69 "We could see . . .": interview with Dr. Hasan, 30 August 1995.

69 "He promised us investors . . .": telephone interview with Robert Dingle, August 1995.

70 "The most brilliant . . .": telephone interview with Robert Daly, August 1995.

70 Qual-Med's strict rules: interview with James Riopelle, 27 August 1995.

70 Qual-Med's takeover of Health Net: The fullest descriptions of this battle appeared in the *Los Angeles Times,* 13 July 1991, 4 August 1992, and 31 August 1993.

71 Greaves's trip to Denver: interview with Roger Greaves, 1 September 1995.

72 "Anyone can pay top dollar . . .": telephone interview with Dr. Hasan, March 1996.

72 "There's nothing I can do . . .": The exact quote was recalled by Health Systems executive Don Prial in an interview, 31 August 1995. Dr. Hasan, in a phone interview in March 1996, confirmed the general thrust of his remarks.

73 Dr. Hasan's defense of his pay: The remark "I get people asking me . . ." was made in a March 1996 phone interview. The comment "We are being innovative . . ." appeared in a *Los Angeles Times* article, 29 August 1995.

73 "When you're a doctor . . .": interview with Dr. Hasan, 30 August 1995.

5. Turning Doctors into Gatekeepers

74 Greenberg's nighttime patient encounter: phone interview with Brian Greenberg, December 1995. Two of Dr. Greenberg's medical school classmates corroborated the story.

75 Description of Dr. Greenberg's practice: firsthand observation, 30 August 1995 and 14 November 1995.

75 Dr. Greenberg's frustrations: interview with Dr. Greenberg, 30 August 1995.

78 Barbara Beeler's concerns: phone interview with Dr. Beeler, July 1995.

79   "On the one hand . . .": Jerome Kassirer, "Managed Care and the Morality of the Marketplace," *NEJM,* 6 July 1995.

80   William Bacigalupo's kidney problems: *Bacigalupo v. Healthshield,* a suit filed in New York state court, Dutchess County, in 1992; Charles R. Hollen, "Legal Briefs," *The Internist,* May 1996; phone interview, May 1996, with Robert Miller, an attorney for Healthshield, a Latham, N.Y., HMO that subsequently changed its name to Community Health Plan.

80   "When I used to encounter an aneurysm": interview with Allan Schwartz, 12 May 1995.

80   David Himmelstein and gag clauses: Dr. Himmelstein's initial remarks were made on *Donahue,* 28 November 1995. He elaborated on his concerns in an article in *NEJM,* 21 December 1995, which carried an editor's note saying that Dr. Himmelstein had been dropped from U.S. Healthcare's network in Massachusetts. In a March 1996 phone interview, U.S. Healthcare medical director Hyman Kahn said that Dr. Himmelstein had been reinstated in the HMO's network.

80   "I want first crack . . .": phone interview with Steven Tamarin, May 1995.

81   Dr. Morrow's views: interview with Robert Morrow, 26 May 1995.

81   Pediatric practice details: in-person interviews with Dr. Greenberg and Robert Barnhard, 30 August 1995 and 14 November 1995; numerous additional phone interviews with Dr. Greenberg in 1995 and 1996.

85   Dr. Greenberg and managed-care contracts: firsthand observation, 31 August 1995.

87   Antibiotics for eye infections: phone interview with Dr. Greenberg, September 1995.

87   The Utah-based HMO clerk: interview with Dr. Greenberg, 30 August 1995.

89   Folders listing specialists: firsthand observation, 14 November 1995.

89   Eosinophilic leukemia case: described by Dr. Greenberg in testimony before the California Senate Committee on Health, 6 June 1995.

90   Children with chronic diseases: phone interview with Dr. Greenberg, June 1995; various articles in *Southern California Medicine,* July-August 1995.

91   Inability to leave managed care: interview with Drs. Barnhard and Greenberg, 14 November 1995.

6. Heart Trouble

92   Accord between HIP and North Shore: Details were announced by HIP in a press release, 11 September 1995. The Long Island retreat beforehand was described by long-time HIP medical director Jesse Jampol in a phone interview, January 1996.

93   Dr. Gold's mortality statistics: cited in *Coronary Artery Bypass Graft Surgery in New York State* (hereafter *CABG/NYS,* New York State Department of Health, June 1995).

93   North Shore's mortality data in the late 1980s: *Newsday,* 11 May 1991.

93   Heart-surgery mortality rates in 1993: as cited in *CABG/NYS.*

93   "I think we've got . . .": phone interview with Anthony Tortolani, January 1996.

94   "I asked him . . .": phone interview with O. Wayne Isom, January 1996.

94   "It's our job . . .": phone interview with Jesse Jampol in February 1996.

94   Treatment methods in 1950s: Sherwin Nuland, *As We Die* (New York: Random House, 1993), p. 11.

96   HMOs and organ transplants: *WSJ*, 16 January 1995.

96   Volume of heart surgeries: data from American Heart Association.

97   *Time*'s tribute to Dr. DeBakey: "The Texas Tornado," *Time*, 28 May 1965.

97   Gerald Kay's work at Good Samaritan: multiple phone interviews with his son, Gregory Kay, January 1996; phone interview with Charles Munger, chairman of Good Samaritan Hospital, February 1996; phone interviews with two other former administrators at Good Samaritan, January 1996; phone interview with Gerald Kay, May 1996.

99   Good Samaritan's mortality rates, 1989–1991: *Medicare Provider Analysis and Review*, annual report (Health Care Financing Administration).

99   Surgery mortality rates, 1991–1993: as cited in *Cardiovascular Procedures* (Aurora, Colo: Healthcare Data Source).

100 "Fully 30 percent . . .": phone interview with Gregory Kay, January 1996.

100 "For a 2 to 3 percent difference . . .": presentation by APM consultant David Anderson at symposium on managed care sponsored by Stanford University, San Francisco, June 15, 1995.

101 "Hospitals are cutting . . .": phone interview with David Perkowski, January 1996.

102 Rates and length of stay at St. Francis: phone interview with Anne Billingsley, January 1996.

102 "If we were as aggressive . . .": interview with Lawrence Yeatman, 6 June 1995.

102 Philadelphia mortality rates: *A Consumer Guide to Coronary Artery Bypass Graft Surgery* (Pennsylvania Health Care Cost Containment Council, 1995).

103 "Mortality data alone . . .": phone interview with Gary Owen, January 1996.

103 "There is no evidence . . .": phone interview with Marc Chassin, January 1996.

104 "They give lip service . . .": phone interview with Janet Monroe, January 1995.

104 Dr. Rose's tussle with U.S. Healthcare: interview with Eric Rose, 12 May 1995; phone interview with Hyman Kahn, July 1996.

104 Patients with high blood pressure: Sheldon Greenfield et al., "Outcomes of Patients with Hypertension and Non-Insulin Dependent Diabetes Mellitus Treated by Different Systems and Specialties," *JAMA*, 8 November 1995; additional comments by Dr. Greenfield in *WSJ*, 8 November 1995.

105 HMOs and cardiac stents: *WSJ*, 23 October 1995; phone interview with Alan Johnson, June 1995.

106 Use of clot-busting drugs: D. S. Lessler and A. L. Alvins, "Cost, Uncertainty and Doctors' Decisions," *Archives of Internal Medicine* 1994.

106 "We tried to reconcile . . .": interview with Joan Ming, 6 June 1995.

107 "These are extremely dangerous . . .": phone interview with James Lock, September 1995.

107   Death rates in pediatric surgery: preliminary research findings presented by
      Kathy Jenkins at the American Heart Association annual meeting, Anaheim,
      California, 13 November 1995.
107   Stuart Kaufman's tussles with managed care: phone interview with Dr. Kauf-
      man, May 1995.
108   Jan Quaegebeur's demeanor: firsthand observation, 9 January 1996.
108   Dr. Quaegebeur's mortality statistics: interview with Dr. Quaegebeur, 9 Jan-
      uary 1996.
109   Trey McPherson's case: firsthand observation of heart surgery, 9 January
      1996; phone interview with Bruce McPherson in January 1996.
109   Bryan Jones's case: *New York Post*, 18 September 1995; *Susan Jones v. U.S.
      Healthcare, et al.*, filed in New York state court for Bronx County, June
      1995.
111   "I'm not denying . . .": phone interview with Dr. Quaegebeur, May 1995.

7. The Breast Cancer Battles

112   Janice Bosworth's background: Bosworth trial testimony December 1993 in
      Jim Fox and estate of Nelene Fox v. Health Net, filed in California state
      court, Riverside County; telephone interview with her husband, Stephen,
      May 1996.
113   Bosworth-Ossorio exchange: Bosworth in her trial testimony recalled spe-
      cific language used by Clifford Ossorio. Dr. Ossorio also testified in the case;
      he recalled reviewing the Bosworth case, but no specific conversations.
114   Duarte's intercession: cited in Ossorio's testimony concerning Bosworth in
      Fox v. Health Net. In an interview 1 September 1995, former Health Net
      chief executive Roger Greaves confirmed that the HMO paid for Bosworth's
      bone marrow transplant, adding that it was done as an employer's gift to her
      rather than as a change in insurance policy.
114   Dr. Ossorio's belief that Bosworth's transplant was futile: In a 30 July 1992
      deposition in *Fox v. Health Net,* Dr. Ossorio said: "As we expected, she
      recurred within weeks after the transplant and did terribly. It was a futile
      kind of treatment." Asked if Bosworth was alive at the time, Dr. Ossorio
      replied, "I don't know." Bosworth was alive; she lived for two and a half
      years after Dr. Ossorio's remarks.
115   Nesmith's plea to Greaves: letter from Joyce Nesmith to Roger Greaves,
      undated, believed to have been mailed on or about 1 September 1993.
116   Odds of becoming disease-free: cited in David Eddy, "High Dose Chemo-
      therapy With Autologous Bone Marrow Transplantation for the Treat-
      ment of Metastatic Breast Cancer," *Journal of Clinical Oncology,* October
      1992.
116   Development of high-dose chemotherapy and BMT: multiple phone inter-
      views with William Peters, a pioneer in the field, from 1994 to 1996, and a
      phone interview with Karen Antman, another leader in the field, December
      1995.
117   Drop in immediate mortality rates: phone interview with Dr. Antman, De-
      cember 1995.

117   Leonard Knapp's background: deposition of Dr. Knapp in *Fox v. Health Net*, 23 February 1993.

118   TAG report and its reception: deposition of Dr. Knapp in *Fox v. Health Net*; telephone interview with Sheila Fifer, president of Technology Assessment Group, December 1996; inspection of the report, which was entered as evidence in *Fox v. Health Net*.

118   Dr. Ossorio's background and views on BMT: deposition of Dr. Ossorio in *Fox v. Health Net*, 30 July 1992; trial testimony by Dr. Ossorio in December 1993.

119   Dr. Ossorio's excitement about changing medical practices: phone interview with Dr. Ossorio, December 1995.

119   "He is a very persuasive individual . . .": deposition of Dr. Knapp in *Fox v. Health Net*.

120   Nelene Fox's declining health: trial testimony by her husband, Jim Fox, in *Fox v. Health Net*, December 1993.

120   "If it was my wife . . .": trial testimony of Stanley Schinke and Jim Fox. Their recollections of the exact language are almost identical; Fox's version appears in the text.

121   Telephone exchange between Drs. Ossorio and Camacho: Both physicians testified in *Fox v. Health Net* in December 1993. Dr. Camacho's recollection was more detailed and referred to a confrontational start; Dr. Ossorio's recollection was less detailed, and he characterized the conversation as educational.

121   "He was quite agitated . . .": trial testimony by Aziz Khan in *Fox v. Health Net*, December 1993.

122   Exchange between Jim Fox and Dr. Camacho: Both men testified in *Fox v. Health Net*, in December 1993, about their recollections of this conversation.

123   Health Net's grid: A copy of the grid was entered as evidence in *Christine and Alan deMeurers v. Health Net et al.*, a dispute submitted in early 1995 to arbitration by the American Arbitration Association.

124   David Eddy's analysis: Eddy, "High-Dose Chemotherapy." Overall Dr. Eddy concluded: "Existing evidence does not demonstrate that HDC/ABMT is superior to conventional-dose chemotherapy for the treatment of metastatic breast cancer. Randomized controlled trials are needed."

125   John Glaspy's views on BMT: in deposition of Dr. Glaspy in *deMeurers v. Health Net*, 25 April 1995.

126   Dennis Slamon's views on the deMeurers case: in deposition of Dr. Slamon in *deMeurers v. Health Net*, 1 May 1995.

129   "This is a hot issue . . .": *WSJ*, 15 February 1994.

130   "I couldn't continue . . .": phone interview with Dr. Ossorio, December 1995.

8. Is This Really an Emergency?

132   Ambiance at the telephone center: firsthand observation, 21 January 1996.

133   Higher cost of emergency-room services: The leading study is Laurence C.

Baker and Linda Schuurman Baker, "Excess Cost of Emergency Department Visits for Nonurgent Care," *Health Affairs,* winter 1994. The authors estimated that nationwide excess charges were $5 billion to $7 billion in 1993.

134 Consumers Union survey: cited in "Are HMOs the Answer?" *Consumer Reports,* 1 August 1992. The magazine reported: "What you think of as an emergency may not be the same as your HMO's definition of an emergency. One-fifth of our readers who had emergencies and were seen by non-HMO doctors said the plan covered only part of the bill. About 10 percent received no payment at all."

134 Comparison with Vietnam war: James Page, ed., *Principles of EMS Systems* (Dallas: American College of Emergency Physicians, 1994), p. 3.

136 "We inherited a system . . .": phone interview with Dr. Owens, January 1996.

138 "We call it a hesitation fee": phone interview with Peter Kilissanly, January 1996.

138 Emergency care and the McGirrs: The account is based on multiple phone interviews in January 1996 with Peter Hackett, director of the Division of Emergency Medical Services for the New York State Health Department, Suffolk County branch, and on phone interview with Mae McGirr, February 1996.

139 Curtis Climer's views: phone interview with Dr. Climer, August 1995; Dr. Climer's letter to the editor, *American Medical News,* 24 July 1995.

140 "If we were really screwing up . . .": phone interview with Richard Cornell, January 1996.

141 Death of Stephen Cummins: described in *Janis O. Cummins et al. v. Kaiser Foundation Health Plan of Georgia Inc.,* a suit filed in Georgia state court, Fulton County, April 1995. Kaiser declined to comment on the allegations while litigation was pending.

141 Darryl Hinthorne's protests: phone interview with Hinthorne, January 1996.

142 Leslie Saxon's heart patient: phone interview with Dr. Saxon, July 1995; interview with Lawrence Yeatman, a UCLA physician, and Joan Ming, a nurse, who were also involved in the patient's care, 6 June 1995.

143 Beatrice Luna's case: phone interview with Luna, January 1996; phone interview with Bruce Janiak, January 1996; phone interview with Hal White, medical director of Medical Value Plan, June 1996.

144 Donna Buehler's case: multiple phone interviews with Mary Burke, the treating physician, in January 1996; phone interview with Todd Buehler, February 1996.

144 Edmund Popiden's case: multiple phone interviews with Popiden, January and February 1996; phone interview with Joe Lucia, January 1996; inspection of Pennsylvania Health Department grievance file on the case.

146 Payment denials at Bellevue: phone interview with Louis Goldfrank, January 1996.

146 John Stamler's files: multiple phone interviews with Dr. Stamler, January 1996; inspection of copies of about 50 of his files.

147 Carbon monoxide poisoning: phone interview with Robert Sweeney, Janu-

ary 1996; phone interview with William Baxt, chairman of emergency medicine at the University of Pennsylvania Medical Center, Philadelphia, February 1996.

147   Keith Ghezzi's proposals: interview with Dr. Ghezzi, 30 January 1996.

148   "If this were easy . . .": phone interview with Barry Wolcott, January 1996.

149   Deb Rogalski's calls: firsthand observation, 21 January 1996.

9. HMOs and Mental Health

150   UBS stance on Rhode Island probe: interview with Don Williams, Linda Johnson, and Alison Woodbine, 8 February 1996; letter from John Chianese, executive director of UBS/Rhode Island, to Johnson, 19 April 1995. Chianese wrote, "UBS's Rhode Island operations underwent a comprehensive Quality Assurance Audit. The audit was conducted on December 6 and 7, 1994" by two UBS executives. "There were no major deficiencies noted," he added. In a phone interview in February 1996, UBS president John Tadich said, "I don't feel we had that many grievous issues. Clearly we were not following the definitions the way they wanted us to. I wish we had."

150   "Our goal . . .": as quoted in *Behavioral Health in Emerging Health Care Systems,* a UBS brochure dated October 1995.

151   Search of UBS medical records: The account is based on an interview with Johnson and Woodbine, 8 February 1996.

152   Manic-depressive case: summary is based on an interview with Johnson and Woodbine, 8 February 1996. In a phone interview in February 1996, UBS medical director Frank Shelp declined to discuss specifics of any cases, citing patient privacy.

152   Handgun-owner case: summary is based on an interview with Johnson and Woodbine, 8 February 1996, and on a February 1996 interview with Ronald Schouten, a Harvard psychiatrist who later reviewed the case.

153   UBS settlement: multiple articles in the *Providence Journal-Bulletin.* The most notable were on 11 June 1995, 12 July 1995, 3 August 1995, and 12 September 1995.

153   Florida weight-loss spas: ChiChi Sileo, "Rip-Offs Depress Mental Health Care," *Insight,* 24 January 1994.

154   Xerox's spending: *WSJ,* 19 December 1995; Joan O'C. Hamilton, "A Furor over Mental Health," *BusinessWeek,* 8 August 1994.

154   Membership in mental-health management companies: Hamilton, "A Furor."

155   Xerox's cost savings: John K. Iglehart, "Health Policy Report: Managed Care and Mental Health," *NEJM,* 11 January 1996.

155   Rand Corporation study: William H. Rogers and Kenneth Wells, "Outcomes for Adult Outpatients with Depression under Prepaid or Fee-for-service Financing," *Archives of General Psychiatry,* December 1994.

155   Iglehart's concerns: *NEJM,* 11 January 1996.

155   "Greed-driven sharks . . .": *WSJ,* 19 December 1995.

155 Iowa's Merit contract: *Des Moines Register,* 31 October 1995.

156 "Neglected stepchild" comparison: Philip Boyle and Daniel Callahan, "Managed Care in Mental Health," *Health Affairs,* fall 1995.

157 Betrayal of confidentiality: Mark Levy, "Why We Should Opt Out of Managed Care," *Psychiatric Times,* July 1995.

157 "The goal is to get . . .": *WSJ,* 1 December 1995.

158 United's desire for a bigger network: phone interview with John Tadich, February 1996.

158 United's spending on mental health: as reported by United Health Plans of New England Inc. in annual reports filed with the Rhode Island Department of Insurance.

158 "I used to tease him . . .": phone interview with Cathy Clark, February 1996.

159 Dr. Harrop's starting pay: phone interview with Tadich, February 1996.

159 Stock options and bonus: interview with Dr. Harrop, 9 February 1996.

159 "I didn't go in thinking . . ." and subsequent details: interview 9 February 1996 with Dr. Harrop.

160 "I remember Dan Harrop . . .": interview with Louis Hafken, 8 February 1996.

160 Decisions upheld more than 80 percent of the time: as cited in a regulatory filing by UBS with the Rhode Island Department of Health, 25 April 1995. That filing listed 91 level-one appeals of UBS's "adverse determination," of which 75 were upheld.

160 Case workers checking the blackboard: based on phone interviews with three former UBS insiders. In a phone interview, February 1996, UBS's Tadich said, "I'm not aware of that particular practice. Triaging patients to providers is part of what we do."

161 "Opposition and resistance can be expected . . .": letter from Harold Davidson to William Corrao, associate medical director, United Health Plans of New England, 17 March 1995.

161 Surge in patient protests and subsequent details: interview with Ruth Glassman and Bill Emmet, 17 March 1995; interview with Jim McNulty, 8 February 1996.

162 Mercer report: Donald Anderson et al., *Report to United Health Plans of New England on the Evaluation of United Behavioral Services of Rhode Island* (William M. Mercer Inc., August 1995).

162 "Their regular practice . . .": *CBS Evening News,* 6 December 1995.

163 "They were only interested . . .": interview with Larry O'Brien, 9 February 1996.

163 Eileen McNamara's concerns: testimony by McNamara at a Rhode Island Department of Health hearing, 13 September 1995.

164 "There was an overstatement . . .": interview with Michael Ingall, 7 February 1996.

164 "I remember one provider . . .": interview with Dr. Harrop, 9 February 1996.

165 Terry Lusignan's sister: description is based on phone interview with Terry Lusignan, February 1996; testimony by Lusignan at a Rhode Island Depart-

ment of Health hearing, 13 September 1995; interview with Glassman, 8 February 1996; and a review of UBS correspondence in the case. Dr. Harrop's letter was written to Alan Gordon, a psychiatrist at Butler Hospital, 4 January 1995.

166 Harvard psychiatrists' assessments: from Dr. Schouten to Alison Woodbine, letter 1 June 1995; *Statement of Deficiencies: United Behavioral Systems,* Rhode Island Department of Health, June 1995.

167 Alleged rape of three-year-old: interview with Johnson, 8 February 1996.

167 "We are absolutely confident . . .": *Minneapolis Star-Tribune,* 13 June 1995.

168 "This can't be good" and subsequent details: interview with Dr. Harrop, who recalled Tadich's words, 9 February 1996. In a phone interview, February 1996, Tadich didn't recall his exact remarks but said Dr. Harrop's account sounded accurate.

169 "We are witnessing . . .": *Minneapolis Star-Tribune,* 12 July 1995.

10. When the Elderly Fall Sick

171 Belva Johnson's nursing-home stay: The account is based on multiple phone interviews with Richard Johnson in early 1996, a brief phone interview with Belva Johnson in March 1996, and phone interviews with Marilyn Blackwood and speech therapist Sadako Yamamoto in March 1996.

172 Health Net sending a messenger to Johnson's bedside and subsequent details: letter to Belva Johnson from Mark N. Saberman M.D., medical director, Health Net, 21 October 1994; legal declaration by Belva Johnson, 14 October 1995; legal declaration by Richard M. Johnson, 15 November 1995.

175 Medicare budget data: *Source Book of Health Insurance Data* (Washington: Health Insurance Association of America, 1994), p. 61.

176 HMOs' upbeat articles: Both examples cited are from *Horizons,* a bimonthly publication of PacifiCare's Medicare HMO.

176 Medicare spending on healthiest versus sickest: The figures for 1993 spending were cited in *NYT,* 18 November 1995. In that article Princeton University economist Uwe Reinhardt said that cost figures almost compelled private plans to seek out the healthy.

178 GAO assessment: as cited in its report *Medicare: Increased HMO Oversight Could Improve Quality and Access to Care,* August 1995.

178 Medicare HMO grievances: The data are compiled from a 1995 summary report (obtained under the federal Freedom of Information Act) by Network Design Group (NDG), Pittsford, New York. NDG adjudicates those grievances under contract from the federal government.

178 Members' ignorance of appeal rights: cited in June Gibbs Brown, *Medicare Risk HMOs: Beneficiary Enrollment and Service Access Problems,* report by the Office of the Inspector General, Department of Health and Human Services, April 1995.

179 Stroke patient outcomes: cited in Randall S. Brown, et al., *The Medicare Risk Program for HMOs,* report by Mathematica Inc., Princeton, N.J.,

February 1993, commissioned by the federal Health Care Financing Administration.

179 Probe of PacifiCare: *Orange County Register,* 1 December 1995; *Los Angeles Times,* 29 November 1995.

180 Pappas case: as described in a legal declaration filed by Norma Pappas in *PacifiCare of California v. Gary S. Mendoza,* filed in California state court in Orange County, July 1995.

180 Davia case: as described in a legal declaration filed by Anne Breck in *PacifiCare v. Mendoza.*

181 "Our philosophy . . .": phone interview with Sam Ho, March 1996.

182 "We used to have a blank check . . .": phone interview with David Powers, March 1996.

183 Grijalva case: as described in *Gregoria Grijalva et al. v. Donna Shalala,* a suit filed in federal district court in Tucson in 1993. Additional details come from the *Arizona Daily Star,* 15 December 1993.

183 "Denials of needed services . . .": phone interviews with Sally Wilson, February and March 1996.

184 "Families sometimes have . . .": phone interview with Jodi Horton, March 1996.

185 "The good death": as discussed in Sherwin Nuland, *How We Die* (New York, Alfred A. Knopf, 1994), pp. xvi–xvii.

186 Patricia Sloan's case: phone interview with Tricia Reis, March 1996; phone interview with Carol Jiminez, Sloan's attorney, March 1996; summary of the case in *Grijalva v. Shalala,* amended complaint.

188 "Beyond the point . . .": Daniel Callahan, *Setting Limits* (New York: Simon & Schuster, 1987), p. 138.

188 "I would reiterate . . .": ibid., p. 153.

11. Poor Patients, Shoddy Care

190 University of Tennessee survey: as cited in *Managed Care and Low-Income Populations,* report on TennCare by Mathematica Policy Research Inc., July 1995.

190 Savanna Zotter's case: phone interview with Carrie Zotter, March 1996; EC interview with Iris Snider, 16–17 February 1995.

193 David Manning's concerns: phone interview with Manning, March 1996.

195 "Medicaid HMOs have made obscene profits": *Fort Lauderdale Sun-Sentinel,* 1 March 1995.

195 Better Health Plan's perks: *Fort Lauderdale Sun-Sentinel,* 12 December 1994.

195 New York state health investigators: *NYT,* 17 November 1995.

196 Dayton, Ohio, problems: *Cleveland Plain Dealer,* 25 June 1995.

196 Complaint against Foundation Health: as cited in *Edward Ivy et al. v. S. Kimberly Belshe et al.,* a suit filed in California state superior court in San Francisco in 1994.

197 Tennessee's Medicaid spending: as cited in Tennessee's formal application for federal approval of TennCare, filed with the federal Department of Health and Human Services, 16 June 1993.

197 McWherter's speech and budget targets: *Atlanta Journal,* 9 April 1993.

198 Triumph turned to mass confusion: EC phone interviews with a half-dozen Tennessee physicians and hospital administrators, February 1996.

198 Twins in different plans: EC phone interview with Mark Gaylord, February 1995.

198 Coby Smith's advice: *NYT,* 2 October 1995.

199 Signing up prison inmates: *Memphis Commercial Appeal,* 22 June 1994, 8 November 1995.

200 Patient costing $300,000: EC phone interview with Don Lighter, former chief medical officer of the University of Tennessee's managed-care plan, February 1996.

200 Bruce Vladeck's doubts: *Atlanta Journal,* 19 November 1993.

200 Ruckhard Welch's worries: *WSJ* (southeast edition), 3 May 1995.

201 "TennCare threatens to cut . . .": letter from Dr. Fernando to state senator Lou Patten, 11 November 1993.

201 Check for $3.94: EC phone interview with Don Lighter, February 1996.

202 "Pediatricians are very compassionate . . .": EC interview with Phil Campbell, 17 February 1996.

202 Iris Snider's practice: EC interviews with Dr. Snider, 16–17 February 1996.

203 Rufus Clifford Jr.'s concerns: memorandum by Dr. Clifford, 4 April 1995.

203 Tennessee's immunization rate: as cited in a news release by the Tennessee Department of Health, 23 August 1995. The rate rose to 80.8 percent in fiscal 1995, up from 78.6 percent a year earlier.

204 Douglas Cobble's frustrations: letter from Dr. Cobble to Access MedPlus, 3 February 1994; EC phone interview with Dr. Cobble, February 1996.

204 Shigellosis epidemic: phone interview with Paulus Zee, February 1996; letter from Dr. Zee to Dr. Snider, 9 March 1994.

205 Coumadin dose problem: letter from John Morgan to Access MedPlus, 28 June 1994.

206 Care of David Owens, Jr.: EC phone interview with Teresa Owens, in February 1996.

207 Destructive ten-year-old boy: EC interview with Brenda Hartgrove, 16 February 1996.

207 TennCare as an election issue: *Knoxville News-Sentinel,* 2 November 1994; *Memphis Commercial Appeal,* 6 November 1994.

208 "You have to be certain . . .": EC phone interview with Yvonne Wood, February 1996.

12. *The Best Lobbyists in America*

210 American Viewpoint's clients: *Los Angeles Times,* 22 February 1996; Associated Press, 4 November 1994.

210 Gary Ferguson's memo: copies of his 28 March 1995 memo were obtained from two separate sources.

212 "Successful lobbies are measured . . .": Donald Barlett and James Steele, *America: What Went Wrong?* (Kansas City: Andrews and McMeel, 1992), p. 190.

212 Phone calls to Turner's office and aftermath: phone interview with Patricia Lucas, March 1996; NY phone interviews with several aides to Texas state senator Jim Turner, March 1996; speech by Turner to the Texas senate, 19 May 1995, in *Dallas Morning News*, 20 May 1995.

213 Guitars at AAHP meetings: interview with Kennett Simmons, 21 February 1995.

214 HMO political donations: *USA Today*, 30 November 1995; *Washington Post*, 17 June 1994.

214 Lobbying battle over Medicare HMOs: *NYT*, 10 December 1995.

214 HMO briefing on grassroots lobbying: personal observation, 28 February 1995.

215 Steve Male's ouster: interview with Male, 3 May 1995; the *Sunday* (Harrisburg) *Patriot-News*, 2 April 1995, disclosed campaign contributions by Leonard Abramson and David Simon.

215 Florida lobbying battle: *Fort Lauderdale Sun-Sentinel*, 5 April 1995.

216 Alberto Gutman's fee and aftermath: *St. Petersburg Times*, 8 February 1996; *Fort Lauderdale Sun-Sentinel*, 11 June 1995.

216 Arkansas bill: *Washington Post*, 22 August 1995.

216 Elizabeth McCaughey's frustration: *NYT*, 31 October 1995.

217 Drafting of Texas doctors' bill: NY phone interviews with five participants in the discussions, including Joe Cunningham, early 1996.

218 "It was pretty darned ugly . . .": NY phone interview with Jeffrey Kloster, in February 1996.

218 "Hospitals . . . are like big oil refineries . . .": NY phone interview with Tom Bond, February 1996.

219 Jeffrey Kloster's tactics: *WSJ* (Texas edition), 19 April 1995; NY phone interview with Kloster, February 1996.

219 TMA lobbyists' maneuvers: *WSJ* (Texas edition) 24 May 1995; NY phone interviews with Connie Barron and Kim Ross, February 1996; phone interview with Laura Johannes, a *WSJ* reporter who covered H.B. 2766 in Texas, March 1996.

220 Nancy Sims's views: NY phone interview with Sims, February 1996.

221 Cost estimate of 1 to 1 1/2 percent: letter from John Rodrigue, president of the Texas Business Group on Health, to members of the Texas house, 9 May 1995.

221 "Watch Your Wallet" ad: *Austin American-Statesman*, 17 May 1995.

221 Bill Gradison's letter: A copy of Gradison's form letter, dated 13 April 1995, was obtained from a recipient; the Health Insurance Association of America confirms mailing about 500 copies.

222 Dane Harris's remarks: David McCormick, "Bad Medicine," *Texas Monthly*, August 1995.

222 Bob Lanier's opposition: as quoted in newspaper advertisements run in May 1995 by the Texas Business Group on Health.

222 "Most of the horror stories . . .": *WSJ* (Texas edition), 24 May 1995.

223 "My idea of what hell . . .": NY phone interview with David Sibley, February 1996.

223 "Baseball-literate governor": phone interview with Tammi Cotten, March 1996.

224 Reactions to Texas veto: *Dallas Morning News,* 17 June 1995; *Austin American-Statesman,* 17 June 1995.

224 Elton Bomer's regulations: *Dallas Morning News,* 16 November 1995 and 28 September 1995; *Houston Chronicle,* 20 June 1995.

225 States debating 100 proposals: as reported in *American Medical News,* 13 November 1995.

225 Model statutes: as cited in Geraldine Dallek et al. *Consumer Protections in State HMO Laws,* (Los Angeles: Center for Health Care Rights, 1995), p. xi.

225 Doctors' use of surrogates: as described in *American Medical News,* 24 July 1995.

226 "This is not a contrived alliance . . .": *American Medical News,* 24 July 1995.

13. A Question of Quality

227 Lonnie Riesman's background and inquiries: phone interview in November 1995 with Dr. Riesman; interview with Dr. Riesman, 6 December 1995.

228 Carlee Christie case: news release, California Department of Corporations, 17 November 1994; interview with Carlee and Harry Christie, 11 June 1995.

230 Howard Viet's concerns: phone interview with Viet, August 1995.

230 NCQA's role in the 1980s: interview with Margaret O'Kane, 13 July 1995; follow-up phone interview with O'Kane and two other executives associated with NCQA's early years, August 1995.

231 California's two full-time employees: *Los Angeles Times,* 27 August 1995.

231 Employers' desire for change: phone interviews with Howard Viet, Daniel Wolfson, Kathleen Angell of Digital Equipment, and three other early participants, August 1995; interview with Helen Darling of Xerox, 10 August 1995.

232 Margaret O'Kane's background: interview with O'Kane, 13 July 1995.

232 NCQA reviews: press release by NCQA, 29 February 1996.

233 *Consumers' Checkbook* survey: Some 89 percent of HMO members in 24 plans with full three-year accreditation from NCQA rated their plans as good, very good, or excellent. That was no better than the 89 percent approval ratings from people in 32 plans with one-year accreditations, or the 90 percent approval ratings from people in 70 plans that hadn't been reviewed. *Consumers' Checkbook* surveyed members in only three plans that flunked the NCQA process; those plans got a 79 percent approval rating.

233 Xerox's dilemma with Mid-Atlantic: interview with Darling, 10 August 1995.

233 Humana's use of consultants: interviews with Christy Bell and Joe Burdell, 8 March 1996; personal observation of the HMO's regional headquarters in Plantation.

234 Live case probes: phone interview with LuAnn Cash, August 1995.

235 Dr. Riesman's findings: interview with Dr. Riesman, 6 December 1995.

236 Mark Smith's concerns: firsthand observation, NCQA meeting, 30 October 1995.

236 Paul Ellwood's background: interview with Dr. Ellwood, 1 May 1995;
     Joseph L. Falkson, *HMOs and the Politics of Health System Reform* (Chi-
     cago: American Hospital Association, 1980), pp. 14–16.
237 Jackson Hole caucus: personal observation, 25–27 June 1995.
238 Judge Stapleton's ruling: as cited in *Cecilia Dukes v. U.S. Healthcare Inc., et
     al.*, a suit reviewed in federal appellate court in 1995.
238 Volume of California calls: multiple phone interviews with Damian Jones, a
     spokesman for the California Department of Corporations, in 1995 and
     1996.
239 Florida Medicare HMO crackdown: phone interview with LaNona Robin-
     son, a vice president of Florida Medical Quality Assurance Inc. (FMQA), the
     state's Medicare review organization, March 1996; *Indications for Cataract
     Surgery*, report issued by FMQA, February 1995.
239 Karin Smith's case: Edward Dolnick, "What Killed Karin Smith," *Glamour*,
     February 1996.
240 Joanna Breen's concerns: phone interview with Breen, March 1996.
240 "I marvel . . .": phone interview with Wes Waller, chief actuary, Foundation
     Health, December 1994.
241 "There are people . . .": phone interview with Susan Pisano, April 1996.
241 Origins of HMO critics' interest: phone interviews with William Sherman
     and Don Wright, March and April 1996.
242 Jeffrey Harris's views on managed care: interview with Harris, 27 June
     1995.
242 Heart surgery for O'Kane's daughter: as described by O'Kane in a briefing
     for journalists in Washington, D.C., 20 December 1995.

14. Building a Better System

248 "If this were China . . .": interview with Robert Brook, 7 June 1995.
252 Medicare contracting rules: *WSJ*, 27 March 1996. Federal rulemakers said
     that doctors or medical groups with fewer than 1,000 Medicare patients
     couldn't be liable for more than $10,000 of specialty-care expenses associ-
     ated with any one patient. Under pressure from HMO lobbyists, federal
     authorities subsequently delayed implementing the new rules for at least
     several months.
253 Independent review boards: Martin Shapiro and Neil Wenger, "Rethinking
     Utilization Review," *NEJM*, 17 November 1995.
261 "We think competition . . .": *Minneapolis Star-Tribune*, 1 August 1995.

Index

11/96

BAKER & TAYLOR